Atlas of
POLYSOMNOGRAPHY

THIRD
EDITION

Atlas of
POLYSOMNOGRAPHY

EDITORS

James D. Geyer, MD, FAASM, FAES
Director, Sleep Program
Alabama Neurology and Sleep Medicine
Neurotexion, LLC
Tuscaloosa, Alabama

Paul R. Carney, MD
Professor and Chief
Department of Neurology
University of North Carolina at Chapel Hill
Chapel Hill, North Carolina

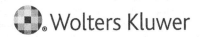 Wolters Kluwer

Philadelphia • Baltimore • New York • London
Buenos Aires • Hong Kong • Sydney • Tokyo

Acquisitions Editor: Chris Teja
Editorial Coordinator: Alexis Pozonsky
Marketing Manager: Rachel Mante-Leung
Production Project Manager: Bridgett Dougherty
Design Coordinator: Holly McLaughlin
Manufacturing Coordinator: Beth Welsh
Prepress Vendor: SPi Global

Third Edition

9 8 7 6 5 4 3 2

Printed in the United States of America

Library of Congress Cataloging-in-Publication Data
Names: Geyer, James D., editor. | Carney, Paul R., editor.
Title: Atlas of polysomnography / editors, James D. Geyer, Paul R. Carney.
Description: 3rd edition. | Philadelphia: Wolters Kluwer, [2018] | Includes bibliographical references and index.
Identifiers: LCCN 2017040692 | ISBN 9781496381088
Subjects: | MESH: Sleep—physiology | Polysomnography | Sleep Wake Disorders | Atlases
Classification: LCC RC547 | NLM WL 17 | DDC 616.8/498—dc23 LC record available at https://lccn.loc.gov/2017040692

MPP0123

To our families and to the memory of Michael Aldrich.

Contributing Authors

Melanie Brown, RPSGT
DCH Northport Sleep Center
Northport, Alabama

Jenna Cooper, CRNP
Alabama Neurology and Sleep Medicine
Tuscaloosa, Alabama

Paul Cox, BSE, MSE
Neurotexion, LLC
Tuscaloosa, Alabama

Emery Geyer
ReflexArc
Tuscaloosa, Alabama

Monica Henderson, RN, RPSGT
Alabama Neurology and Sleep Medicine
Tuscaloosa, Alabama

Teresa Kizzire, RPSGT
The Sleep Center at Pickens County Medical Center
Carrollton, Alabama

Lori May, RPSGT
DCH Northport Sleep Center
Northport, Alabama

Jennifer Parr, RPSGT
DCH Northport Sleep Center
Northport, Alabama

Craig Schumacher, RPSGT
Tombigbee Sleep Center
Demopolis, Alabama

Prefaces

PREFACE to the Third Edition

Sleep medicine continues to evolve rapidly as a subspecialty with numerous disorders now recognized and an ever-changing set of diagnostic criteria and protocols. The criteria used for the evaluation of polysomnography have changed several times in just the past few years. This edition of the atlas contains many new images utilizing the most recent staging and scoring criteria. There are, however, some images using the older montages, which still convey important and valid teaching points.

This atlas is designed to aid the sleep medicine specialist and those training in sleep medicine. It also serves as a reference and training tool for technologists. The atlas covers normal polysomnographic features of wakefulness and the various stages of sleep as well as polysomnographic findings characteristic of sleep-related breathing disorders, sleep-related movements, and parasomnias. In addition, examples of cardiac arrhythmias, nocturnal seizures, and artifacts are included. A variety of time scales are used to illustrate their value.

PREFACE to the Second Edition

Sleep medicine continues to evolve rapidly as a subspecialty with numerous disorders now recognized and an ever-changing set of diagnostic criteria and protocols. As with any medical discipline, accurate diagnosis is an essential prerequisite for a rational approach to management. Polysomnography, the recording of multiple physiologic functions during sleep, was developed in the 1970s and is the most important laboratory test used in sleep medicine. Polysomnography complements the clinical evaluation and assists with diagnosis and management of a variety of sleep disorders.[1]

Digital amplifiers and computerized signal processing are now the standard of care and provide many advantages over older analog amplifiers and paper recording. This is especially true for the evaluation of brief electroencephalographic (EEG) transients such as epileptiform sharp waves and spikes and their differentiation from artifacts and benign EEG waveforms. This section of the book has been significantly expanded. Digitized data can also be displayed using a variety of montages depending on the purpose at hand; for example, the display can be limited to EEG, electrooculogram (EOG), and chin electromyogram (EMG) during sleep staging, and then expanded to include respiratory and leg movement channels during scoring of these functions. Filters and sensitivities can be altered during review to assist with interpretation of the study.

While digital polysomnography provides a number of advantages as described above, features related to signal acquisition, display resolution, and printer resolution must be understood by the technologist and interpreter. For digital signal acquisition, the analog signal generated by the transducer must be converted to digitized information. A critical variable is the rate at which the signal is sampled and digitized. For slowly varying signals, such as thoracic motion, a sampling rate of 20 Hz may be sufficient; for rapidly varying signals, such as EEG and EMG, the sampling rate must be much higher, usually 250 Hz or more. If the sampling rate is inadequate, waveforms are distorted and scoring and interpretation may be erroneous. For example, if the sampling rate for eye movement channels is too low, the sharp deflection associated with a rapid eye movement may appear as a slower deflection characteristic of a slow eye movement.

Because of differences in signal acquisition and display parameters, not all digital recordings have the same appearance. In addition, although transducers used for recording of EEG, EOG, and EMG are largely standardized, EEG and EOG montages vary among laboratories. Furthermore, transducers and recording techniques for assessment of respiration during sleep vary widely among sleep laboratories.[2] For example, airflow can be monitored directly with a pneumotachograph, thermistor, thermocouple, or indirectly with recordings of tracheal sound or by summation of signals from thoracic and abdominal inductance recordings. Respiratory effort can be assessed with respiratory inductance plethysmography, stretch-sensitive transducers (strain gauges), diaphragmatic EMG, intrathoracic (esophageal) pressure, or nasal pressure. Scoring of sleep stages has been standardized for many years[3] and has recently been updated.[4] The new scoring and staging criteria are discussed in detail in the text, and the waveforms are presented in the appropriate chapters.

As a result of these variations, the overall appearance of the polysomnographic display may be markedly different from one laboratory to the next. No atlas can provide examples of normal and abnormal polysomnography using all of the displays and transducers used in accredited sleep laboratories. For this atlas, the illustrations were prepared from several sleep centers and electrodiagnostic/neurophysiology laboratories in order to introduce the reader to several of the possible formats.

This atlas is designed to aid the sleep medicine specialist and those training in sleep medicine. It also serves as a reference and training tool for technologists. The atlas covers normal polysomnographic features of wakefulness and the various stages of sleep as well as polysomnographic findings characteristic of sleep-related breathing disorders, sleep-related movements, and parasomnias. In addition, examples of cardiac arrhythmias, nocturnal seizures, and artifacts are included. A variety of time scales are used to illustrate their value.

1. American Academy of Sleep Medicine. *International Classification of Sleep Disorders: Diagnostic and Coding Manual*. 2nd Ed. Westchester, IL: American Academy of Sleep Medicine, 2005.
2. Parisi RA, Santiago TV. Respiration and respiratory function: Technique of recording and evaluation. In: Chokroverty S, ed. *Sleep Disorders Medicine: Basic Sciences, Technical Considerations, and Clinical Aspects*. Boston, MA: Butterworth-Heinemann, 1994:127–139.
3. Rechtschaffen A, Kales A. *A manual of Standardized Terminology, Techniques, and Scoring system for Sleep Stages of Human Subjects*. Los Angeles, CA: Brain Information Service/Brain Research Institute, 1968.
4. Iber C, Ancoli-Israel S, Chesson A, Quan SF; for the American Academy of Sleep Medicine. *The AASM Manual for the Scoring of Sleep and Associated Events: Rules, Terminology and Technical Specifications*. 1st Ed. Westchester, IL: American Academy of Sleep Medicine, 2007.

PREFACE to the First Edition

Sleep medicine is a relatively new medical subspecialty that is rapidly expanding as the prevalence, and importance of sleep disorders has become apparent. As with any medical discipline, accurate diagnosis is an essential prerequisite for a rational approach to management. Polysomnography, the recording of multiple physiologic functions during sleep, was developed in the 1970s and is the most important laboratory test used in sleep medicine. Polysomnography complements the clinical evaluation and assists with diagnosis and management of a wide range of sleep disorders.[1]

As the array of sleep diagnoses has expanded, the techniques and equipment used for sleep recordings have become more sophisticated. While sleep studies in the 1970s used analog amplifiers and bulky paper recordings that rarely consisted of more than eight channels, computer technology of the late 1990s permits recording of dozens of channels using sensitive noninvasive or minimally invasive transducers, digital amplifiers, electronic displays, and compact data storage on magnetic or optical media.[2]

Digital amplifiers and computerized signal processing provide many advantages over older analog amplifiers and paper recording. For example, digitized data can be displayed using a compressed time scale that makes slow rhythms more readily identifiable, such as the regular occurrence of periodic leg movements at 20- to 30-second intervals. Alternatively, an expanded time scale can be used that permits easier identification of brief electroencephalographic (EEG) transients such as epileptiform sharp waves and spikes and their differentiation from artifacts and benign EEG waveforms. Digitized data can also be displayed using a variety of montages depending on the purpose at hand; for example, the display can be limited to EEG, electrooculogram (EOG), and chin electromyogram (EMG) during sleep staging, and then expanded to include respiratory and leg movement channels during scoring of these functions. Filters and sensitivities can be altered during review to assist with interpretation of the study.

In addition to digital polysomnography, several other technical advances have improved the diagnostic value of sleep recordings. Polysomnography can be combined with video recording (video-polysomnography); the simultaneous analysis of behavior and polysomnographic findings assists with diagnosis of parasomnias, nocturnal seizures, and other sleep-related behaviors. To assist with diagnosis of sleep-related breathing disorders, intrathoracic pressure can be monitored with intraesophageal pressure sensors that are easily inserted and well tolerated. With the availability of 16 to 32 or more channels for a recording, esophageal pH, end-tidal carbon dioxide level, and transcutaneous CO_2 monitoring can be included in selected situations without sacrificing standard channels.

While digital polysomnography provides a number of advantages as described above, features related to signal acquisition, display resolution, and printer resolution must be understood by the technologist and interpreter. For digital signal acquisition, the analog signal generated by the transducer must be converted to digitized information. A critical variable is the rate at which the signal is sampled and digitized. For slowly varying signals, such as thoracic motion, a sampling rate of 20 Hz may be sufficient; for rapidly varying signals, such as EEG and EMG, the sampling rate must be much higher, usually 250 Hz or more. If the sampling rate is inadequate, waveforms are distorted and scoring and interpretation may be erroneous. For example, if the sampling rate for eye movement channels is too low, the sharp deflection associated with a rapid eye movement may appear as a slower deflection characteristic of a slow eye movement.

Display resolution is based on the characteristics of the computer and display monitor and the software used for data acquisition and display. The array of pixels in the screen determines the maximum resolution; for example, a 1024 × 768 display provides lower resolution than a 1600 × 1200 display. While the lower-resolution display may be sufficient for assessment of slowly varying signals such as respiration, it may be inadequate for identification of rapid EEG transients.

Printer resolution is based on the characteristics of the printer, computer, and software. In some cases, waveforms that are not adequately displayed on the monitor can be better analyzed if a high-resolution printout is obtained.

Because of differences in signal acquisition and display parameters, not all digital recordings have the same appearance. In addition, although transducers used for recording of EEG, EOG, and EMG are largely standardized, EEG and EOG montages vary among laboratories. Furthermore, transducers and recording techniques for assessment of respiration during sleep vary widely among sleep laboratories.[3] For example, airflow can be monitored directly with a pneumotachograph, thermistor, thermocouple, or indirectly with recordings of tracheal sound or by summation of signals from thoracic and abdominal inductance recordings. Respiratory effort can be assessed with respiratory inductance plethysmography, stretch-sensitive transducers (strain gauges), diaphragmatic EMG, intrathoracic (esophageal) pressure, or nasal pressure. Furthermore, although scoring of sleep stages has been standardized for many years,[4] no consensus has been reached at this writing concerning scoring criteria for respiratory events.

As a result of these variations, the overall appearance of the polysomnographic display may be markedly different from one laboratory to the next. No atlas can provide examples of normal and abnormal polysomnography using all of the displays and transducers used in accredited sleep laboratories. For this atlas, all of the illustrations were prepared from sleep studies performed at the University of Michigan Sleep Disorders Center, or, in a few cases, from neonatal EEG studies performed in the University of Michigan Electrodiagnostic Laboratory. The studies were recorded using digital equipment manufactured by the Telefactor Corporation (Conshohocken, PA). The montages, filter settings, sensitivities, and A-D sampling rates used to generate the displays are specified in the Technical Introduction.

The illustrations were prepared based on 1600 × 1200 screen displays and printed with a Hewlett-Packard Laser Jet printer on 8.5 × 11–inch paper at 600 dot per inch resolution.

The EEG electrodes were placed according to the International 10 to 20 system.

The EOG electrodes were placed 1 cm superior and lateral to the right outer canthus and 1 cm inferior and lateral to the left outer canthus.

One chin EMG electrode was placed on the chin (mental), and two electrodes were placed under the chin (submental). The submental electrode placement is generally at the mandible. Generally, there is a 3–cm distance between electrodes.

The EKG was recorded with one electrode each placed 2 to 3 cm below the left and right clavicles midway between the shoulder and neck.

Many of the recordings also include a second EKG channel recorded from a left leg EMG channel and left ear electrode.

Airflow was recorded with a single channel nasal/oral thermocouple from Pro-Tech (Woodinville, WA). This thermocouple has sensors for each nostril and another that is located over the mouth.

Thoracic and abdominal motion was recorded with respiratory effort sensors utilizing piezoelectric crystal sensors from EPM Systems (Midlothian, VA). These sensors are attached to a belt that is placed around the patient.

For many of the recordings, an additional system was used to assess respiratory effort. This system, labeled *backup* in the montages, was also recorded with piezoelectric crystal sensors from EPM Systems (Midlothian, VA). This backup belt was placed between the thoracic and abdominal belts.

Snoring sound was recorded with piezoelectric crystal sensors from EPM Systems (Midlothian, VA). This sensor is placed either 2 cm to the left or right of the trachea, midway down the neck.

Oximetry was recorded with an Ohmeda model 3740 (Louisville, CO). Oximetry was recorded from a finger site.

Many of the illustrations were obtained from studies of patients who were undergoing a treatment trial of continuous positive airway pressure (CPAP) or bilevel positive airway pressure (BPAP) and include recordings of mask flow and tidal volume. The CPAP and BPAP equipment that generated these signals included models manufactured by Respironics, Inc., and Healthdyne.

This atlas is designed to aid the sleep medicine specialist and those training in sleep medicine. It also serves as a reference and training tool for technologists. The atlas covers normal polysomnographic features of wakefulness and the various stages of sleep as well as polysomnographic findings characteristic of sleep-related breathing disorders, sleep-related movements, and parasomnias. In addition, examples of cardiac arrhythmias, nocturnal seizures, and artifacts are included. While most of the figures use a 30-second time base, a variety of shorter and longer time scales are used to illustrate their value.

1. American Sleep Disorders Association. *International Classification of Sleep Disorders, Revised: Diagnostic and Coding Manual*. Rochester, MN: American Sleep Disorders Association, 1997.
2. Gotman J. The use of computers in analysis and display of EEG and evoked potentials. In Daly DD, Pedley TA, eds. *Current Practice of Clinical Electroencephalography*, 2nd Ed. New York: Raven Press, 1990:51–83.
3. Parisi RA, Santiago TV. Respiration and respiratory function: Technique of recording and evaluation. In: Chokroverty S, ed. *Sleep Disorders Medicine: Basic Sciences, Technical Considerations, and Clinical Aspects*. Boston, MA: Butterworth-Heinemann, 1994:127–139.
4. Rechtschaffen A, Kales A. *A Manual of Standardized Terminology, Techniques, and Scoring System for Sleep Stages of Human Subjects*. Los Angeles, CA: Brain Information Service/Brain Research Institute, 1968.

Acknowledgments

ACKNOWLEDGMENTS to the Third Edition

We again thank all those members of the technical and support staff without whose diligent help we could neither care for our patients nor produce this text.

A special thanks goes to Alexis Pozonsky, Chris Teja, Nicole Dernoski, Kel McGowan, Jamie Elfrank, Rebecca Gaertner, Remya Divakaran, V. Venkatesan (SPi Global), and the other members of the editorial and production staff at Wolters Kluwer Health who provided important suggestions and support.

Finally, a special thanks goes to our wives and families for their continued and unwavering support.

ACKNOWLEDGMENTS to the Second Edition

As in all projects of this type, thanks must go to the technical and support staff at each of our Sleep Centers: The DCH Sleep Center, The University of Florida, and The St. Cloud Hospital Sleep Center.

A special thanks goes to Leanne McMillan, Tom Gibbons, Fran DeStefano, Lisa McAllister, and the other members of the editorial and production staff at Lippincott Williams & Wilkins who provided important suggestions and support.

Finally, a special thanks goes to our wives and families for their unwavering support.

ACKNOWLEDGMENTS to the First Edition

Ronald Chervin, MD, and Beth Malow, MD, were invaluable contributors to this project. The other faculty members of the University of Michigan Department of Neurology Clinical Neurophysiology Laboratory; Ivo Drury, MBBCh; Ahmad Beydoun, MD; Linda Selwa, MD; Robert MacDonald, MD, PhD; Jaideep Kapur, MD, PhD; Erasmo Passaro, MD; and Wassim Nasreddine, MD, were vital to both the fellowship program in sleep medicine and the production of this text.

The other members of the fellowship training programs in sleep medicine and clinical neurophysiology provided support, ideas, and interesting studies. We therefore thank and acknowledge the contributions of Sarah Nath, MD; L. John Greenfield, MD, PhD; Kirk Levy, MD; and Willie Anderson, MD.

As in all projects of this type, a special thanks must go to the technical and support staff. In particular, we would like to thank Ken Morton, RPSGT, sleep laboratory supervisor at the University of Michigan, and Brenda Livingston, clinic coordinator in the University of Michigan Sleep Disorders Center.

A special thanks goes to Anne Sydor, PhD, and the other members of the editorial and production staff at Lippincott Williams & Wilkins who provided important suggestions and support.

Finally, a special thanks goes to our families for their unwavering support.

Contents

Additional neonatal polysomnographs found in online eBook version

Introduction to Sleep and Polysomnography

James D. Geyer, MD and Paul R. Carney, MD

Overview of Sleep Stages and Cycles

The monitoring of sleep is complex and requires a distinct skill set including a detailed knowledge of electroencephalographic (EEG), respiratory monitoring and EKG. Expertise in only one of these areas does not confer the ability to accurately interpret a polysomnogram. On the contrary, understanding only one facet of recording can engender a false sense of mastery.

Sleep is not homogeneous. It is quite heterogeneous and divided into various stages based on EEG, electrooculographic (EOG) or eye movements, and electromyographic (EMG) activity (1–3). The basic terminology and methodology involved in monitoring each type of activity will be reviewed in detail. Sleep is composed of nonrapid eye movement (NREM) and rapid eye movement (REM) sleep. NREM sleep is further divided into stages N1, N2, and N3. Stages N1 and N2 are called light sleep, and stage N3 is called deep, delta, or slow-wave sleep. There are usually four or five cycles of sleep in a typical night, each composed of a segment of NREM sleep followed by REM sleep. Periods of wake may also interrupt sleep during the night but should be brief and self-limited in the normal adult. As the night progresses, the length of the REM sleep period in each cycle usually increases. The hypnogram is a convenient method of graphically displaying large amounts of information about the organization of sleep. Each stage of sleep is characterized by a level on the vertical axis of the graph with time of night on the horizontal axis.

Because sleep monitoring was traditionally recorded by paper polygraph recording systems, the night was divided into epochs of time that corresponded to the length of each paper page. Based on the standard paper speed for sleep recording of 10 mm per second, a 30-cm page represented 30 seconds. Each 30-second page was referred to as an epoch. Though modern polysomnography is performed digitally, the convention of scoring sleep in 30-second epochs remains the standard. When a shift in sleep stage occurs during a given epoch, the stage present for the majority of that epoch defines the stage scored for that epoch.

Sleep Architecture Definitions

The term sleep architecture describes the structure of sleep. Common terms used in sleep monitoring are listed in **Table 1-1**. The total monitoring time or total recording time (TRT) is also called total bedtime (TBT). This is the time duration from lights out (start of recording) to lights on (termination of recording). The total amount of time spent in sleep stages N1, N2, N3, and R is termed the *total sleep time* (TST). The time from the first sleep until the final awakening is called the *sleep period time* (SPT). SPT encompasses all sleep as well as periods of wake after sleep onset (WASO) and before the final awakening of the study; SPT = TST + WASO. The time from the start of sleep monitoring (or lights out) until the first epoch of sleep is called the *sleep latency*. The time from the first epoch of sleep until the first REM sleep is called the *REM latency*. It is useful not only to determine the total minutes of each sleep stage but also to characterize the relative proportion of time spent in each sleep stage. Stages N1 to N3 and R can also be displayed as a percentage of total sleep time (%TST). Alternatively, the various sleep stages and WASO can be calculated as a percentage of the

TABLE 1-1 Sleep Architecture Definitions

- Lights out—start of sleep recording
- Light on—end of sleep recording
- TBT (total bedtime)—time from lights out to lights on
- TST (total sleep time) = minutes of stages 1, 2, 3, and REM
- WASO (wake after sleep onset)—minutes of wake after first sleep but before the final awakening
- SPT (sleep period time) = TST + WASO
- Sleep latency—time from lights out until the first epoch of sleep
- REM latency—time from first epoch of sleep to the first epoch of REM sleep
- Sleep efficiency—(TST × 100)/TBT
- Stage N1, 2, 3, and REM as %TST—percentage of TST occupied by each sleep stage
- Stage N1, 2, 3, and REM, WASO as %SPT—percentage of SPT occupied by sleep stages and WASO
- Arousal index

TABLE 1-2 Representative Changes in Sleep Architecture

	20-Year-Old	60-Year-Old	Severe Sleep Apnea[a]
WASO% SPT	5	15	20
Stage N1% SPT	5	5	10
Stage N2% SPT	50	55	60
Stage N3% SPT	20	5	0
Stage R% SPT	25	20	10

[a]High interpatient variability.

sleep period time (%SPT). Sleep efficiency (in percent) is usually defined as either the TST × 100/SPT or TST × 100/TBT.

The normal range of the percentage of sleep spent in each sleep stage varies with age (2,3) and is affected by sleep disorders (**Table 1-2**). In adults there is a decrease in stage N3 sleep with increasing age, while the amount of REM sleep remains fairly constant over time. The changes in stage N3 are related in part to a lowering of the voltage of the delta activity secondary to the filtering effects of the skull with advancing age. The amounts of stage N1 sleep and WASO also increases with age. Severe obstructive sleep apnea (OSA) can result in dramatically diminished amounts of stage N3 and stage R. Chronic insomnia (difficulty initiating or maintaining sleep) is characterized by a long sleep latency or increased WASO. The amount of time in stages N3 and R sleep is commonly decreased as well. The REM latency is also affected by sleep disorders and medications. A short REM latency (usually < 70 minutes) may occur in some cases of sleep apnea, depression, narcolepsy, prior REM sleep deprivation, or the withdrawal of REM suppressant medications. An increased REM latency can be seen with REM suppressants (ethanol and many antidepressants), an unfamiliar or uncomfortable sleep environment, sleep apnea, or any significant sleep disturbance.

Electroencephalographic Terminology and Monitoring

Standard sleep monitoring requires monitoring of frontal, central, and occipital EEG activity (preferably bilaterally), which are referenced to mastoid electrodes. Alpha activity is more prominent in occipital tracings. The terminology for the electrodes adheres to the International 10–20 nomenclature, which guides the exact placement of the electrodes. Even subscripts refer to electrodes on the right and odd subscripts to electrodes on the left side of the head. The usual derivations use the recording electrodes referenced to the opposite mastoid electrode (e.g., C4-M1). Use of greater interelectrode distances increases the voltage difference between electrodes, yielding more easily distinguished waveforms. Full EEG montage recording enhances the ability to identify EEG abnormalities.

EEG activity is characterized by the signal amplitude (voltage), direction of major deflection (polarity), and frequency in cycles per second or hertz (Hz). Standard frequency ranges include delta (<4 Hz), theta (4 to 7 Hz), alpha (8 to 13 Hz), and beta (>13 Hz). Alpha activity is commonly noted during relaxed wakefulness with eyes closed. This activity is best recorded from the occipital derivations but may spread temporally in some individuals. Alpha activity should attenuate when the eyes are open. Bursts of alpha waves also are seen during brief arousals from sleep. Alpha activity can also be seen during REM sleep but is typically several Hz slower than the alpha activity recorded during wakefulness. Alpha activity decreases with the onset of stage N1 sleep. Vertex *sharp waves* are high-amplitude, centrally predominant negative waves (upward deflection on EEG tracings) with a short duration occurring during the transition from Stage N1 to N2 sleep. A sharp wave is defined as deflection lasting between 70 and 200 milliseconds (**Table 1-3**).

Sleep spindles, which are characteristic of stage N2 sleep, are sinusoidal oscillations of 12 to 14 Hz with a duration lasting between 0.5 and 1.5 seconds. They may persist into stage N3 but usually do not occur in stage R. The K complex is a high-amplitude, biphasic wave lasting at least 0.5 second and consisting of an initial sharp, negative voltage followed by a positive deflection slow wave. Spindles frequently are superimposed on K complexes. Sharp waves differ from K complexes in that they are narrower, not biphasic, and usually of lower amplitude.

As sleep deepens, slow waves or delta activity appears. These are high-amplitude, broad waves. In contrast to the EEG definition of delta activity as less than 4 Hz, delta slow-wave activity is defined for sleep staging purposes as waves less than 2 Hz (longer than 0.5-second duration waveforms) with a peak-to-peak amplitude of greater than 75 μV and is measured utilizing the frontal derivations (1). Because a K complex resembles slow-wave activity, differentiating the two can be challenging in some instances. However, by definition, a K complex should stand out or be distinct from the lower-amplitude, background EEG activity. Therefore, a continuous

TABLE 1-3 Standard Sensitivity and Filter Settings

	Sensitivity	Low Filter	High Filter
EEG	50 μV = 1 cm; 100 μV = 1 channel width	0.3[a]	35[a]
EOG	50 μV = 1 cm; 100 μV = 1 channel width	0.3	35
EMG	50 μv = 1 cm; 100 μV = 1 channel width	10	100
EKG		0.3	70
Airflow (thermistor)	Variable	0.1	15
Chest	Variable	0.1	15
Abdomen	Variable	0.1	15
Sao$_2$ (%)	1 Volt = 0%–100% or 50%–100%	DC	15
Nasal pressure machine flow	Variable	DC or AC with low filter setting of 0.03	15 100 to see snoring
PAP flow		DC	DC
Snoring		10	10

[a]Note that these filter settings are different from traditional EEG monitoring settings.

series of high-voltage slow (HVS) waves would not be considered to be a series of K complexes.

Sawtooth waves are notched–jagged waves of frequency in the theta range (3 to 7 Hz) that may occur during stage R sleep. These waveforms are not required for stage R, but their presence can help confirm its presence.

 Eye Movement Recording

Eye movement recording is possible because an electrical potential difference exists across the eyeball: front positive (+), back negative (–). Two things can confound this standardized approach: asymmetric or dysconjugate eye movements and an artificial eye.

There are two common patterns of eye movements. Slow eye movements (SEMs), also called slow-rolling eye movements, are pendular, oscillating movements seen in drowsy (eyes closed) wakefulness and stage N1 sleep. By stage N2 sleep, SEMs usually have disappeared. REMs are sharper (narrower deflections), which are typical of eyes-open wake and REM sleep. Reading eye movements occur with a slow movement in one direction followed by a fast recovery in the other direction. These movements are usually rhythmic and recurring.

In the two-tracing method of eye movement recording, large-amplitude EEG activity or artifact reflected in the EOG tracings usually causes in-phase defections. This is commonly seen with K complexes and stage N3 sleep delta activity.

The main purpose of recording eye movements is to identify the scanning or reading eye movements of wakefulness, slow rolling eye movements of drowsiness, and REM sleep. EOG (eye movement) electrodes typically are placed at the outer corners of the eyes—at the right outer canthus (ROC) and the left outer canthus (LOC). In a common approach, two eye channels are recorded, and the eye electrodes are referenced to the opposite mastoid (ROC-M1 and LOC-M2). In pediatric recording, alternative eye leads referenced to FPz may be more easily tolerated (4,5).

The electric dipole of the eye, with the cornea being positive in relation to the retina, allows for the recording of eye movements with surface electrodes (4,6). Eye movements are typically conjugate, with both eyes moving toward one eye electrode and away from the other.

High-amplitude EEG activity or artifact occurring in the EOG tracings usually causes *in-phase defections* and not the *out-of-phase deflections* seen with conjugate eye movements.

 Electromyographic Recording

Usually, three EMG leads are placed in the mental and submental areas. The voltage between two of these three is monitored (e.g., EMG1-EMG3). If either of these leads fails, the third lead can be substituted. The gain of the chin EMG is adjusted so that some activity is noted during wakefulness. The chin EMG is an essential element only for identifying stage R sleep. In stage R, the chin EMG is relatively reduced, with the amplitude being equal to or lower than the lowest EMG amplitude in NREM sleep. The chin EMG may also reach the REM level long before the onset of REMS or an EEG meeting criteria for stage R. Depending on the gain, a reduction in the chin EMG amplitude from wakefulness to sleep and often a further reduction on transition from stage N1 to N3 may be seen. However, a reduction in the chin EMG is not required for stages N2 to N3. The reduction in the EMG amplitude during REM sleep is a reflection of the generalized skeletal-muscle hypotonia present in this sleep stage. Brief EMG activity bursts, referred to as phasic activity, may be seen during REM sleep, especially when there is vigorous eye movement. The combination of REMs, a relatively reduced chin EMG, and a low-voltage mixed-frequency EEG is consistent with stage R.

 Sleep Stage Characteristics

The basic rules for sleep staging are summarized in **Table 1-4**. Note that some characteristics are required and some are helpful but not required to stage a particular epoch. The typical patterns associated with each sleep stage are discussed below.

Stage Wake

During eyes-open wake, the EEG is characterized by high-frequency, low-voltage activity. The EOG tracings typically show REMs, and the chin EMG activity is relatively high, allowing differentiation from Stage R sleep. During eyes-closed drowsy wake,

TABLE 1-4 Summary of Sleep Stage Characteristics

Stage	EEG	EOG	EMG
		Characteristics[a,b]	
Wake (eyes open)	Low-voltage, high-frequency, attenuated alpha activity	Eye blinks, REMs	Relatively high
Wake (eyes closed)	Low-voltage, high-frequency >50% alpha activity	Slow-rolling eye movements	Relatively high
Stage N1	Low-amplitude mixed-frequency **<50% Alpha activity No spindles, K complexes**	Slow-rolling eye movements	May be lower than wake
	Sharp waves near transition to stage N2		
Stage N2	**At least one sleep spindle or K complex <20% Slow-wave activity**[b]		May be lower than wake
Stage N3	**>20% Frontally predominant slow-wave activity**	[c]	Usually low
Stage R	**Low-voltage mixed-frequency**	**Episodic REMs**	**Relatively reduced** (equal or lower than the lowest in NREM)
	Sawtooth waves—may be present		

[a]Required characteristics in bold.
[b]Slow wave activity, frequency < 2 Hz; peak to peak amplitude > 75 µV; >50% means slow wave activity present in more than 50% of the epoch; REMs, rapid eye movements.
[c]Slow waves usually seen in EOG tracings.

the EEG is characterized by prominent alpha activity (>50% of the epoch). Both slow, scanning and rapid irregular eye movements are usually present. The level of muscle tone is usually relatively high. The epoch should be scored as stage W when more than 50% of the epoch consists of alpha rhythm or findings consistent with stage W, such as eye blinks (conjugate vertical eye movements with a frequency between 0.5 and 2 Hz), reading eye movements (series of repetitive movements with a slow phase followed by a rapid or return phase), or REMs with a high chin EMG tone. Caution should be used in scoring stage W with REMs and a high chin EMG tone since this may also occur in REM sleep behavior disorder (RBD).

The alpha rhythm is composed of 8- to 13-Hz waves over the posterior head regions during relaxed wakefulness with eyes closed. The lower limit of 8 Hz is typically attained by 8 years of age. The frequency of the alpha rhythm in adults is typically between 9 and 11 Hz, decreasing slightly with advancing age. A posteriorly dominant rhythm of less than 8 Hz during wakefulness in an adult is abnormal. Identifying the waking background activity is vital for correct sleep staging. The frequency and morphology of the alpha rhythm should be similar over the two hemispheres. An interhemispheric asymmetry of the alpha rhythm of 1 Hz or greater is

also abnormal. Importantly, in some individuals, no waking alpha rhythm can be identified. The individual may have a low-amplitude fast background during wakefulness.

In referential montages, the distribution of the alpha rhythm is usually maximal at the occipital electrodes (O1, O2). In some cases, the amplitude of the alpha rhythm may be highest in the parietal or posterior temporal regions and occasionally is more diffusely distributed. The voltage of the alpha rhythm in adults is in the range of 15 to 45 µV. Higher voltages are observed in younger individuals. The voltage decreases with advancing age, secondary to changes in bone density and increased electrical impedance of intervening tissue. A mild voltage asymmetry is common, with the right hemisphere typically being of a somewhat higher amplitude. Voltage asymmetries are considered significant when the interhemispheric amplitude difference is greater than 50%.

Stage N1

The stage N1 EEG is characterized by low-voltage, mixed-frequency activity (4 to 7 Hz). Stage N1 is scored when less than 50% of an epoch contains alpha waves and criteria for deeper stages of sleep are not met. SEMs are conjugate, repetitious, sinusoidal eye movements with an initial deflection usually lasting at least 500 milliseconds. Slow-rolling eye movements often are present in the eye movement tracings, and the level of muscle tone (EMG) is equal or diminished compared to that in the awake state. Some patients do not exhibit prominent alpha activity, making detection of sleep onset difficult. In stage N1, the EEG is mixed frequency with activity in the 4- to 7-Hz theta range. One staging method to determine sleep onset in difficult cases is to find the first epoch of unequivocal sleep (usually stage N2) and then stage backwards to an epoch of definite wakefulness.

Vertex waves commonly occur in stage N1 sleep and are defined by a sharp configuration maximal over the central derivations. Vertex waves should clearly stand out from the background activity.

Positive occipital sharp transients (POSTs) are surface-positive triangular waves occasionally followed by a lower-voltage negative phase that can be seen in light sleep, especially in children. POSTs often occur in runs of bilaterally synchronous 4- to 5-Hz waves, Asymmetries are common. These waveforms first appear in drowsiness but may persist into deeper stages of NREM sleep. POSTs are not identified in all individuals.

Stage N2

Stage N2 sleep is characterized by the presence of one or more K complexes or sleep spindles. To qualify as stage N2, the majority of an epoch must meet criteria for stage N2 sleep with less than 20% slow (delta) wave EEG activity (<6 seconds of a 30-second epoch). Stage N2 occupies the greatest proportion of the TST for most individuals, accounting for approximately 40% to 50% of sleep. Stage N2 sleep ends with a sleep stage transition, or an arousal.

Although frequency changes associated with arousals and sleep spindles are more typically noted in the central and occipital EEG derivations, these findings should be used to score sleep even if they are only identified in the frontal derivations. These findings include one or more K complexes unassociated with arousals and one or more sleep spindles.

The EOG usually shows no eye movement activity during stage N2 sleep, but SEMs may persist in some individuals. This is especially true for those individuals taking SSRI antidepressants and neuroleptics, among other medications.

Stage N3

Stage N3 sleep is called slow-wave, delta, or deep sleep. Stage N3 is scored when frontally predominant slow-wave activity (frequency < 2 Hz and amplitude > 75 μV peak-to-peak) is present for greater than 20% of the epoch. Pathologic wave forms that meet the slow wave activity criteria, such as those generated by metabolic encephalopathies, epilepsies, or epileptiform activity, are not counted as slow-wave activity of sleep. Similarly, waveforms produced by artifact or those of noncerebral origin should not be included in the scoring of slow waves. Spindles may be present in the EEG. The high-voltage EEG activity is usually easily identified in the eye leads, and since the activity is in-phase, it should not be mistaken for eye movements. The EMG during stage N3 sleep is usually lower than that seen during stages N1 and N2 sleep, but this is inconsistent. Typically, stage N3 occurs mostly in the early portions of the night.

Stage R

Stage R sleep is characterized by a low-voltage, mixed-frequency EEG, the presence of episodic REMs, and a relatively low-amplitude chin EMG. Sawtooth waves also may occur in the EEG. REMs consist of conjugate, irregular, sharply peaked eye movements with an initial deflection usually lasting less than 500 milliseconds. Sawtooth waves are commonly seen in stage R sleep. These waveforms are somewhat more difficult to identify on digital recordings since they become more obvious when viewed upside down.

Transient muscle activity consists of short irregular bursts of EMG activity usually with duration less than 0.25 seconds superimposed on low EMG baseline tone. The activity may be seen in the chin or anterior tibial EMG derivations, as well as in EEG or EOG deviations. The activity is maximal in association with REMs (phasic activity).

There usually are three to five episodes of REM sleep during the night, which tend to increase in length as the night progresses. The number of eye movements per unit time (REM density) also increases during the night. Not all epochs of REM sleep contain REMs. Epochs of sleep otherwise meeting criteria for stage R and contiguous with epochs of unequivocal stage R (REMs present) are scored as stage R. Bursts of alpha waves can occur during REM sleep, but the frequency is often 1 to 2 Hz slower than during stage W.

Stage R is associated with many unique, physiologic changes, such as widespread skeletal muscle hypotonia and sleep-related erections. Skeletal muscle hypotonia is a protective mechanism to prevent the acting out of dreams. In RBD, muscle tone is present, and body movements and even violent behavior can occur during REM sleep. This condition is commonly seen in association with tauopathies including Parkinson disease and can even presage onset of clinical manifestations by years.

Arousals

Arousal from sleep denotes a transition from a state of sleep to wakefulness. Frequent arousals can cause daytime sleepiness by shortening the total amount of sleep. Even if arousals are brief (1 to 5 seconds) with a rapid return to sleep, daytime sleepiness may result, although the TST may remain relatively normal (7). Thus, the restorative function of sleep depends on continuity as well as duration. Many disorders that are associated with excessive daytime sleepiness also are associated with frequent, brief arousals, including OSA and periodic limb movements.

Atypical Sleep Patterns

Several special cases can make sleep staging difficult by atypical EEG, EOG, and EMG patterns. In alpha sleep, prominent alpha activity persists into NREM sleep. The presence of spindles, K complexes, and slow-wave activity allows sleep staging despite prominent alpha activity. Causes of the pattern include pain, psychiatric disorders, chronic pain syndromes, and any cause of nonrestorative sleep (8,9). Patients taking benzodiazepines may have very prominent "pseudo-spindle" activity (14 to 16 rather than the usual 12 to 14 Hz) (10). SEMs are usually absent by the time stable stage N2 sleep is present. However, patients on some serotonin reuptake inhibitors (fluoxetine and others) may have prominent slow and rapid eye movements during NREM sleep (11). While a reduction in the chin EMG is required for staging REM sleep, patients with the RBD may have high chin activity during what otherwise appears to be REM sleep (12).

Sleep Staging in Infants and Children

Newborn term infants do not have the well-developed adult EEG patterns to allow staging according to standard adult criteria.

The following is a brief description of terminology and sleep staging for the newborn infant according to the state determination of Anders et al. (13). Infant sleep is divided into active sleep (corresponding to REM sleep), quiet sleep (corresponding to NREM sleep), and indeterminant sleep, which is often a transitional sleep stage. Behavioral observations are critical. Wakefulness is characterized by crying, quiet eyes open, and feeding. Sleep is often defined as sustained eye closure. Newborn infants typically have periods of sleep lasting 3 to 4 hours interrupted by feeding, and total sleep in 24 hours is usually 16 to 18 hours. They have cycles of sleep with a 45- to 60-minute periodicity with about 50% active sleep. In newborns, the presence of REM (active sleep) at sleep onset is the norm. In contrast, the adult sleep cycle is 90 to 100 minutes, REM occupies about 20% of sleep, and NREM sleep is noted at sleep onset.

The EEG patterns of newborn infants have been characterized as low-voltage irregular (LVI), tracé alternant (TA), high-voltage slow (HVS), and mixed (M) (**Table 1-5**). Eye movement monitoring is used as in adults. An epoch is considered to have high or low EMG

TABLE 1-5 EEG Patterns Used in Infant Sleep Staging

EEG Pattern	
Low-voltage irregular (LVI)	Low-voltage (14–35 µV),[a] little variation Theta (5–8 Hz) predominates
	Slow activity (1–5 Hz) also present
Tracé alternant (TA)	Bursts of high-voltage slow waves (0.5–3 Hz) with superimposition of rapid low-voltage sharp waves 2–4 Hz
	In between the high-voltage bursts (alternating with them) is low-voltage mixed-frequency activity of 4–8 seconds in duration
High-voltage slow (HVS)	Continuous moderately rhythmic medium-to high-voltage (50–150 µV) slow waves (0.5–4 Hz)
Mixed (M)	High-voltage slow- and low-voltage polyrhythmic activity
	Voltage lower than in HVS

[a]µV, microvolts.

TABLE 1-6 Characteristics of Active and Quiet Sleep

	Active Sleep	**Quiet Sleep**	**Indeterminant**
Behavioral	Eyes closed	Eyes closed	Not meeting criteria for active or quiet sleep
	Facial movements: smiles, grimaces, frowns	No body movements except startles and phasic jerks	
	Burst of sucking	Sucking may occur	
	Body—small digit or limb movements		
EEG	LVI, M, HVS (rarely)	HVS, TA, M	
EOG	REMs	No REMs	
	A few SEMs and a few dysconjugate movements may occur		
EMG	Low	High	
Respiration	Irregular	Regular	
		Postsigh pauses may occur	

if over one-half of the epoch shows the pattern. The characteristics of active sleep, quiet sleep, and indeterminant sleep are listed in **Table 1-6**. The change from active to quiet sleep is more likely to manifest indeterminant sleep. Nonnutritive sucking commonly continues into sleep.

As children mature, more typical adult EEG patterns begin to appear. Sleep spindles begin to appear at 2 months and are usually seen after 3 to 4 months of age (14). K complexes usually begin to appear at 6 months of age and are fully developed by 2 years of age (15). The point at which sleep staging follows adult rules is not well defined but usually is possible after age 6 months. After about 3 months, the percentage of REM sleep starts to diminish and the intensity of body movements during active (REM) sleep begins to decrease. The pattern of NREM at sleep onset begins to emerge, but the sleep cycle period does not reach the adult value of 90 to 100 minutes until adolescence.

Note that the sleep of premature infants is somewhat different from term infants (36 to 40 weeks' gestation). In premature infants, quiet sleep usually shows a pattern of tracé discontinu (16). This differs from TA as there is electrical quiescence (rather than a reduction in amplitude) between bursts of high-voltage activity. In addition, delta brushes (fast waves of 10 to 20 Hz) are superimposed on the delta waves. As the infant matures, delta brushes disappear and TA pattern replaces tracé discontinue.

There is no precise upper age boundary for pediatric sleep staging rules. Not all sleep waveforms are well developed by 2 months postterm. Sleep spindles may be seen by age 6 weeks to 3 months postterm and are present in all normal infants by age 2 to 3 months postterm. At this age the spindles are asynchronous between the hemispheres but become more synchronous over the first year of life. K complexes are usually present by age 3 to 6 months postterm.

EEG activity of 0.5 to 2 Hz with a typical amplitude of 100 to 400 μV in the frontal regions may first appear by 2 months of age and is usually present by age 4 to 5 months postterm. The criteria for slow-wave activity in infants are the same as those for adults (amplitude $\geq$ 75 μV of 0.5 to 2 Hz). NREM sleep can be scored as stage N1, N2, or N3 in most infants by age 5 to 6 months postterm and occasionally in infants as young as 4 months postterm.

In infants younger than 6 months postterm, non-EEG parameters are helpful in distinguishing NREM sleep from REM sleep. In REM sleep these parameters include the presence of irregular respiration, loss of chin muscle tone, transient muscle activity (muscle twitches), and REMs. In NREM sleep, they consist of regular respiration, absence of eye movements, and preserved chin muscle tone.

Identifying stage wake is more challenging in children than in adults. The posterior-dominant rhythms evolve with maturation. The posterior-dominant rhythm in infants and children typically contains intermixed slower EEG rhythms. Posterior slow waves of youth (PSW) are intermittent runs of bilateral but often asymmetric 2.5 to 4.5 Hz slow waves superimposed on the posterior-dominant rhythm. These waveforms are typically less than 120% of the background voltage, block with eye opening, and disappear with drowsiness and sleep. PSW are uncommon in children less than 2 years of age and are most commonly seen between ages 8 to 14 years.

Another commonly seen slow wave activity during wakefulness in children is random or semirhythmic occipital slowing. This finding consists of less than 100 µV, 2.5 to 4.5 Hz rhythmic or arrhythmic activity lasting less than 3 seconds. It is a normal finding in EEGs of children ages 1 to 15 years and is especially prominent in children ages 5 to 7 years.

Posterior-Dominant Rhythm

Frequency of 3.5–4.5 Hz	3–4 months postterm
Frequency of 5–6 Hz	5–6 months postterm
Frequency of 7.5–9.5 Hz	3 years
Mean frequency of 9 Hz	9 years
Mean frequency of 10 Hz	15 years
Vertex sharp waves	4–6 months postterm
Hypnagogic hypersynchrony (HH)	3–6 months postterm

Respiratory Monitoring

The major components of respiratory monitoring during sleep are snoring, airflow, respiratory effort, and arterial oxygen saturation (17,18). For selected cases, exhaled or transcutaneous PCO_2 may also be monitored (and is required for pediatric monitoring).

Monitoring of nasal pressure with a small nasal cannula connected to a pressure transducer is the standard modality for assessing airflow (15,16). The nasal pressure system tends to underestimate airflow at low flow rates and overestimate it at higher flow rates. In the midrange of typical flow rates during sleep, the nasal pressure signal varies fairly linearly with flow. In addition to changes in magnitude, changes in the morphology or shape of the nasal pressure signal can provide useful information. A flattened profile usually means that there is a limitation of airflow (15,16). The only significant disadvantage of nasal pressure monitoring is that mouth breathing is not adequately detected. This disadvantage can be ameliorated by adding a nasal–oral thermistor to the nasal pressure monitor.

In pediatric polysomnography, exhaled CO_2 or transcutaneous CO_2 monitoring is required. Apnea usually causes an absence of fluctuations in this signal. Small expiratory puffs rich in CO_2 can complicate interpretation (6). The end-tidal PCO_2 (value at the end of exhalation) provides a fairly accurate estimate of arterial PCO_2. During long periods of hypoventilation that are common in children with sleep apnea, the end-tidal PCO_2 will be elevated (>45 mm Hg) (14). The degree of hypoventilation can be underestimated when there is frequent obstruction or mouth breathing, and these issues should be noted in the report when they occur.

Esophageal pressure monitoring (reflecting changes in pleural pressure) is the most sensitive method of detecting respiratory effort. This approach is rarely used in clinical practice because of its invasive nature (16). Respiratory inductance plethysmography (RIP) has replaced the use of strain gauge–based belt systems that monitored chest and abdominal movement. Changes in the sum of the ribcage and abdomen RIP signals correspond to changes in tidal volume (17,18). The inductance of each coil varies with changes in the area enclosed by the bands. During upper-airway narrowing or total occlusion, the chest and abdominal bands may move paradoxically. Changes in body position may affect the ability of RIP belts to detect chest or abdominal movement. Furthermore, obese patients may exhibit minimal chest or abdominal wall movement even with significant effort. Nevertheless, diagnosing central apnea based on only on surface detection of inspiratory effort can be challenging.

Arterial oxygen saturation (SaO_2) is measured during sleep studies using pulse oximetry (finger or ear probes). The term SpO_2 indicates that the SaO_2 was obtained via pulse oximetry. An oxygen desaturation is typically defined as a decrease in SaO_2 of 4% or more from baseline. The maximum drop in SaO_2 usually trails the respiratory event, whether apnea or hypopnea, termination by approximately 6 to 8 seconds, or longer. This delay is secondary to a combination of factors including the blood circulation time and instrumental delay caused by the oximeter averaging time. Movement artifact can result in erroneous oxygen desaturation readings. Furthermore, systems with long averaging times impair the detection of brief or lower amplitude oxygen desaturations.

Adult Respiratory Definitions

In adults and children above 18 years of age, apnea is defined as absence of airflow for ≥10 seconds (13,14). Adult scoring criteria may be used for children over 13 years of age at the discretion of the sleep specialist (17,18). An obstructive apnea is cessation of airflow with persistent inspiratory effort. In central apnea, there is an absence of inspiratory effort. Mixed apnea is defined as an apnea with both central and obstructive components. A hypopnea is a reduction in airflow for 10 seconds or longer (17). The apnea + hypopnea index (AHI) is the total number of apneas and hypopneas per hour of sleep. In adults, an AHI of less than 5 is considered normal.

Hypopneas can be further classified as obstructive, central, or mixed. If the upper airway narrows significantly, airflow can fall (obstructive hypopnea). Alternatively, airflow can fall from a decrease in respiratory effort (central hypopnea). In a mixed hypopnea, there is a decrease in respiratory effort and an increase in upper airway resistance. However, unless accurate measures of airflow and esophageal or supraglottic pressure are obtained, such differentiation is difficult.

The new requirements for an event to be classified as a hypopnea are as follows. A hypopnea should be scored only if all of the following criteria are present.

- The nasal pressure signal excursions (or those of the alternative hypopnea sensor) drop by greater than 30% of baseline.
- The event duration is at least 10 seconds.
- There is a greater than 4% oxygen desaturation from preevent baseline.
- At least 90% of the event's duration must meet the amplitude reduction of criteria for hypopnea.

Alternatively, a hypopnea can also be scored if all of these criteria are present.

- The nasal pressure signal excursions (or those of the alternative hypopnea sensor) drop by greater than 50% of baseline.
- The duration of the event is at least 10 seconds.
- There is a greater than 3% oxygen desaturation from preevent baseline or the event is associated with arousal.
- At least 90% of the event's duration must meet the amplitude reduction of criteria for hypopnea.

Respiratory events that do not meet criteria for either apnea or hypopnea can induce arousal from sleep. Such events have been called upper-airway resistance events (UARE), after the upper-airway resistance syndrome (UARS) (19). An AASM task force recommended that such events be called respiratory effort–related arousals (RERAs). The recommended criteria for a RERA is a respiratory event of 10 seconds or longer followed by an arousal that does not meet criteria for an apnea or hypopnea but is associated with a crescendo of inspiratory effort (esophageal monitoring) or a flattened waveform on nasal pressure monitoring (20). Typically, following arousal, there is a sudden drop in esophageal pressure deflections. The exact definition of hypopnea that one uses will often determine whether a given event is classified as a hypopnea or an RERA. RDI = AHI + RERA index, where the RERA index is the number of RERAs per hour of sleep, and RERAs are arousals associated with respiratory events not meeting criteria for apnea or hypopnea.

Monitoring hypoventilation is optional according to the latest scoring criteria but is a very important component of patient management. Hypoventilation may be scored if either an increase in the arterial P_{CO_2} (or surrogate) to a value >55 mm Hg for ≥10 minutes occurs or there is ≥10 mm Hg increase in arterial P_{CO_2} (or surrogate) during sleep in comparison to an awake supine value to a value exceeding 50 mm Hg for ≥10 minutes.

Cheyne-Stokes breathing is scored when there are episodes of ≥3 consecutive central apneas and/or central hypopneas separated by a crescendo and decrescendo change in breathing amplitude with a cycle length of ≥40 seconds. There must be ≥5 central apneas and/or central hypopneas per hour of sleep associated with the crescendo/decrescendo breathing pattern recorded over ≥2 hours of monitoring. Furthermore, central apneas that occur within a run of Cheyne-Stokes breathing should be scored as individual apneas as well.

Pediatric Respiratory Definitions

Periodic breathing is defined as three or more respiratory pauses of at least 3 seconds in duration separated by less than 20 seconds of normal respiration. Periodic breathing is seen primarily in premature infants and mainly during active sleep (21). Although this is controversial, some feel that the presence of periodic breathing for greater than 5% of TST or during quiet sleep in term infants is abnormal. Central apnea in infants is thought to be abnormal if the event is greater than 20 seconds in duration or associated with arterial oxygen desaturation or significant bradycardia (21–24).

In children, a cessation of airflow of any duration (usually two or more respiratory cycles) is considered an apnea when the event is obstructive (21–24), that is, the 10-second rule for adults does not apply. Of note, the respiratory rate in children (20 to 30 per minute) is greater than in adults (12 to 15 per minute). In fact, 10 seconds in an adult is usually the time required for two to three respiratory cycles. Obstructive apnea is very uncommon in normal children. Therefore, an obstructive AHI > 1 is considered abnormal. In children with OSA, the predominant event during NREM sleep is obstructive hypoventilation rather than a discrete apnea or hypopnea. Obstructive hypoventilation is characterized by a long period of upper-airway narrowing with a stable reduction in airflow and an increase in the end-tidal P_{CO_2}. There is usually a mild decrease in the arterial oxygen desaturation. The ribcage is not completely calcified in infants and young children. Therefore, some paradoxical breathing is not necessarily abnormal. However, worsening paradox during an event would still suggest a partial airway obstruction. Nasal pressure monitoring is being used more frequently in children, and periods of hypoventilation are more easily detected (reduced airflow with a flattened profile). Normative values have been published for the end-tidal P_{CO_2}. One paper suggested that a peak end-tidal P_{CO_2} > 53 mm Hg or end-tidal P_{CO_2} > 45 mm Hg for more than 60% of TST should be considered abnormal (22).

Central apnea in infants was discussed previously. The significance of central apnea in older children is less certain. Most do not consider central apneas following sighs (big breaths) to be abnormal. Some central apnea is probably normal in children, especially during REM sleep. In one study, up to 30% of normal children had some central apnea. Central apneas, when longer than 20 seconds, or those of any length associated with SaO_2 below 90%, are often considered abnormal, although a few such events have been noted in normal children (25). Therefore, most would recommend observation alone unless the events are frequent.

Leg Movement Monitoring

The EMG of the anterior tibial muscle (anterior lateral aspect of the calf) of both legs is monitored to detect leg movements (LMs) (26).

Two electrodes are placed on the belly of the upper portion of the muscle of each leg about 2 to 4 cm apart. An electrode loop is taped in place to provide strain relief. Usually each leg is displayed on a separate channel. However, if the number of recording channels is limited, one can link an electrode on each leg and display both leg EMGs on a single tracing. Recording from both legs is required to accurately assess the number of movements. During biocalibration, the patient is asked to dorsiflex and plantar flex the great toe of the right and then the left leg to determine the adequacy of the electrodes and amplifier settings. The amplitude should be at least one-half of the channel width on digital recording. The use of 60-Hz (notch) filters should be avoided. Impedances need to be less than 5,000 Ω. Sensitivity limits of –100 and +100 µV (upper/lower) are preferred.

A significant LM event is defined by an absolute increase in µV above resting baseline for the anterior tibialis EMG. This requires a stable resting EMG for the relaxed anterior tibialis whose absolute signal should be no greater than +10 µV between negative and positive deflection (±5 µV) or +5 µV for rectified signals. A limb movement should not be scored if it occurs less than 0.5 seconds preceding or following an apnea, hypopnea, RERA, or sleep-disordered breathing event. The minimum duration of an LM event is 0.5 seconds, and the maximum duration of an LM event is 10 seconds. The minimum amplitude of an LM event is an 8-µV increase in EMG voltage above resting EMG.

The timing of the onset of an LM event is defined as the point at which there is an 8-µV increase in EMG voltage above resting EMG, and the ending of a LM event is defined as the start of a period lasting at least 0.5 seconds during which the EMG does not exceed 2 µV above the resting EMG.

An arousal and a limb movement that occur in a periodic LM (PLM) series should be considered associated with each other if they occur simultaneously or when there is less than 0.5 seconds between the end of one event and the onset of the other event regardless of which is first.

When periodic limb movements occur with an interval of less than 10 seconds and each is associated with a 3-second arousal, only the first arousal should be scored though both limb movements may be scored. Therefore, the arousal index and PLM index with arousal, but not the Periodic Limb Movement Index, would be influenced by not scoring the second "arousal."

To be considered a PLM, the movement must occur in a group of four or more movements, each separated by more than 5 and less than 90 seconds (measured onset to onset). To be scored as a periodic LM in sleep, an LM must be preceded by at least 10 seconds of sleep. In most sleep centers, LMs associated with termination of respiratory events are not counted as PLMs. Some may score and tabulate this type of LM separately. The PLM index is the number of periodic LMs divided by the hours of sleep (TST in hours). Rough guidelines for the PLM index are >5 to <25 mild, >25 to <50 moderate, and ≥50 per hour severe (27). A PLM arousal is an arousal that occurs in association with (within 1 to 2 seconds) a PLM. The PLM arousal index is the number of PLM arousals per hour of sleep. LMs that occur during wake or after an arousal are either not counted or tabulated separately. For example, the PLMW (PLMwake) index is the number of PLMs per hour of wake. Of note, frequent LMs during wake, especially at sleep onset, may suggest the presence of the restless legs syndrome. The latter is a clinical diagnosis made on the basis of patient symptoms.

Alternating Leg Muscle Activation (ALMA) likely represents a benign movement which has particular associated EMG patterns. The duration is of the muscle activation 100 to 500 milliseconds. Four discrete and alternating leg EMG activity bursts are required to score an ALMA series. The minimum frequency of the alternating EMG bursts in ALMA must occur with a frequency between 0.5 Hz and 3.0 Hz.

Hypnagogic Foot Tremor (HFT) is a benign movement phenomenon associated with characteristic EMG patterns. Hypnagogic foot tremor typically lasts 250 to 1000 milliseconds. There must be at least four EMG bursts to create a HFT series. The frequency of the EMG bursts in a HFT is 0.3 to 4.0 Hz.

Excessive Fragmentary Myoclonus (EFM) appears to be a benign sleep-related movement associated with characteristic EMG patterns. Typically, no visible movements are present. The usual maximum EMG burst duration seen in fragmentary myoclonus is 150 milliseconds. In order to score EFM, there must be at least 20 minutes of NREM sleep with EFM, containing at least 5 EMG potentials per minute.

During sleep, masticatory muscle contractions frequently occur. These muscle contractions can take 2 forms. One is a sustained tonic contraction or jaw clenching. The other occurs as a series of repetitive brief phasic muscle contractions termed rhythmic masticatory muscle activity (RMMA).

Bruxism is scored when there are elevations of chin EMG activity that are at least twice the amplitude of background EMG. Brief episodes of bruxism occur with a duration between 0.25 and 2 seconds and if at least 3 such elevations occur in a regular sequence. Sustained bruxism occurs with an event duration of more than 2 seconds. A period of at least 3 seconds of stable background chin EMG must occur before a new episode of bruxism can be scored.

Rhythmic Movement Disorder diagnosis requires a combination of EMG and video monitoring. The frequency of movements ranges between 0.5 and 2.0 Hz and at least four movements are required to make a cluster of rhythmic movements. An individual rhythmic EMG burst must be at least twice the amplitude of the resting background EMG activity.

Biocalibrations and Technical Issues

In addition to the standard physiologic parameters monitored in polysomnography, body position (using low-light video monitoring) and treatment level (CPAP, bilevel pressure) are usually added in comments by the technologists. In most centers, a video recording is also made on traditional video tape or digitally as part of the digital recording. It is standard practice to perform amplifier calibrations at the start of recording. In traditional paper recording, a calibration voltage signal (square wave voltage) was applied and the resulting pen deflections, along with the sensitivity, polarity, and filter settings on each channel, were documented on the paper. Similarly, in digital recording, a voltage is applied, although it is often a sine-wave voltage. The impedance of the head electrodes is also checked prior to recording. The electrical impedance should be less than 5,000 Ω. Electrodes with higher impedances should be inspected and the problems corrected.

A biocalibration procedure is performed (**Table 1-7**) while signals are acquired with the patient connected to the monitoring equipment (4,5). This procedure permits checking of amplifier settings and integrity of monitoring leads/transducers. It also provides a baseline record of the patient's EEG and eye movements during wakefulness with eyes closed and open. A summary of typical commands and their utility is listed in **Table 1-7.**

TABLE 1-7 Biocalibration Findings and Procedures

A. Biocalibration Findings

Eyes closed	EEG: Alpha EEG activity
	EOG: slow eye movements
Eyes open	EEG: attenuation of alpha rhythm
	EOG: REMs, blinks
Look right, look left, look up, look down	Integrity of eye leads, polarity, amplitude
	Eye movements should cause out-of-phase deflections
Grit teeth	Chin EMG
Breathe in, breathe out	Airflow, chest, abdomen movements adequate gain? Tracings in phase? (polarity of inspiration is usually upward).
Deep breath in, hold breath	Apnea detection
Wiggle right toe, left toe	Leg EMG, amplitude reference to evaluate LMs

B. Biocalibration Procedure

1. Perform and document an impedance check of the EEG, EOG, and EMG electrodes
2. Record a minimum of 30 seconds of EEG with patient awake lying quietly with eyes open
3. Record a minimum of 30 seconds of EEG with patient lying quietly with eyes closed
4. Ask the patient to look up and down without moving head (×5)
5. Ask the patient to look left and right without moving head (×5)
6. Ask the patient to blink (×5)
7. Ask the patient to grit teeth and/or chew (5 seconds)
8. Ask the patient to simulate a snore or hum (5 seconds)
9. Ask the patient to breathe normally and assure that airflow and effort channel signals are synchronized
10. Ask the patient to perform a breath hold (10 seconds)
11. Ask the patient to breathe normally and upon instruction to take a breath in and out—check polarity and mark the record IN and OUT accordingly
12. Ask the patient to breathe through the nose only (10 seconds)
13. Ask the patient to breathe through the mouth only (10 seconds)
14. Ask the patient to take a deep breath and exhale slowly (prolonged expiration—10 seconds)
15. Ask the patient to flex the left foot/raise toes on left foot (×5)
16. Ask the patient to flex the right foot/raise toes on right foot (×5)
17. Ask the patient to flex/extend the fingers on the left hand, as appropriate, if upper extremity EMG is recorded
18. Ask the patient to flex/extend the fingers on the right hand, as appropriate, if upper extremity EMG is recorded

REFERENCES

1. Rechtschaffen A, Kales A, eds. *A Manual of Standardized Terminology Techniques and Scoring System for Sleep Stages of Human Sleep*. Los Angeles, CA: Brain Information Service/Brain Research Institute, UCLA, 1968.
2. Williams RL, Karacan I, Hursch CJ. *Electroencephalography of Human Sleep: Clinical Applications*. New York: Wiley, 1974.
3. Caraskadon MA, Rechschaffen A. Monitoring and staging human sleep. In: Kryger MH, Roth T, Dement WC, eds. *Principles and Practice of Sleep Medicine*. Philadelphia, PA: WB Saunders, 2000:1197–1215.
4. Keenan SA. Polysomnographic techniques: An overview. In: Chokroverty S, ed. *Sleep Disorders Medicine*. Boston, MA: Butterworth-Heinemann, 1999:151–169.
5. Butkov N. Polysomnography. In: Lee-Chiong TL, Sateia MJ, Carskadon MA, eds. *Sleep Medicine*. Philadelphia, PA: Hanley and Belfus, 2002:605–637.
6. Berry RB. *Sleep Medicine Pearls*. 2nd Ed. Philadelphia, PA: Hanley and Belfus, 2003.
7. Bonnet MH. Performance and sleepiness as a function of frequency and placement of sleep disruption. *Psychophysiology* 1986;23:263–271.
8. Butkov N. Atlas of clinical polysomnography, Ashland OR. *Synapse Media* 1996;110–112.
9. Hauri P, Hawkins DR. Alpha-delta sleep. *Electroencephalogr Clin Neurophysiol* 1973;34:233–237.
10. Johnson LC, Spinweber CL, Seidel WR, et al. Sleep spindle and delta changes during chronic use of short acting and long acting benzodiazepine hypnotic. *Electroencephalogr Clin Neurophysiol* 1983;55:662–667.
11. Armitage R, Trivedi M, Rush AJ. Fluoxetine and oculomotor activity during sleep in depressed patients. *Neuropsychopharmacology* 1995;12:159–165.
12. Schenck CH, Bundlie SR, Patterson AL, et al. Rapid eye movement sleep behavior disorder. *JAMA* 1987;257:1786–1789.
13. Anders T, Emde R, Parmalee A. *A Manual of Standardized Terminology, Techniques and Criteria for Scoring of State of Sleep and Wakefulness in Newborn Infants*. Los Angeles, CA: Brain Information Service, University of California Los Angeles, 1971.
14. Tanguay P, Ornitz E, Kaplan A, et al. Evolution of sleep spindles in childhood. *Electroencephalogr Clin Neurophysiol* 1975;38:175.
15. Metcalf D, Mondale J, Butler F. Ontogenesis of spontaneous K complexes. *Psychophysiology* 1971;26:49.
16. Sheldon SH, Riter S, Detrojan M. *Atlas of Sleep Medicine in Infants and Children*. Armonk, NY: Futura, 1999.
17. Block AJ, Boysen PG, Wynne JW, et al. Sleep apnea, hypopnea, and oxygen desaturation in normal subjects: A strong male predominance. *N Engl J Med* 1979;330:513–517.
18. Kryger MH. Monitoring respiratory and cardiac function. In: Kryger MH, Roth T, Dement WC, eds. *Principles and Practice of Sleep Medicine*. Philadelphia, PA: WB Saunders, 2000:1217–1230.
19. Guillemenault C, Stoohs R, Clerk A, et al. A cause of excessive daytime sleepiness: The upper airway resistance syndrome. *Chest* 1993;104:781–787.
20. Berry RB, Brooks R, Gamaldo CE, et al.; for the American Academy of Sleep Medicine. *The AASM Manual for the Scoring of Sleep and Associated Events: Rules, Terminology and Technical Specifications, Version 2.4*. www.aasmnet.org. Darien, IL: American Academy of Sleep Medicine, 2017.
21. American Thoracic Society. Standards and indication for cardiopulmonary sleep studies in children. *Am J Respir Crit Care Med* 1996;153:866–878.
22. Marcus CL, Omlin KJ, Basinki J, et al. Normal polysomnographic values for children and adolescents. *Am Rev Respir Dis* 1992;146:1235–1239.
23. American Thoracic Society. Cardiorespiratory studies in children: Establishment of normative data and polysomnographic predictors of morbidity. *Am J Respir Crit Care Med* 1999;160:1381–1387.
24. Marcus CL. Sleep-disordered breathing in children—State of the art. *Am J Respir Crit Care Med* 2001;164:16–30.
25. Weese-Mayer DE, Morrow AS, Conway LP, et al. Assessing clinical significance of apnea exceeding fifteen seconds with event recording. *J Pediatr* 1990;117:568–574.
26. ASDA Task Force. Recording and scoring leg movements. *Sleep* 1993;16:749–759.
27. Diagnostic and Classification Steering Committee; Thorpy MJ, Chairman. *International Classification of Sleep Disorders: Diagnostic and Coding Manual*. Rochester, MN: American Sleep Disorders Association, 1990:65–71.

Sleep Staging

James D. Geyer, MD and Paul R. Carney, MD

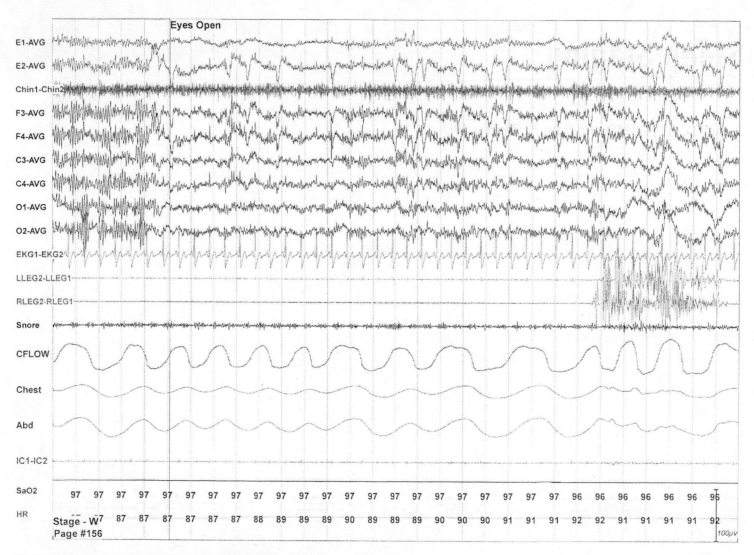

FIGURE 2-1   **Polysomnogram: CPAP montage; 30 second page.**
Clinical: 29-year-old man.
Staging: Stage wake. There is a well-modulated alpha rhythm. The alpha rhythm is dramatically attenuated with eye opening. The alpha rhythm is most prominent posteriorly, but its scalp topography varies across individuals. In this patient, the alpha rhythm is well represented in the central derivations. (Copyright JNP Enterprises, 2017.)

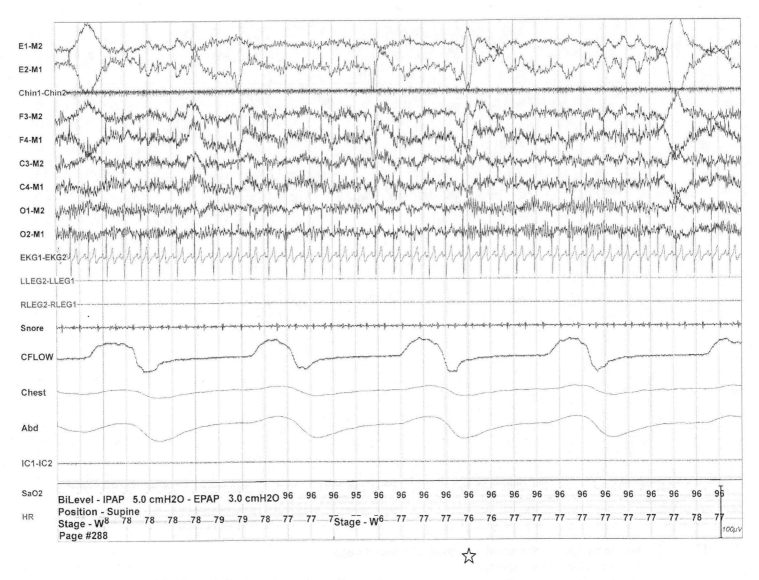

☆

FIGURE 2-2 **Polysomnogram: CPAP montage; 30 second page.**
Clinical: 29-year-old man.
Staging: Stage wake. There is a well-modulated alpha rhythm. The alpha rhythm increases with eye closure (*star*). The alpha rhythm is most prominent posteriorly, but its scalp topography varies across individuals. In this patient, the alpha rhythm is well represented in the central derivations. (Copyright JNP Enterprises, 2017.)

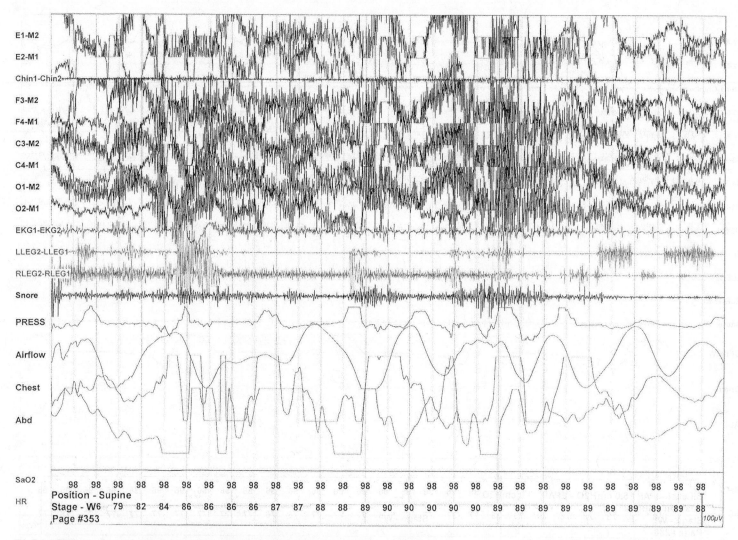

FIGURE 2-3 **Polysomnogram: Standard montage; 30 second page.**
Clinical: 35-year-old woman.
Staging: Stage wake. There is prominent motion artifact obscuring the EEG and EOG derivations.
(Copyright JNP Enterprises, 2017.)

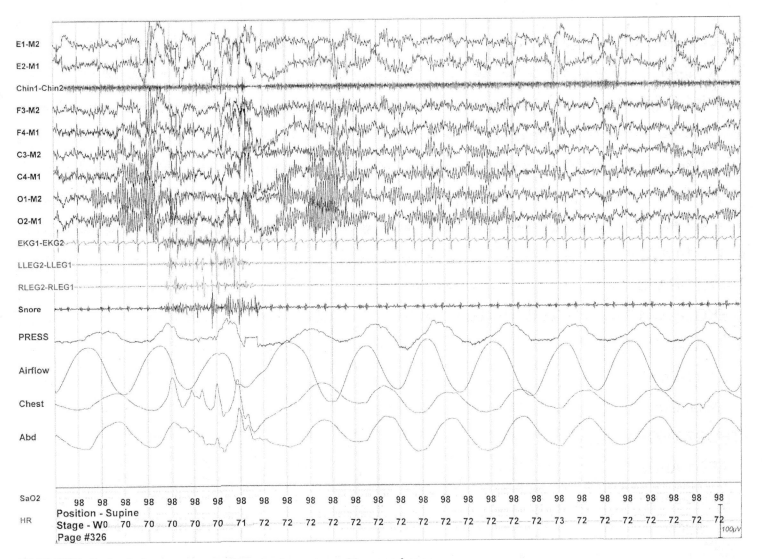

FIGURE 2-4 **Polysomnogram: Standard montage; 30 second page.**
Clinical: 31-year-old man.
Staging: Stage wake. There is partial obscuration of the background rhythms, but the well-modulated alpha rhythm can still be identified. (Copyright JNP Enterprises, 2017.)

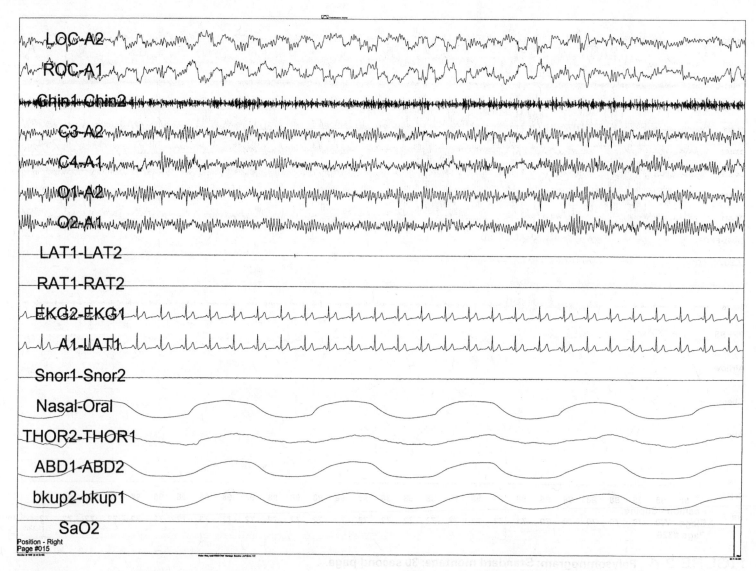

Position - Right
Page #015

FIGURE 2-5   **Polysomnogram: Standard montage (prior recording/display montage); 30 second page.**
Clinical: 17-year-old man.
Staging: Stage wake. There is a well-modulated 8-Hz alpha rhythm. The alpha rhythm is most prominent posteriorly, but its scalp topography varies across individuals. In this patient, the alpha rhythm is well represented in the central derivations.

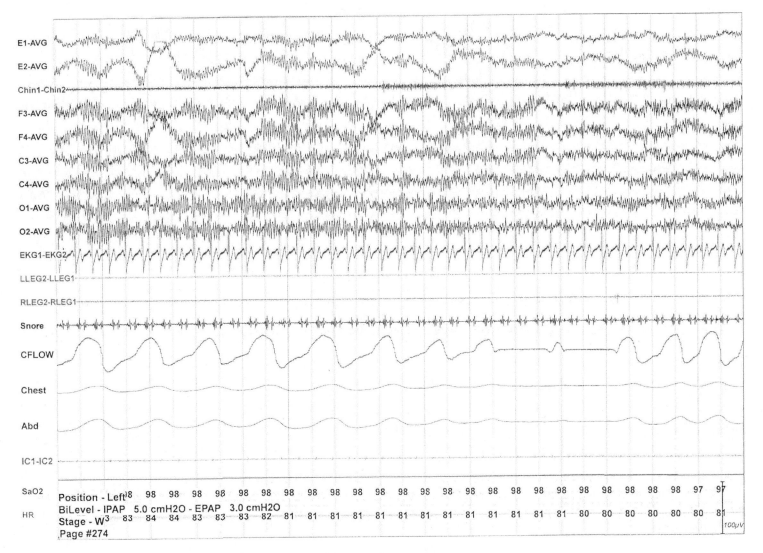

FIGURE 2-6 **Polysomnogram: CPAP montage; 30 second page.**
Clinical: 33-year-old man.
Staging: Stage wake. There is a well-modulated alpha rhythm. The alpha rhythm begins to slow in the second half of the epoch. Furthermore, there is slowing of the eye movements. This suggests the transition into drowsiness toward light sleep. (Copyright JNP Enterprises, 2017.)

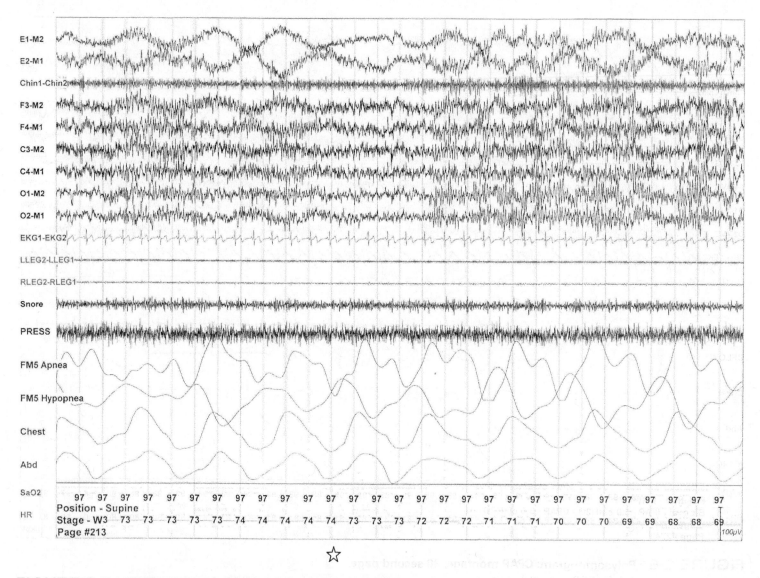

☆

FIGURE 2-7   **Polysomnogram: Standard montage; 30 second page.**
Clinical: 25-year-old man.
Staging: Stage wake. There is a well-modulated alpha rhythm. There is slowing of the eye movements
(*star*). This suggests the transition into drowsiness.
Technical: There is artifact in the pressure transducer channel (PRESS) secondary to the transducer
becoming dislodged. (Copyright JNP Enterprises, 2017.)

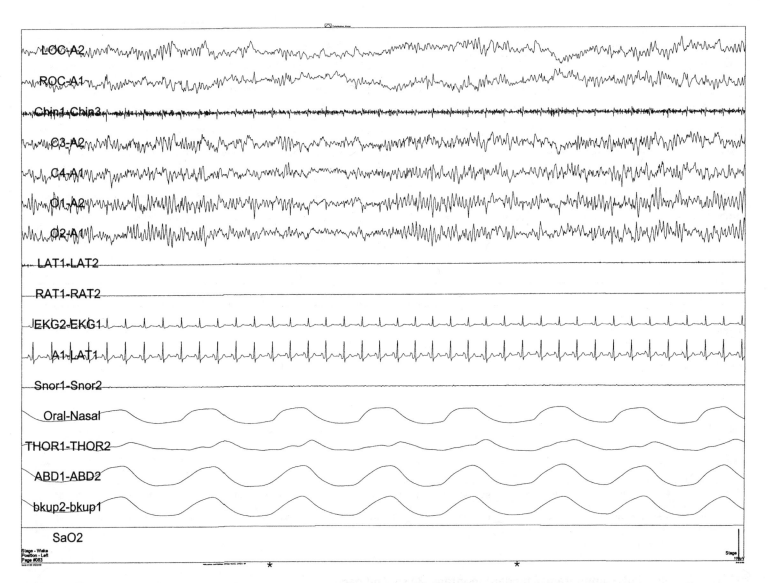

FIGURE 2-8 **Polysomnogram: Standard montage (prior recording/display montage); 30 second page.**
Clinical: 39-year-old woman.
Staging: Stage wake. Although alpha activity is present during the majority of the epoch, intermittent prominent theta activity (*) is consistent with brief episodes of sleep (microsleep).

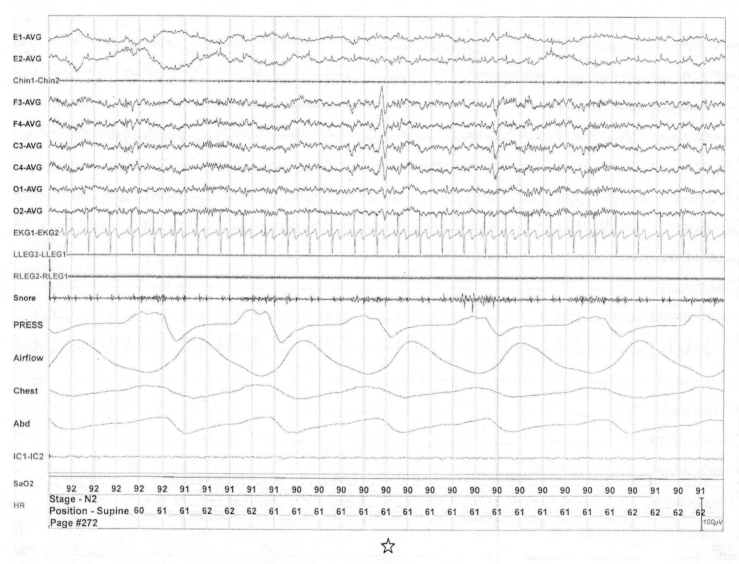

FIGURE 2-9   **Polysomnogram: Standard montage; 30 second page.**
Clinical: 44-year-old woman.
Staging: Stage N1. There are some slow eye movements, which diminish during the epoch. The alpha rhythm has attenuated. There is a vertex wave (*star*). (Copyright JNP Enterprises, 2017.)

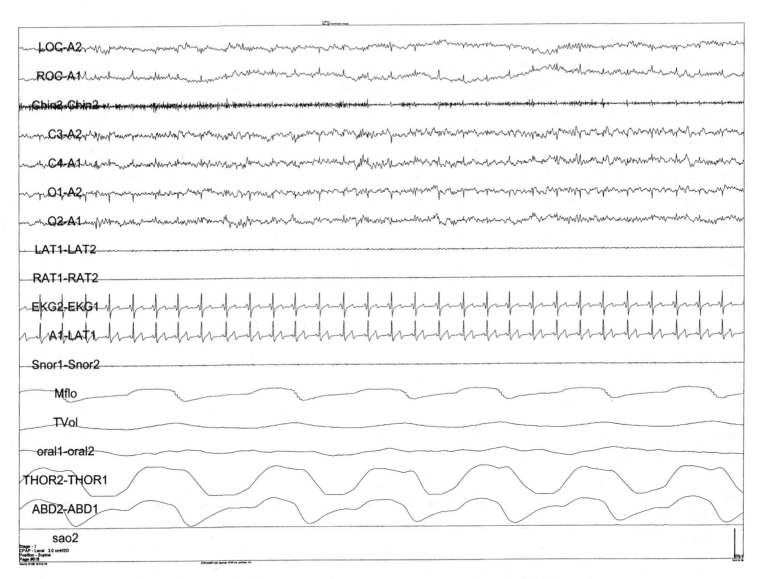

FIGURE 2-10   **Polysomnogram: CPAP montage (prior recording/display montage); 30 second page.**
Clinical: 37-year-old man.
Staging: Stage N1 sleep with prominent theta activity. There are slow eye movements and a gradual reduction of EMG activity.

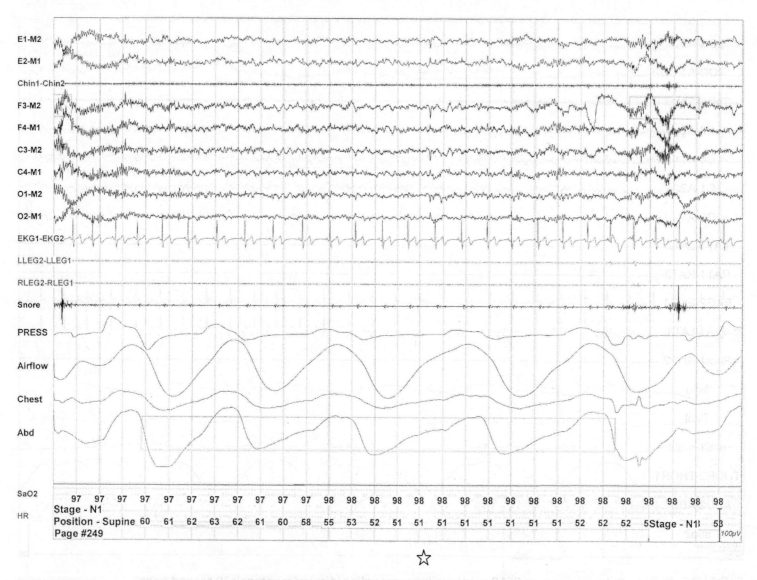

FIGURE 2-11   **Polysomnogram: Standard montage; 30 second page.**
Clinical: 28-year-old man.
Staging: Stage N1. The alpha rhythm is attenuated. There is an asymmetric (left greater than right) vertex wave (*star*). (Copyright JNP Enterprises, 2017.)

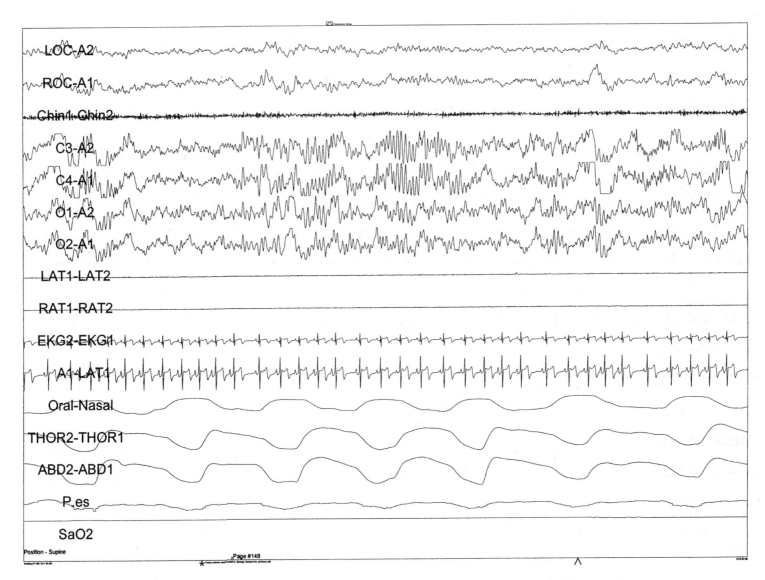

FIGURE 2-12 **Polysomnogram: Standard montage (prior recording/display montage); 30 second page.**
Clinical: 5-year-old girl.
Staging: Stage N1 sleep.
EEG: Rhythmic moderate- to high-amplitude 4- to 5-Hz activity, referred to as hypnagogic hypersynchrony (*), is a prominent feature of drowsy wakefulness and stage 1 sleep between the ages of 6 months and 6 years. It becomes less prominent during late childhood and adolescence. Near the end of the epoch, a K-complex (^) indicates the transition to stage 2 sleep.

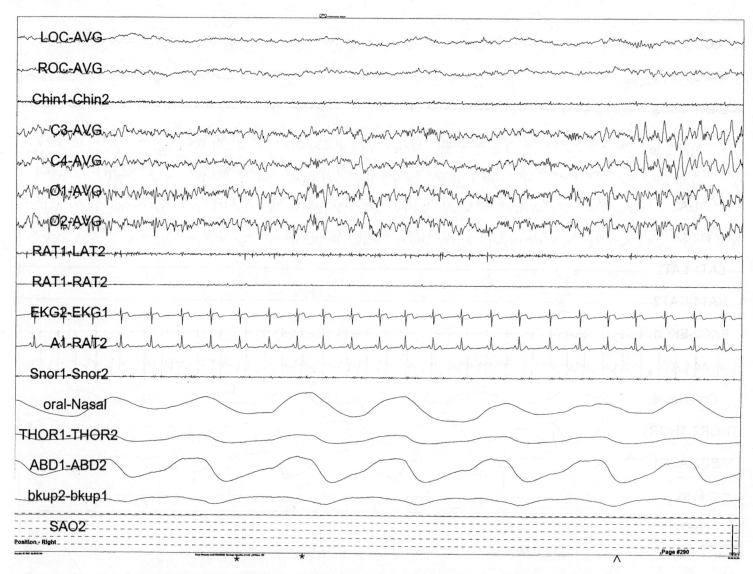

FIGURE 2-13   **Polysomnogram: Standard montage (prior recording/display montage); 30 second page.**
Clinical: 55-year-old man.
Staging: Stage N1 sleep. There are positive occipital sharp transients (POSTs) (*) and vertex waves (^).
These transients are seen in most persons during stage 1 sleep and occasionally during stage 2 sleep.

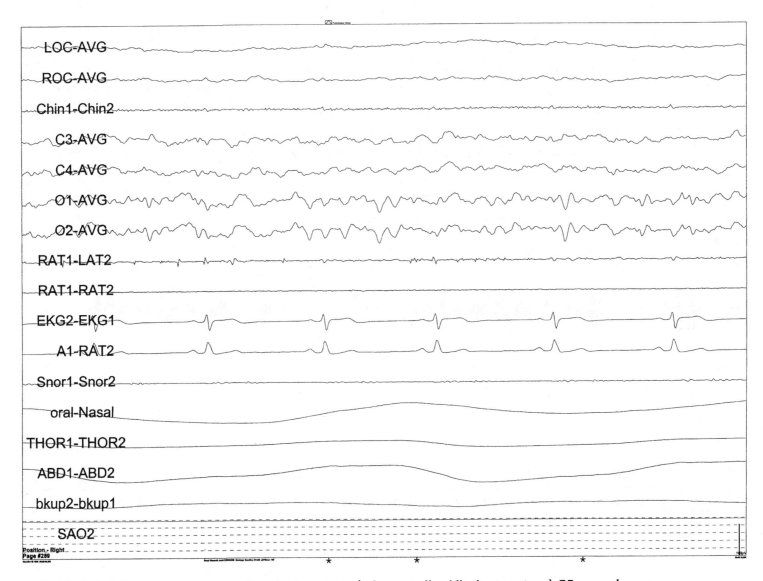

FIGURE 2-14 **Polysomnogram: Standard montage (prior recording/display montage); 7.5 second page.**
Clinical: 55-year-old man.
Staging: Stage N1 sleep with several POSTs and vertex waves (*).

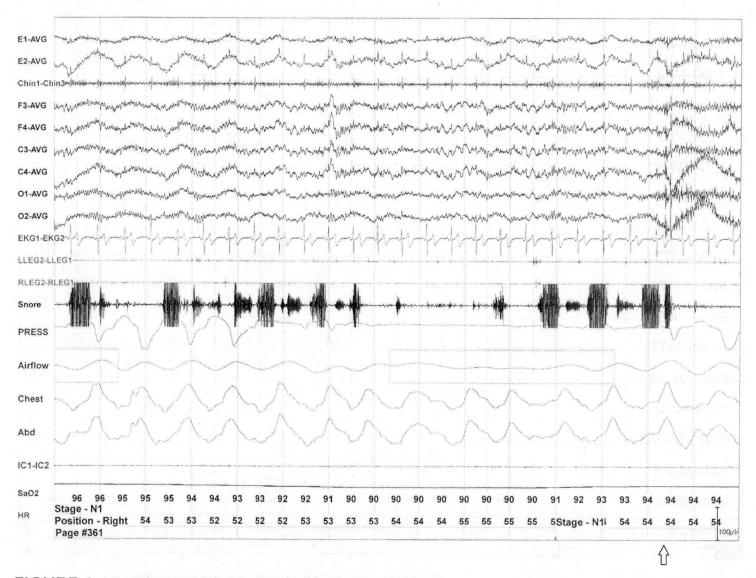

FIGURE 2-15   **Polysomnogram: Standard montage; 30 second page.**
Clinical: 52-year-old man.
Staging: Stage N1 with an arousal (*arrow*). There is a respiratory event resulting in an arousal from stage N1 sleep toward the end of the epoch. There is associated motion artifact in the EEG derivations. (Copyright JNP Enterprises, 2017.)

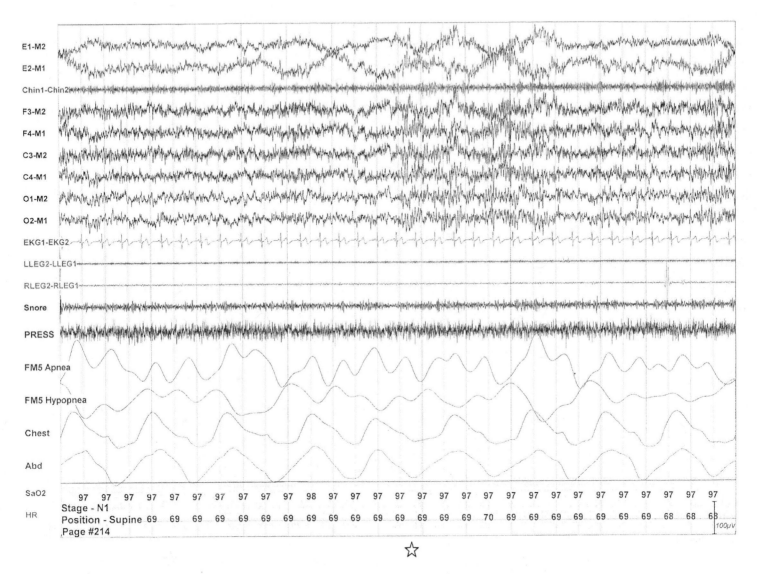

FIGURE 2-16 **Polysomnogram: Standard montage; 30 second page.**

Clinical: 25-year-old man.

Staging: Stage N1. There is an arousal (*star*) with an associated increase in the alpha rhythm. The speed of the eye movements also increases.

Technical: There is artifact in the pressure transducer channel (PRESS) secondary to the transducer becoming dislodged. (Copyright JNP Enterprises, 2017.)

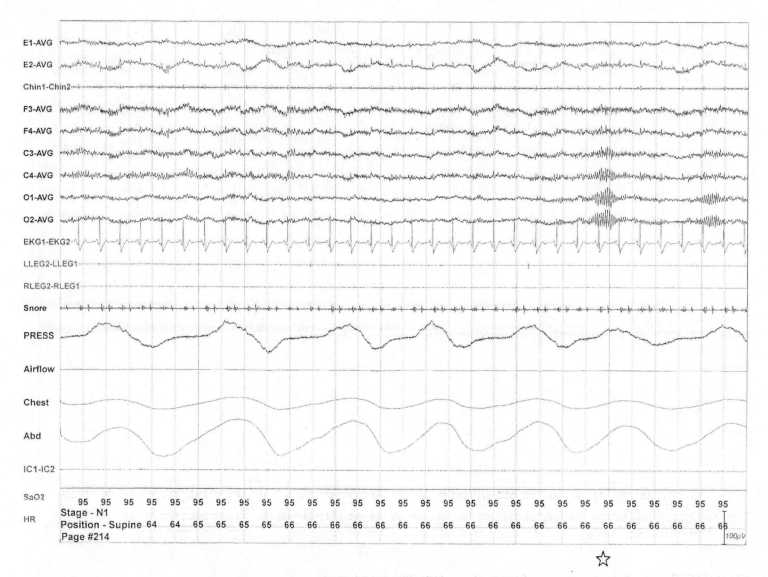

FIGURE 2-17 **Polysomnogram: Standard montage; 30 second page.**
Clinical: 52-year-old man.
Staging: Stage N1 with a transition to stage N2 toward the end of the epoch (*star*). There is a sleep spindle at this point. (Copyright JNP Enterprises, 2017.)

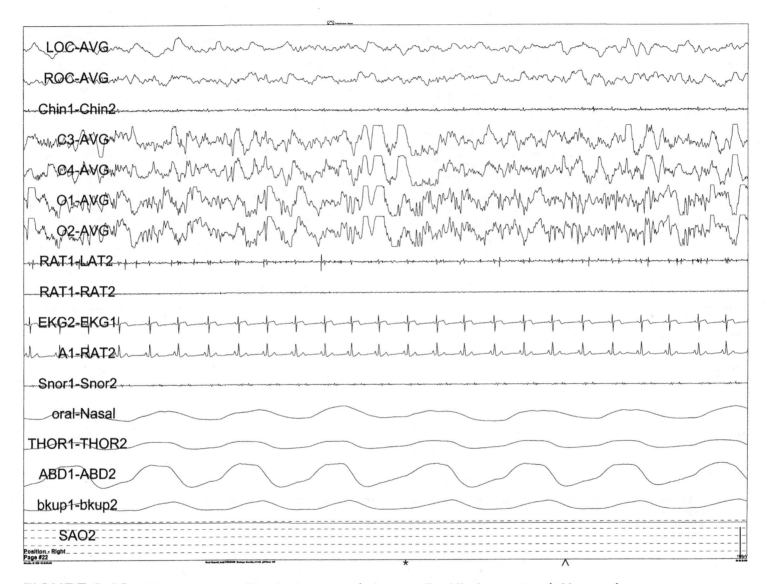

FIGURE 2-18   **Polysomnogram: Standard montage (prior recording/display montage); 30 second page.**
Clinical: 62-year-old man.
Staging: Stage N2 sleep with a K-complex (*) and repetitive POSTs (^).

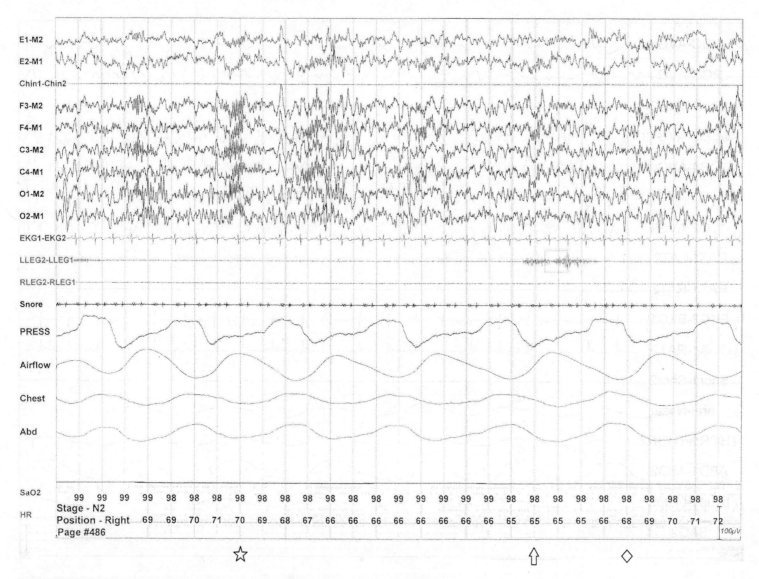

FIGURE 2-19 **Polysomnogram: Standard montage; 30 second page.**
Clinical: 41-year-old woman.
Staging: Stage N2 with sleep spindles (*star*), vertex waves (*arrow*), and POSTs (*diamond*). (Copyright NeuroTexion, 2017.)

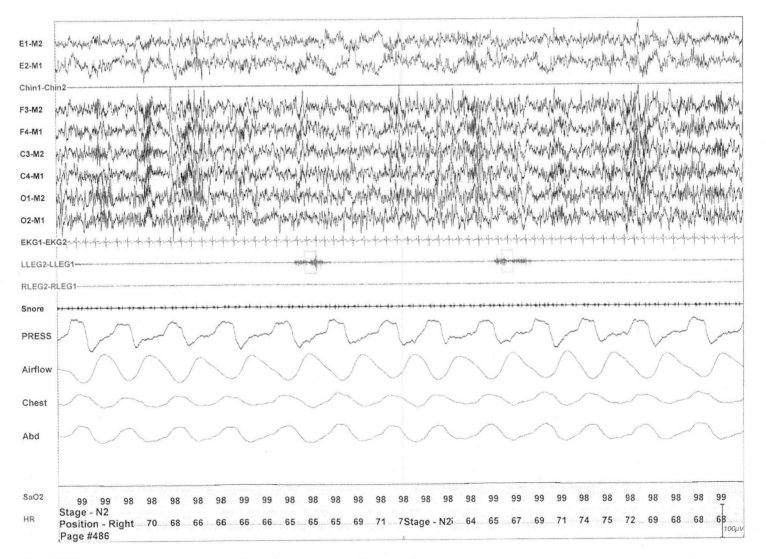

FIGURE 2-20   Polysomnogram: Standard montage; 60 second page.
Clinical: 41-year-old woman.
Staging: Stage N2 with sleep spindles, vertex waves, and POSTs. The time compression makes it more difficult to identify the waveforms. (Copyright NeuroTexion, 2017.)

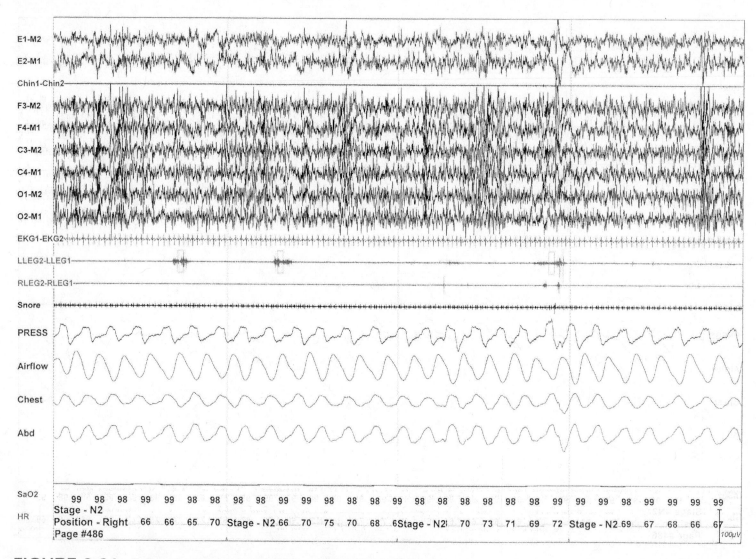

FIGURE 2-21   Polysomnogram: Standard montage; 120 second page.
Clinical: 41-year-old woman.
Staging: Stage N2 with sleep spindles, vertex waves, and POSTs. The time compression makes distinguishing the waveforms extremely difficult. (Copyright NeuroTexion, 2017.)

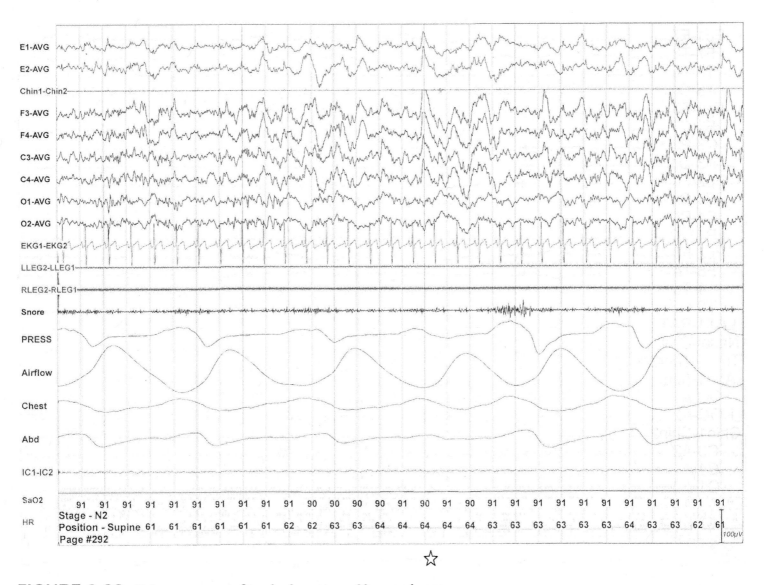

FIGURE 2-22   **Polysomnogram: Standard montage; 30 second page.**
Clinical: 39-year-old man.
Staging: Stage N2 with repetitive K-complexes (*star*). (Copyright NeuroTexion, 2017.)

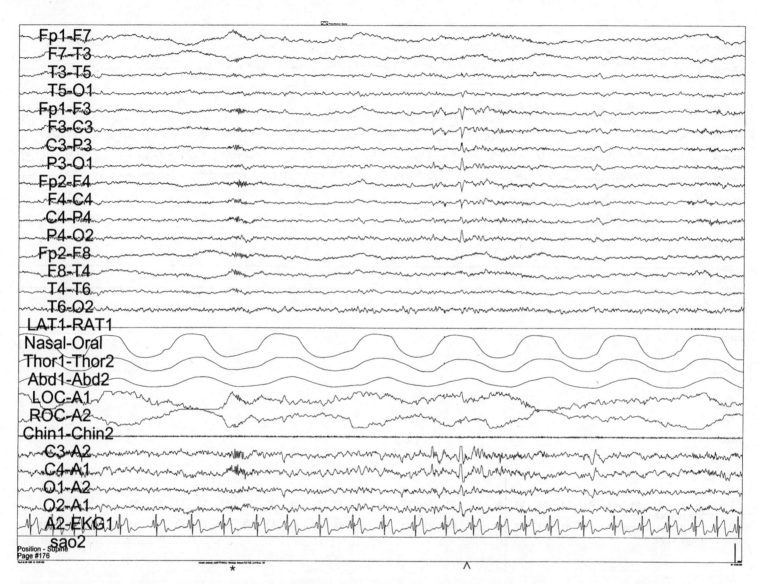

FIGURE 2-23   **Polysomnogram: Expanded EEG montage (prior recording/display montage); 30 second page.**
Clinical: 24-year-old man.
Staging: Stage N2 sleep with a sleep spindles (*) and a vertex wave (^). The expanded EEG montage demonstrates the frontocentral topography of the sleep spindle and the parasagittal topography of the vertex wave.

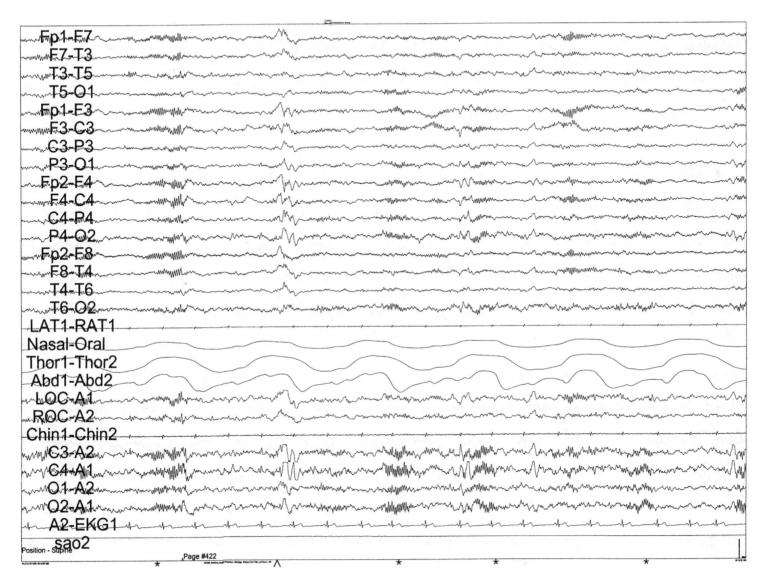

FIGURE 2-24   **Polysomnogram: Expanded EEG montage (prior recording/display montage); 30 second page.**
Clinical: 24-year-old man.
Staging: Stage N2 sleep with frequent sleep spindles (*) and K-complexes (^).

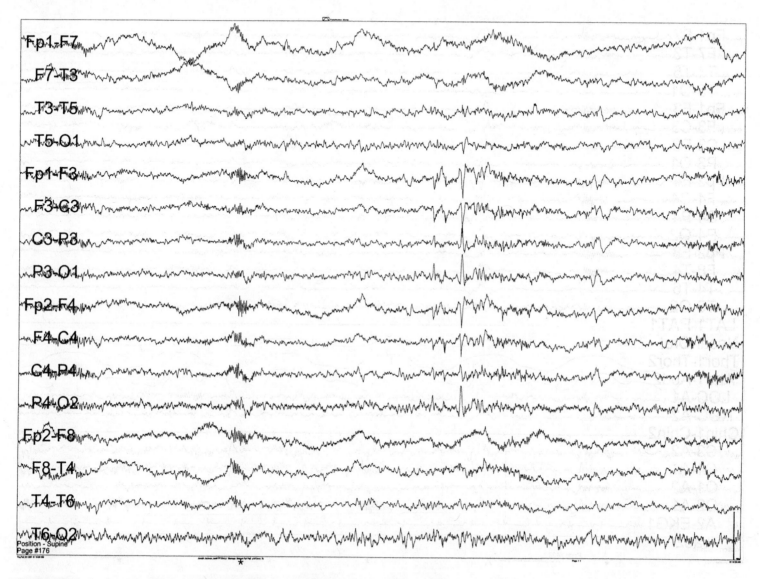

FIGURE 2-25 **Polysomnogram: EEG channels only; 30 second page.**
Clinical: 24-year-old man.
Staging: Stage N2 sleep with sleep spindles and vertex waves. The asymmetric topography of the initial spindle (*), with greater amplitude in the right temporal derivations than in the left temporal derivations, is within normal limits.

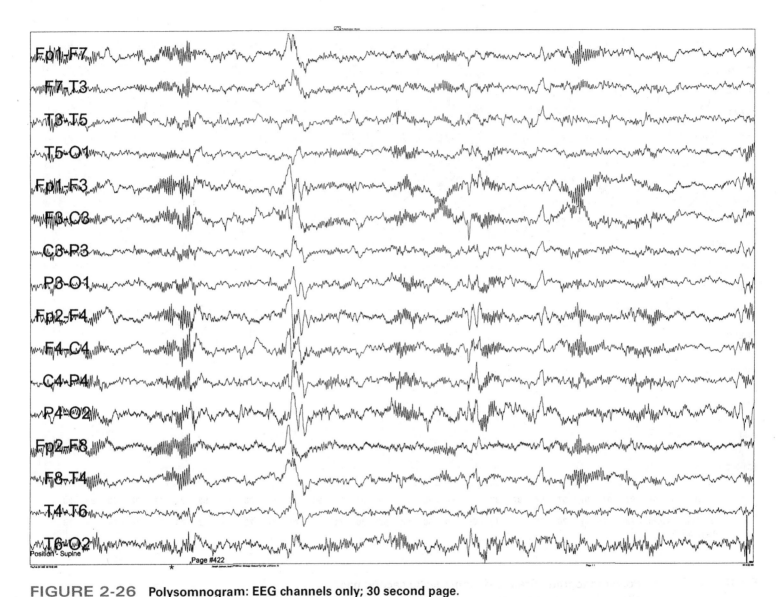

FIGURE 2-26 **Polysomnogram: EEG channels only; 30 second page.**
Clinical: 24-year-old man.
Staging: Stage N2 sleep with sleep spindles and K-complexes. Some spindles (*) are better represented in temporal derivations than in other derivations.

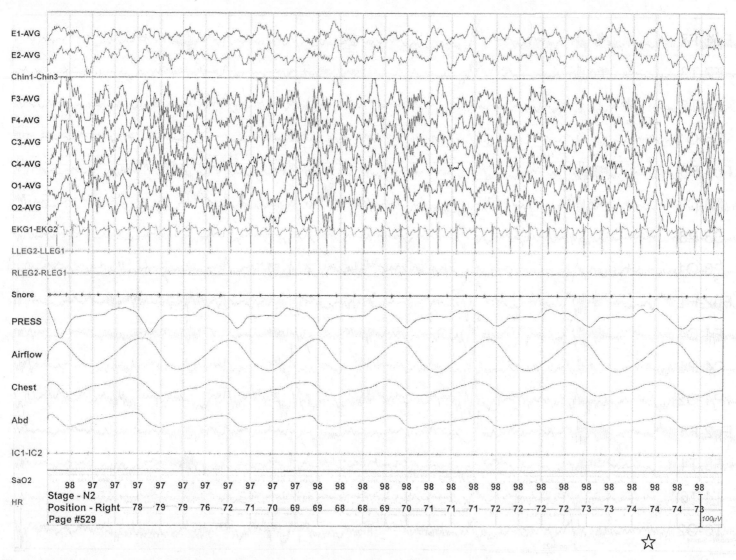

FIGURE 2-27   **Polysomnogram: Standard montage; 30 second page.**
Clinical: 67-year-old man.
Staging: Stage N2 sleep with K-complexes and sleep spindles. The presence of delta waves (*star*) presages the transition to stage N3 sleep. (Copyright NeuroTexion, 2017.)

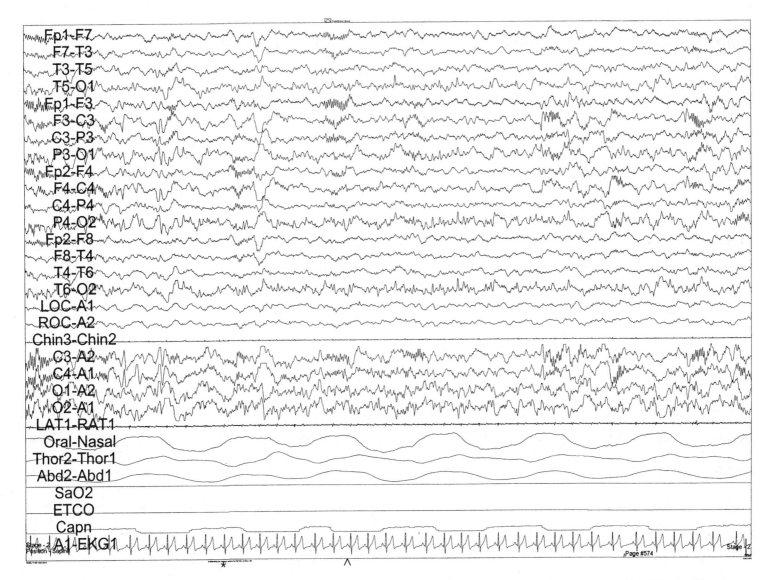

FIGURE 2-28   **Polysomnogram: Expanded EEG montage with CO_2 monitoring (prior recording/display montage); 30 second page.**

Clinical: 68-year-old man with excessive daytime sleepiness and chronic obstructive pulmonary disease (COPD).

Staging: Stage N2 sleep.

Respiratory: Normal respirations.

EEG: Asymmetric sleep spindles occurring first on the right (*) and then on the left (^). Other features of stage N2 sleep are present including K-complexes and POSTs.

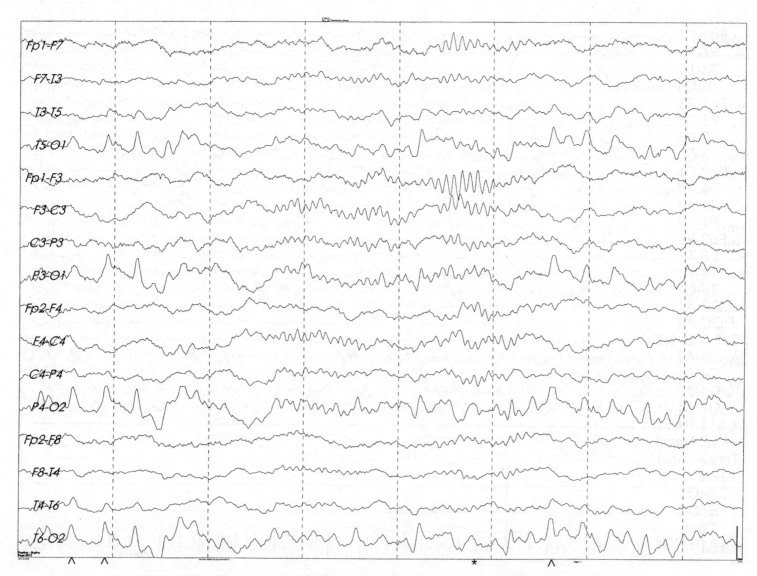

FIGURE 2-29   **EEG channels from an expanded EEG montage polysomnogram; 10 second page.**
Clinical: 68-year-old man with excessive daytime sleepiness and COPD.
Staging: Stage N2 sleep.
EEG: Asymmetric sleep spindles (*) most prominent over the left hemisphere especially channels Fp1-F3 and F3-C3. POSTs (^) are prominent in the occipital derivations.

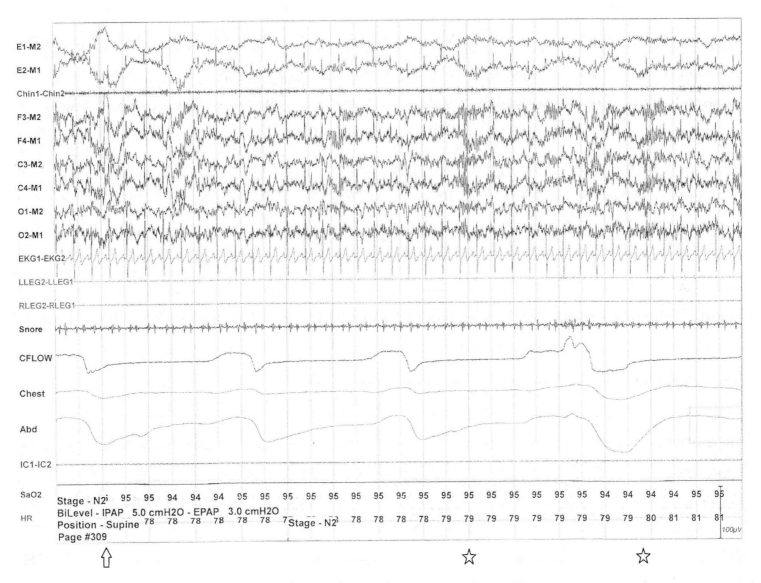

FIGURE 2-30 **Polysomnogram: CPAP montage; 30 second page.**
Clinical: 55-year-old man taking an SSRI.
Staging: Stage N2 with sleep spindles (*star*) and a K-complex (*arrow*). There are persistent eye movements, which can commonly be seen with the use of SSRI medications. (Copyright NeuroTexion, 2017.)

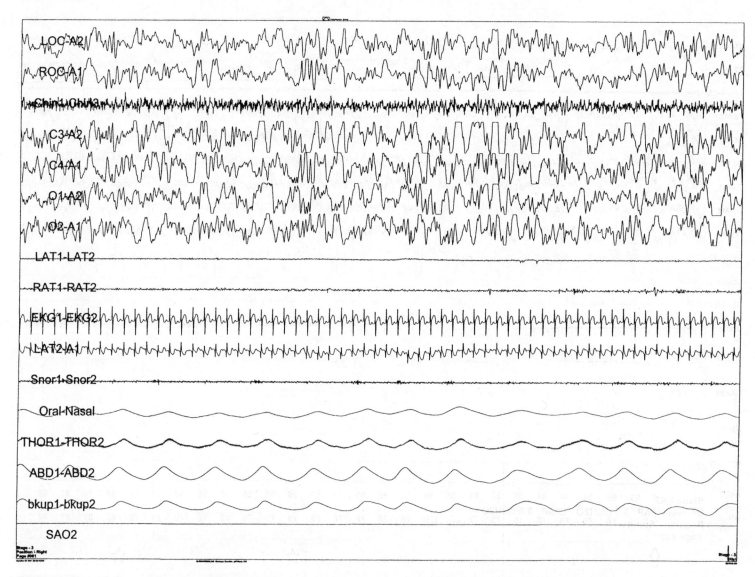

FIGURE 2-31 **Polysomnogram: Standard montage (prior recording/display montage); 30 second page.**
Clinical: 10-month-old girl.
Staging: Stage N3 sleep. The delta waves, characteristic of slow wave sleep, are prominent by the end of the first year of life.

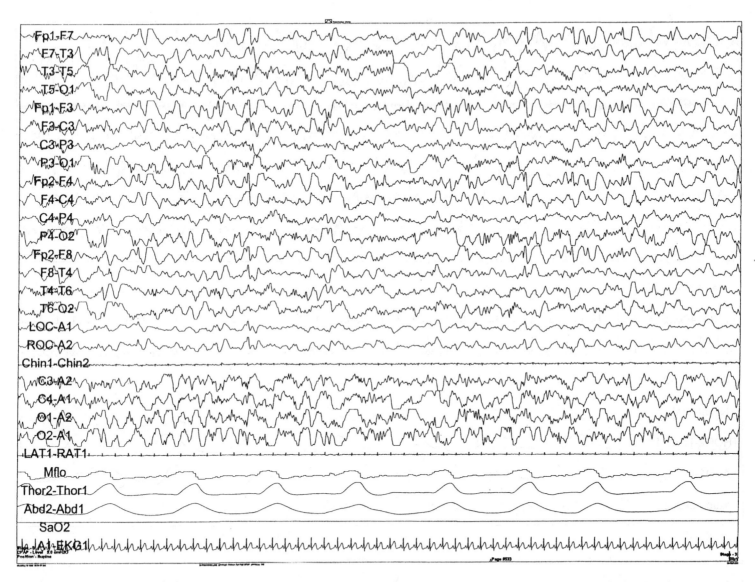

FIGURE 2-32 Polysomnogram: Expanded EEG montage (prior recording/display montage); 30 second page.
Clinical: 2-year-old boy.
Staging: Stage N3 sleep.

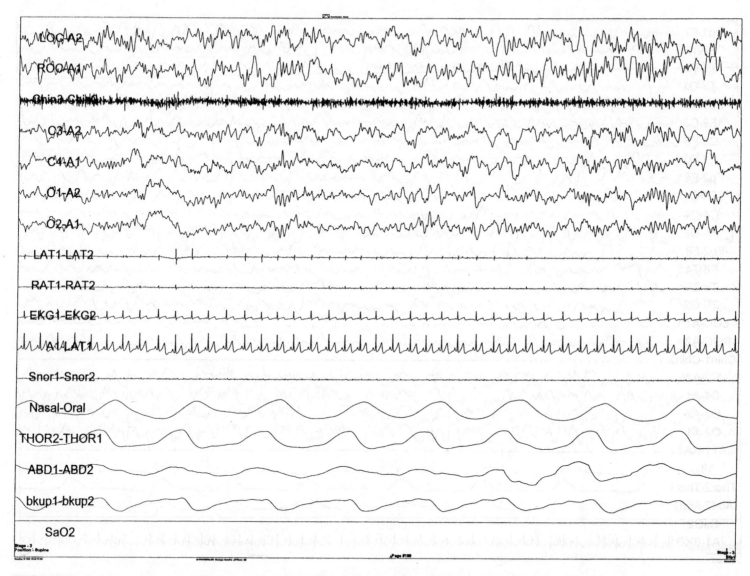

FIGURE 2-33   **Polysomnogram: Standard montage (prior recording/display montage); 30 second page.**
Clinical: 4-year-old boy.
Staging: Stage N3 sleep.

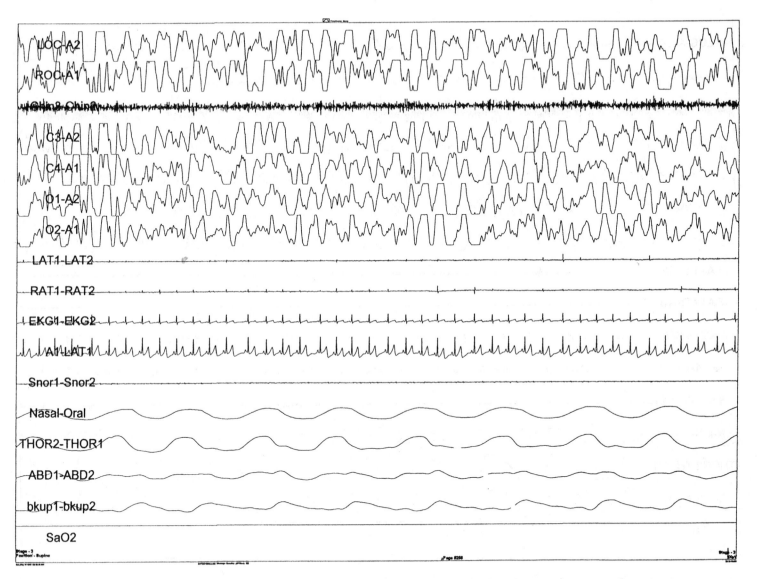

FIGURE 2-34 **Polysomnogram: Standard montage (prior recording/display montage); 30 second page.**
Clinical: 4-year-old boy.
Staging: Stage N3 sleep.

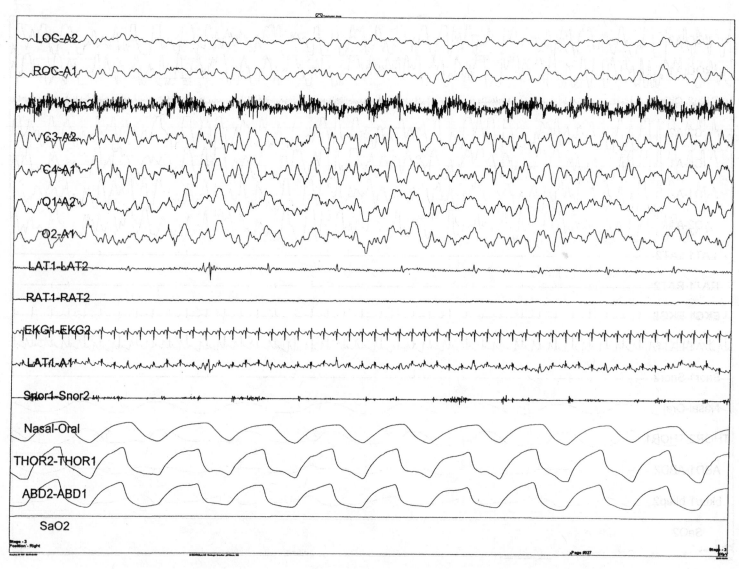

FIGURE 2-35 **Polysomnogram: Standard montage (prior recording/display montage); 30 second page.**
Clinical: 6-year-old boy.
Staging: Stage N3 sleep.

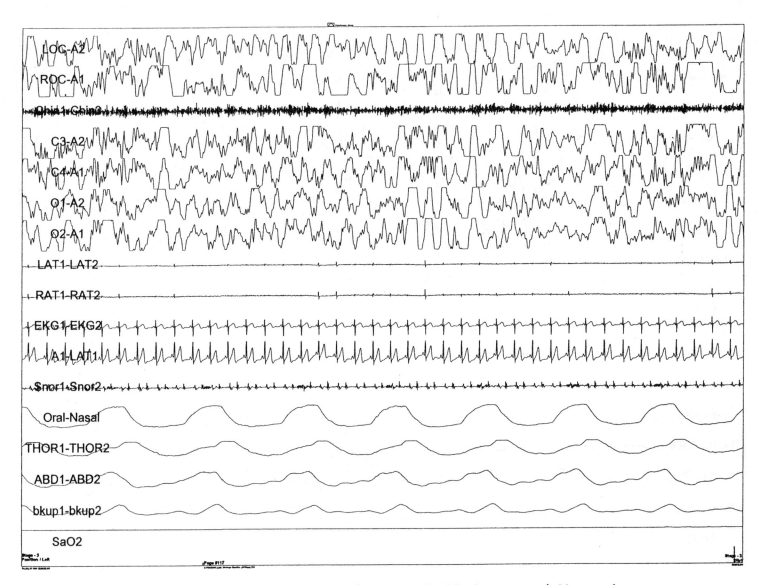

FIGURE 2-36 **Polysomnogram: Standard montage (prior recording/display montage); 30 second page.**
Clinical: 8-year-old girl.
Staging: Stage N3 sleep.

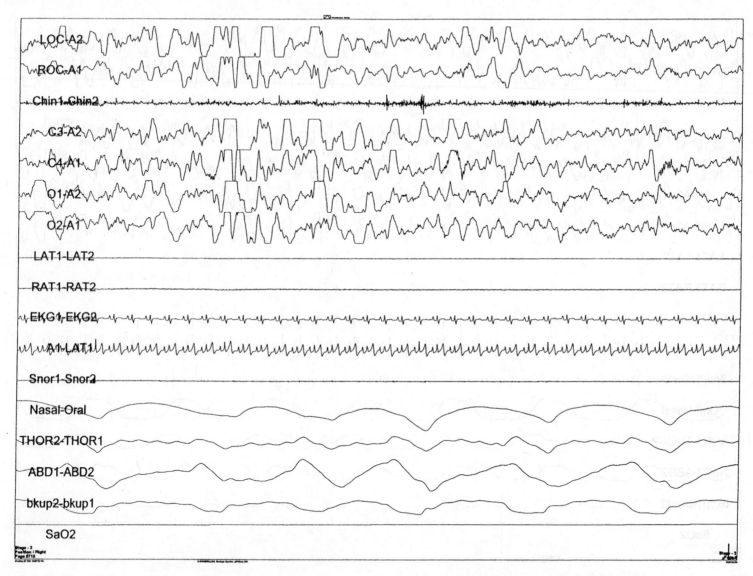

FIGURE 2-37 **Polysomnogram: Standard montage (prior recording/display montage); 30 second page.**
Clinical: 10-year-old boy.
Staging: Stage N3 sleep.

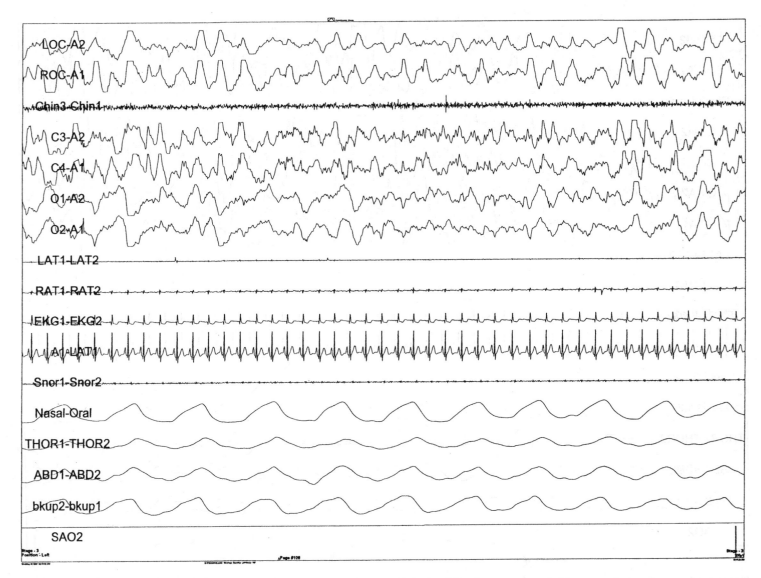

FIGURE 2-38   **Polysomnogram: Standard montage (prior recording/display montage); 30 second page.**

Clinical: 18-year-old man.

Staging: Stage N3 sleep.

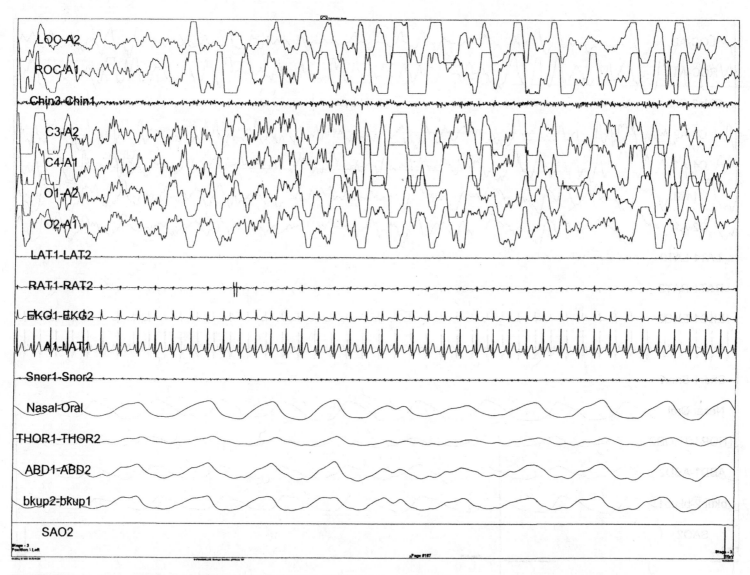

FIGURE 2-39 **Polysomnogram: Standard montage (prior recording/display montage); 30 second page.**
Clinical: 18-year-old man.
Staging: Stage N3 sleep.

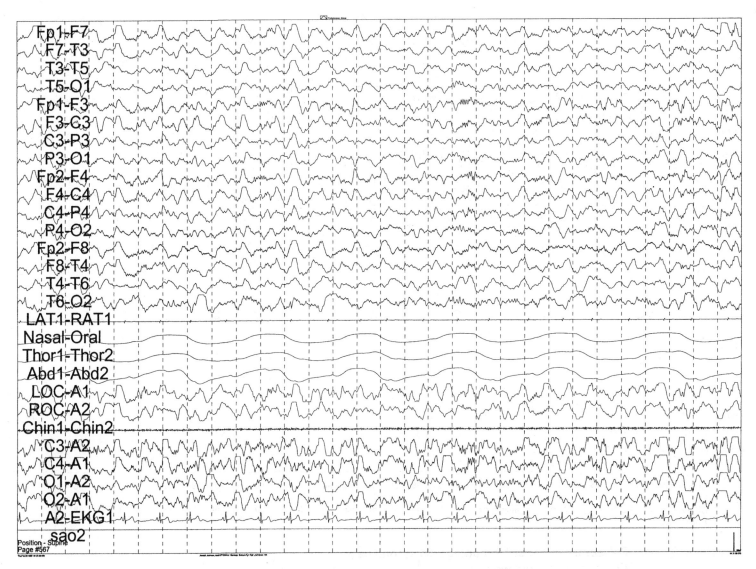

FIGURE 2-40 **Polysomnogram: Expanded EEG montage (prior recording/display montage); 30 second page with 1 second lines.**

Clinical: 29-year-old man.

Staging: Stage N3 sleep with delta activity. The delta waves are diffusely distributed with greater amplitude in anterior derivations.

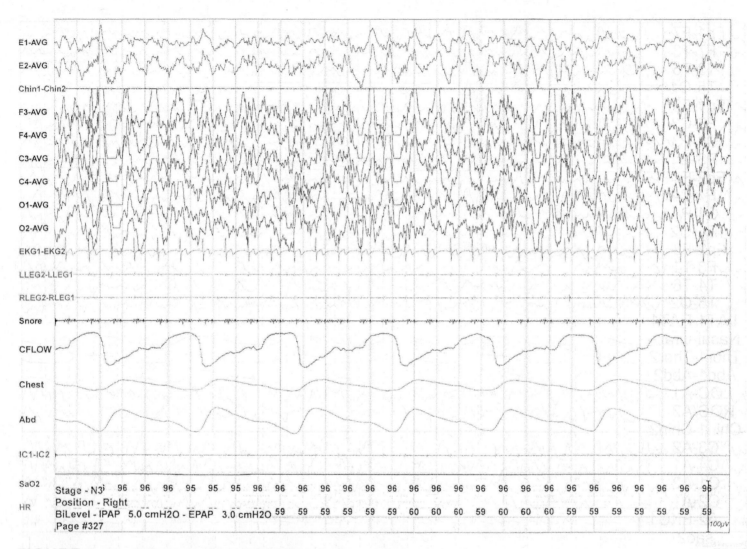

FIGURE 2-41   Polysomnogram: CPAP montage; 30 second page.

Clinical: 35-year-old woman.

Staging: Stage N3 with prominent delta activity visible in the EOG derivations. (Copyright NeuroTexion, 2017.)

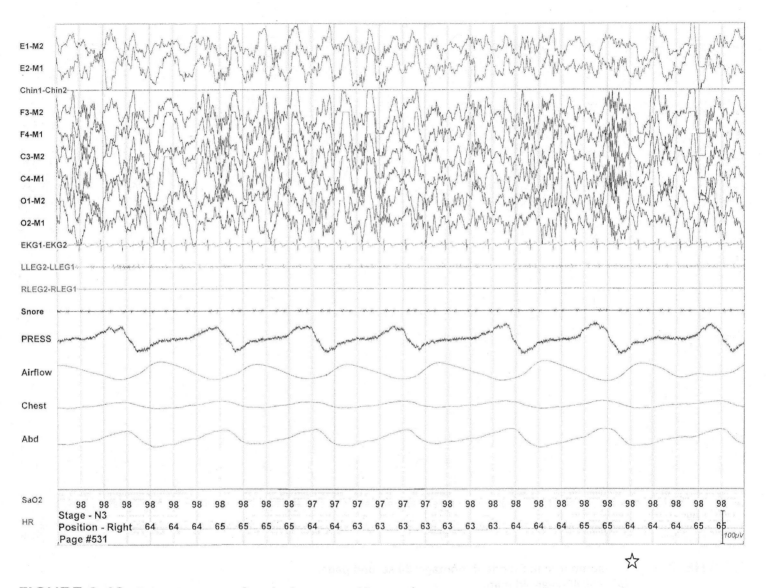

FIGURE 2-42   **Polysomnogram: Standard montage; 30 second page.**
Clinical: 40-year-old man.
Staging: Stage N3 with a rare sleep spindles (*star*). (Copyright NeuroTexion, 2017.)

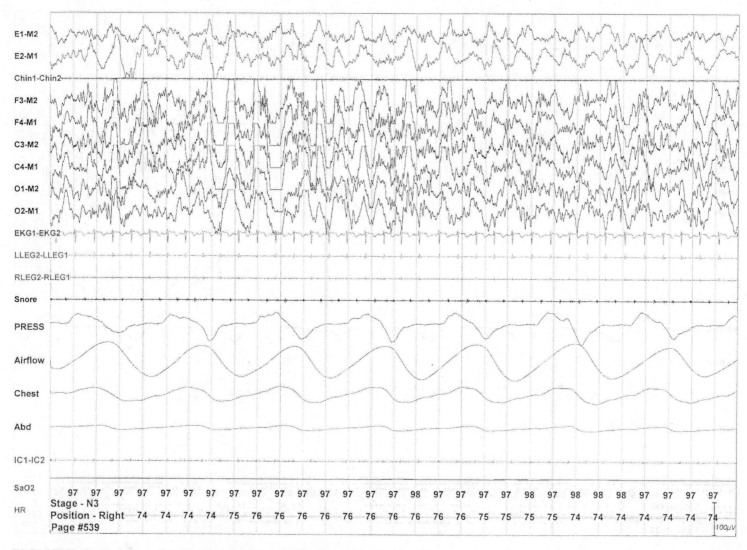

FIGURE 2-43   **Polysomnogram: Standard montage; 30 second page.**
Clinical: 40-year-old man.
Staging: Stage N3 with alpha intrusion evident in the EEG and EOG derivations. (Copyright NeuroTexion, 2017.)

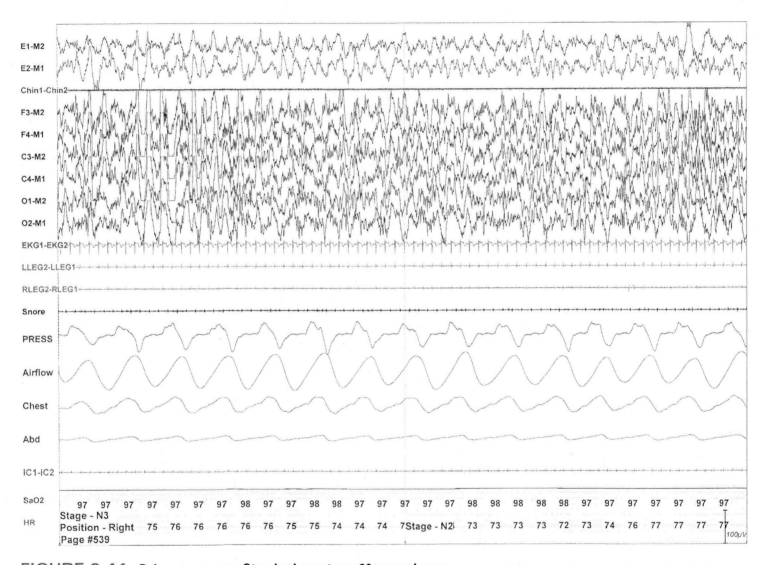

FIGURE 2-44   **Polysomnogram: Standard montage; 60 second page.**
Clinical: 40-year-old man.
Staging: Stage N3 with alpha intrusion evident in the EEG and EOG derivations. (Copyright NeuroTexion, 2017.)

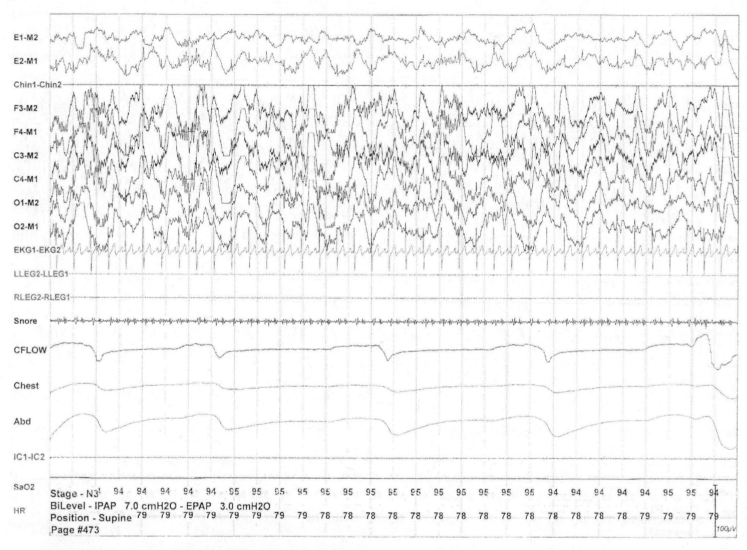

FIGURE 2-45 **Polysomnogram: CPAP montage; 30 second page.**
Clinical: 28-year-old woman who has been prescribed an SSRI.
Staging: Stage N3 sleep. There is delta activity evident in the EOG channels with occasional eye movements. (Copyright NeuroTexion, 2017.)

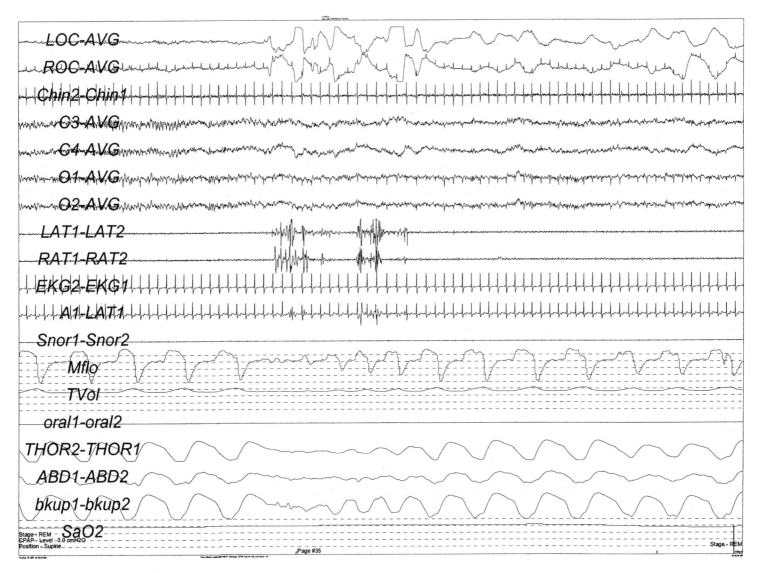

FIGURE 2-46 **Polysomnogram: CPAP montage (prior recording/display montage); 60 second page.**
Clinical: 35-year-old woman.
Staging: Stage R sleep. Several rapid eye movements occur in a cluster accompanied by limb twitches and irregular respirations. Epochs containing such clusters of rapid eye movements and muscle twitches are sometimes referred to as *phasic REM sleep.*

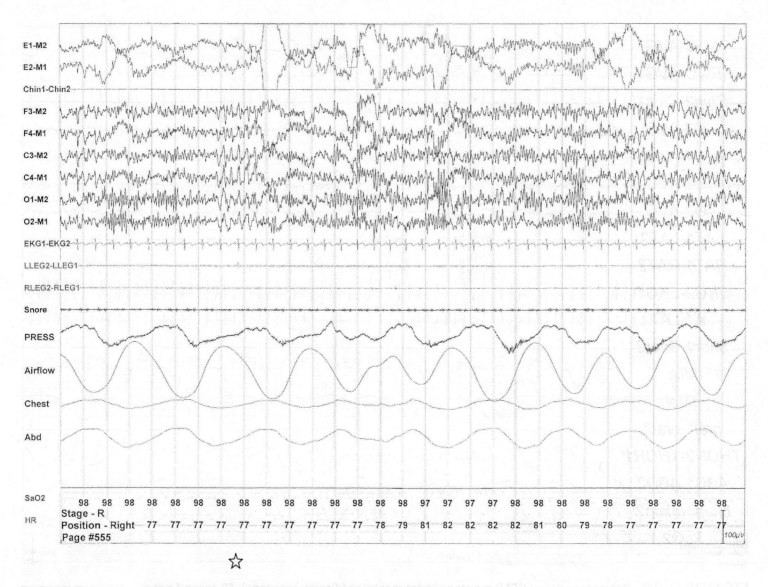

FIGURE 2-47   Polysomnogram: Standard montage; 30 second page.
Clinical: 36-year-old man.
Staging: Stage R with rapid eye movements, decreased EMG tone, and sawtooth waves (*star*). There is also some alpha activity, which was slightly slower than the patient's typical waking alpha rhythm. (Copyright NeuroTexion, 2017.)

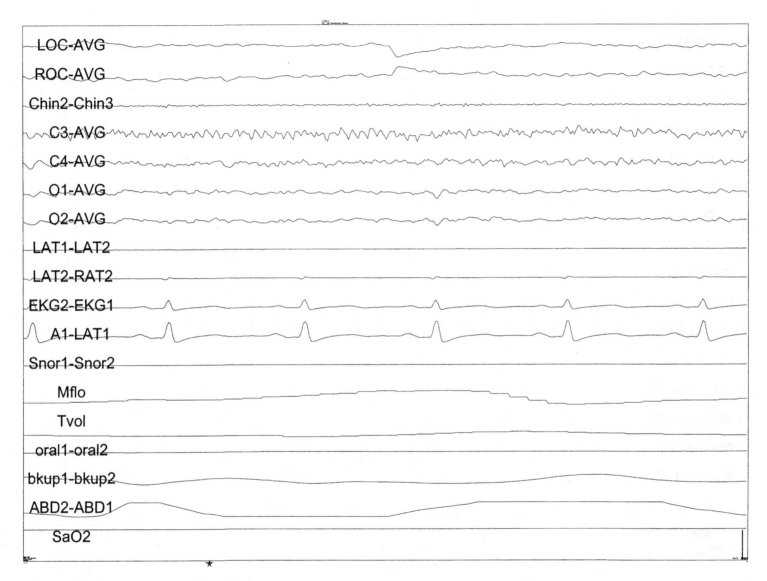

FIGURE 2-48   **Polysomnogram: CPAP montage (prior recording/display montage); 7.5 second page.**
Clinical: 64-year-old man.
Staging: Stage R sleep with sawtooth waves (*).

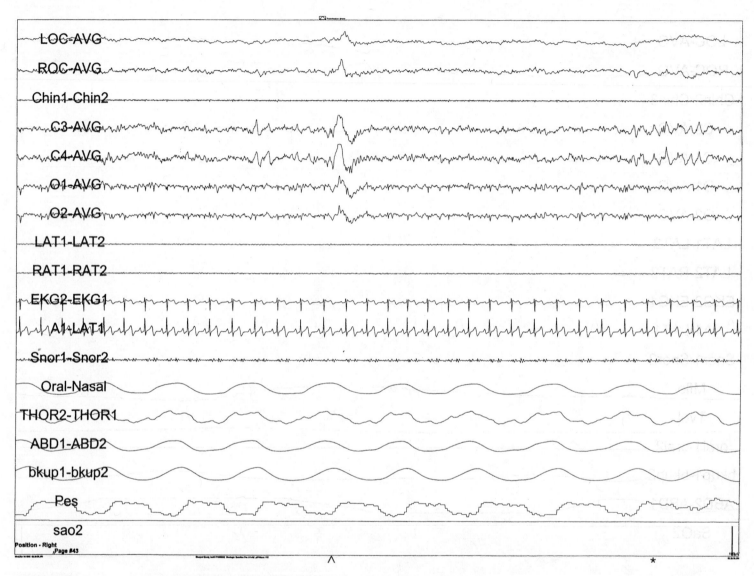

FIGURE 2-49   **Polysomnogram: Standard montage with intrathoracic pressure monitoring (prior recording/display montage); 30 second page.**

Clinical: 39-year-old woman.

Staging: Stage R sleep with sawtooth waves (*). Although a single K-complex (^) is present, rapid eye movements were present in preceding and succeeding epochs, indicating that this epoch should be scored as REM sleep.

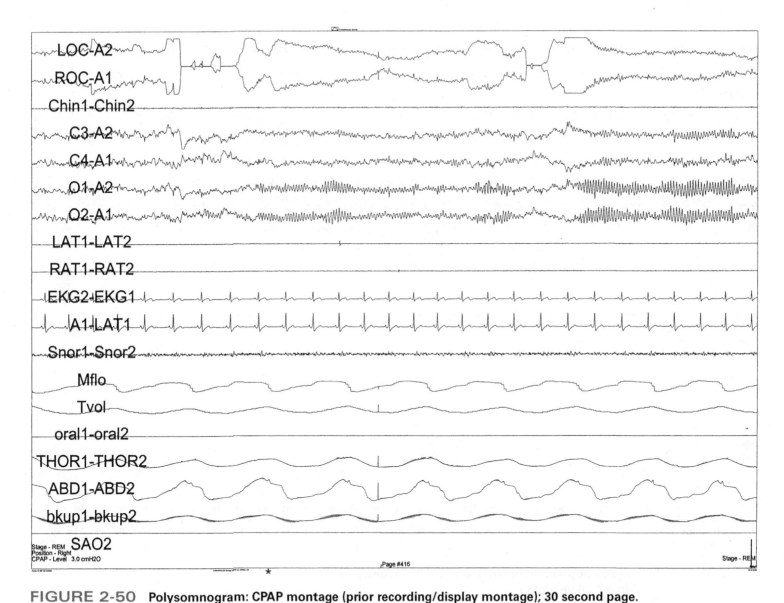

FIGURE 2-50 **Polysomnogram: CPAP montage (prior recording/display montage); 30 second page.**
Clinical: 41-year-old man.
Staging: Stage R sleep with alpha activity (*). The amount of posterior dominant alpha activity during REM sleep varies widely among individuals.

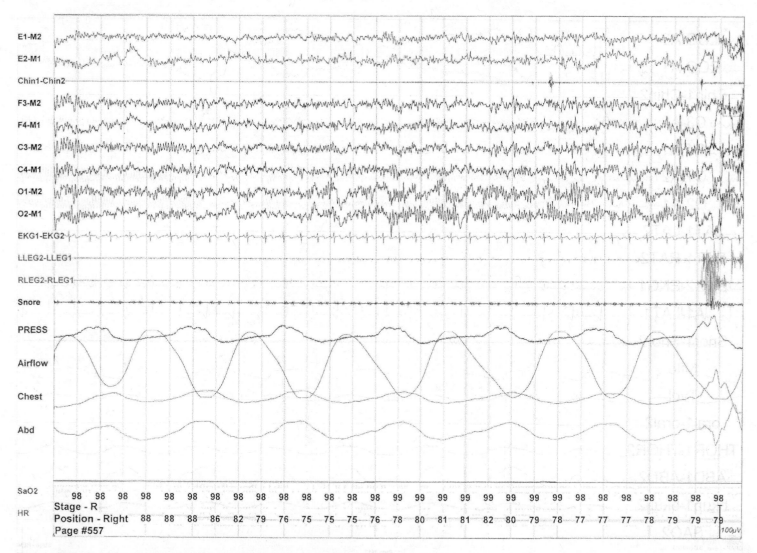

FIGURE 2-51   **Polysomnogram: Standard montage; 30 second page.**
Clinical: 36-year-old man.
Staging: Stage R without rapid eye movements (tonic REM sleep). There is an alpha rhythm and some poorly formed sawtooth activity. (Copyright NeuroTexion, 2017.)

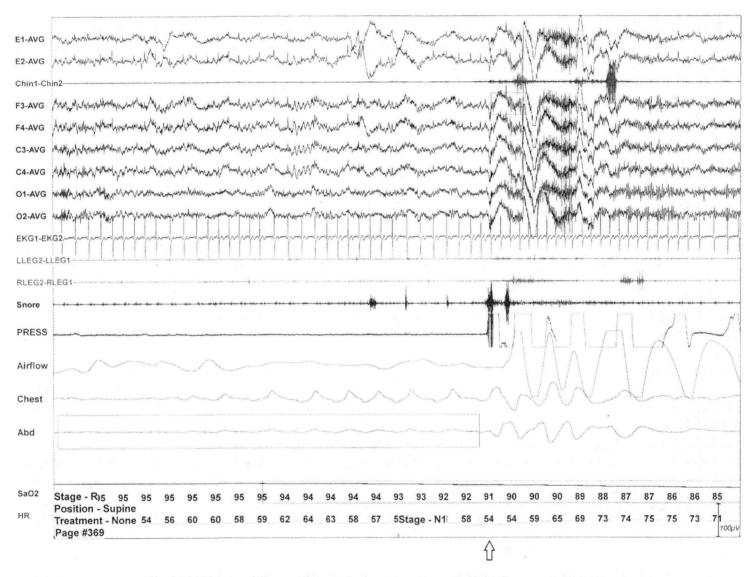

FIGURE 2-52   **Polysomnogram: Standard montage; 30 second page.**
Clinical: 40-year-old man.
Staging: Stage R with an arousal (*arrow*) with increased muscle tone as well as associated myogenic and motion artifact.
Respiratory: There is a respiratory event preceding the arousal. (Copyright NeuroTexion, 2017.)

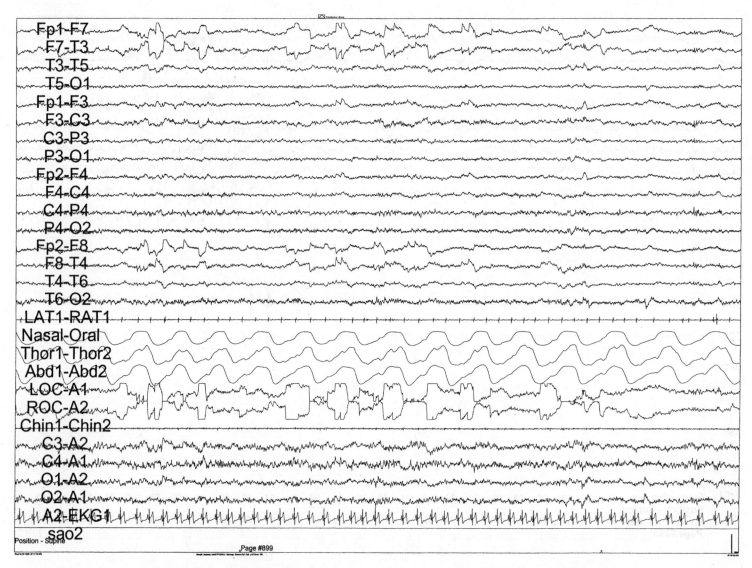

FIGURE 2-53   **Polysomnogram: Expanded EEG (prior recording/display montage); 60 second page.**
Clinical: 38-year-old man.
Staging: Stage R sleep with representation of rapid eye movements in channels Fp1-F7 and Fp2-F8. The potentials produced by rapid eye movements are recorded by the lateral frontal electrodes, F7 and F8. Horizontal rapid eye movements, such as these, are often recorded by lateral frontal or anterior temporal (T1 and T2) electrodes, while vertical eye movements may be recorded by prefrontal (Fp1 and Fp2) electrodes.

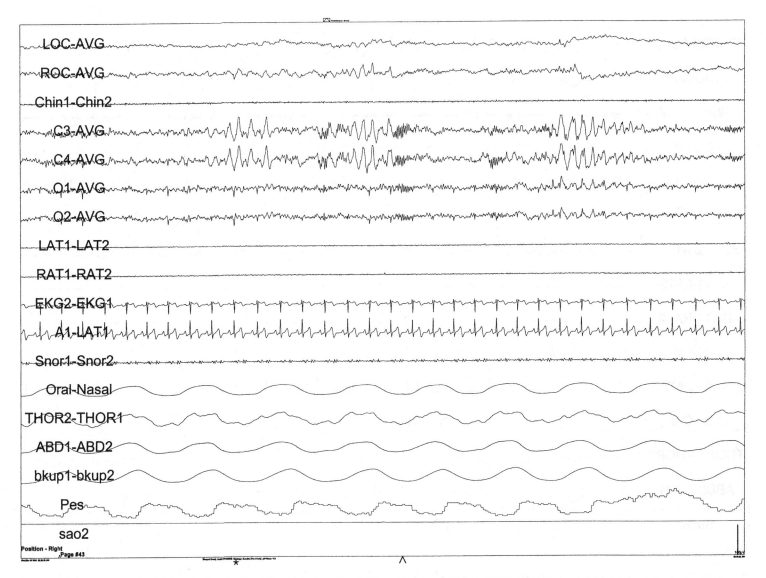

FIGURE 2-54 **Polysomnogram: Standard montage with intrathoracic pressure monitoring (prior recording/display montage); 30 second page.**

Clinical: 28-year-old man.

Staging: Transition from NREM sleep to REM sleep. There are elements of REM sleep including sawtooth waves (*) and decreased muscle tone. There are also several sleep spindles (^). Features of REM and NREM sleep are often intermixed for a few seconds or minutes before and after a period of REM sleep.

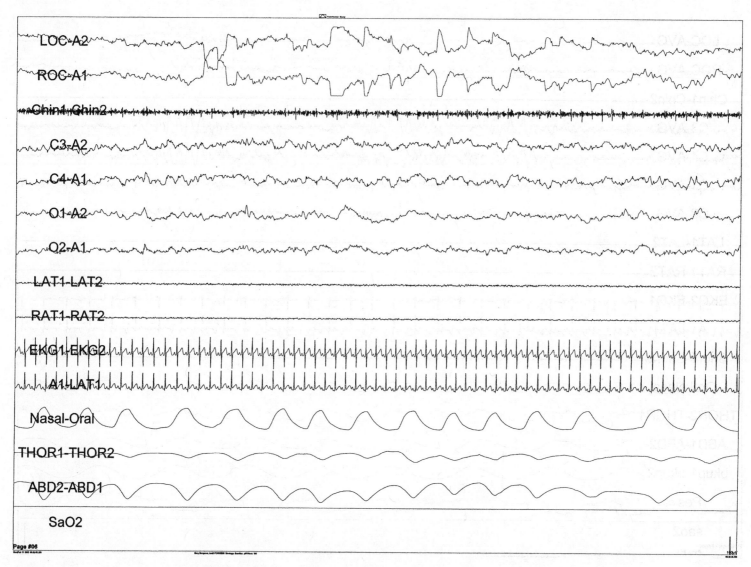

FIGURE 2-55   **Polysomnogram: Standard montage (prior recording/display montage); 60 second page.**
Clinical: 5-week-old girl.
Staging: Stage R sleep with incomplete atonia.
Respiratory: Irregular respirations during REM sleep. Such variations in frequency and amplitude of respirations are normal at this age during REM sleep.

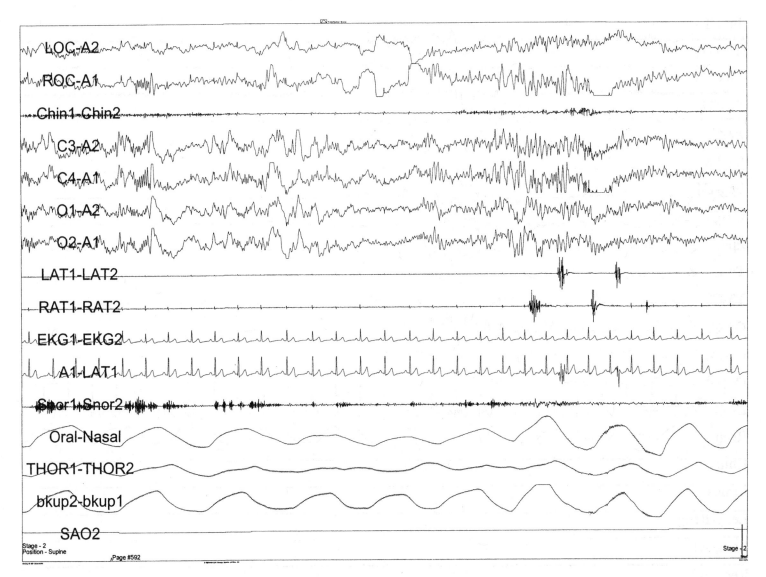

FIGURE 2-56   **Polysomnogram: Standard montage (prior recording/display montage); 30 second page.**
Clinical: 55-year-old man.
Staging: Elements of stage N2 sleep, stage N3 sleep, REM sleep, and an arousal.
Respiratory: Hypopnea with an associated arousal.

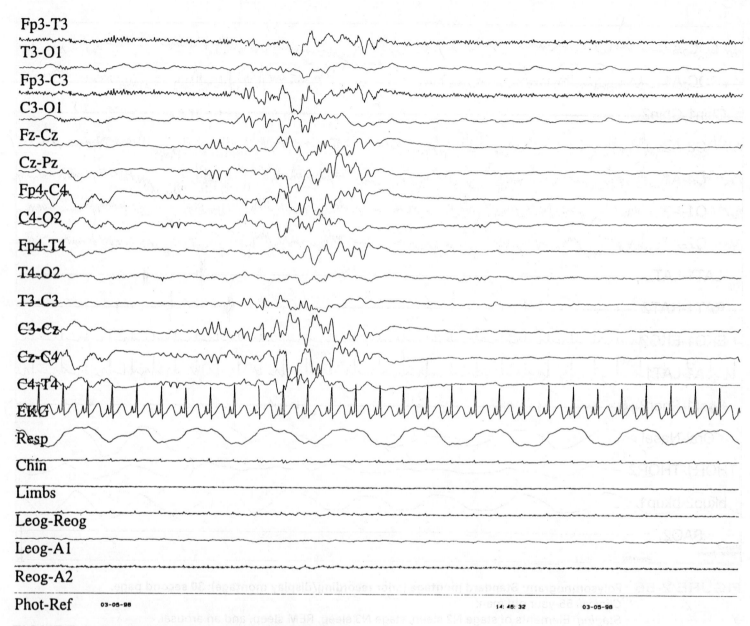

Fp3-T3
T3-O1
Fp3-C3
C3-O1
Fz-Cz
Cz-Pz
Fp4-C4
C4-O2
Fp4-T4
T4-O2
T3-C3
C3-Cz
Cz-C4
C4-T4
EKG
Resp
Chin
Limbs
Leog-Reog
Leog-A1
Reog-A2
Phot-Ref   03-05-98   14:46:32   03-05-98

FIGURE 2-57   Neonatal recording; 30 second page.
Clinical: 30-week conceptional age patient.
Respiratory: Normal respirations.
EEG: Tracé discontinue with delta brushes. This discontinuous EEG pattern is a normal feature of NREM sleep (quiet sleep) at this age.

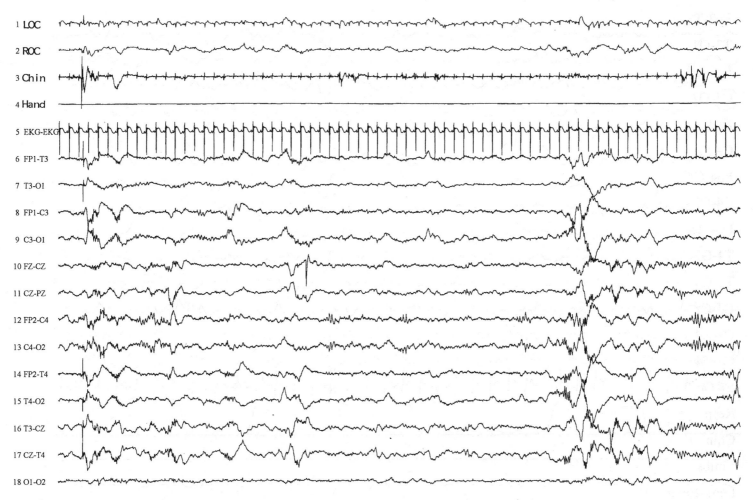

FIGURE 2-58   **Neonatal recording; 30 second page.**

Clinical: 30-week conceptional age patient.

Respiratory: Normal respirations.

EEG: Tracé discontinue with delta brushes during NREM sleep.

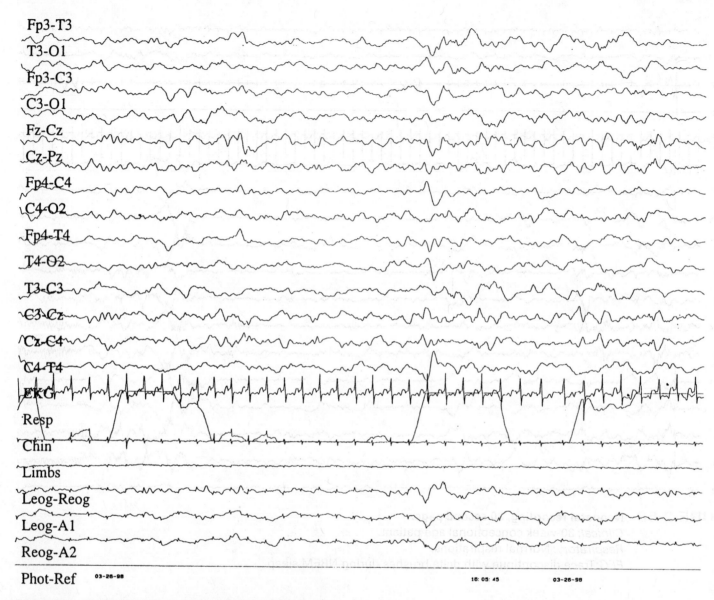

Fp3-T3
T3-O1
Fp3-C3
C3-O1
Fz-Cz
Cz-Pz
Fp4-C4
C4-O2
Fp4-T4
T4-O2
T3-C3
C3-Cz
Cz-C4
C4-T4
EKG
Resp
Chin
Limbs
Leog-Reog
Leog-A1
Reog-A2
Phot-Ref   03-26-98   16: 05: 45   03-26-98

FIGURE 2-59   **Neonatal recording; 30 second page.**
Clinical: 42-week conceptional age patient in NREM sleep.
Respiratory: Partially obscured by artifact.
EEG: Tracé alternant with bursts of higher-amplitude delta and theta activity separated by periods of moderate-amplitude–mixed frequency activity. The tracé alternant pattern is a normal feature of NREM sleep at this age.

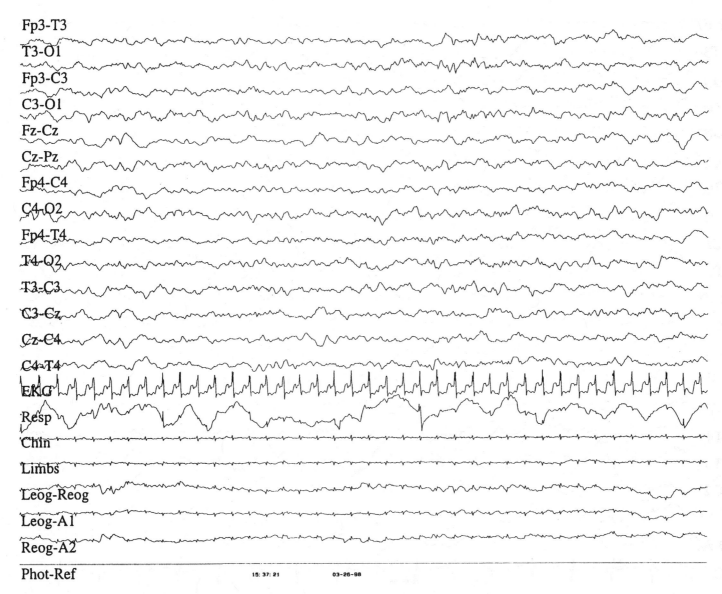

Fp3-T3
T3-O1
Fp3-C3
C3-O1
Fz-Cz
Cz-Pz
Fp4-C4
C4-O2
Fp4-T4
T4-O2
T3-C3
C3-Cz
Cz-C4
C4-T4
EKG
Resp
Chin
Limbs
Leog-Reog
Leog-A1
Reog-A2
Phot-Ref

15: 37: 21   03-26-98

FIGURE 2-60   **Neonatal recording; 30 second page.**
Clinical: 30-week conceptional age patient in REM sleep (active sleep).
Respiratory: Slightly irregular respirations.
EEG: Continuous mixed frequency background activity.
REM sleep is the most common sleep onset pattern in neonates and makes up about 50% of newborn sleep.

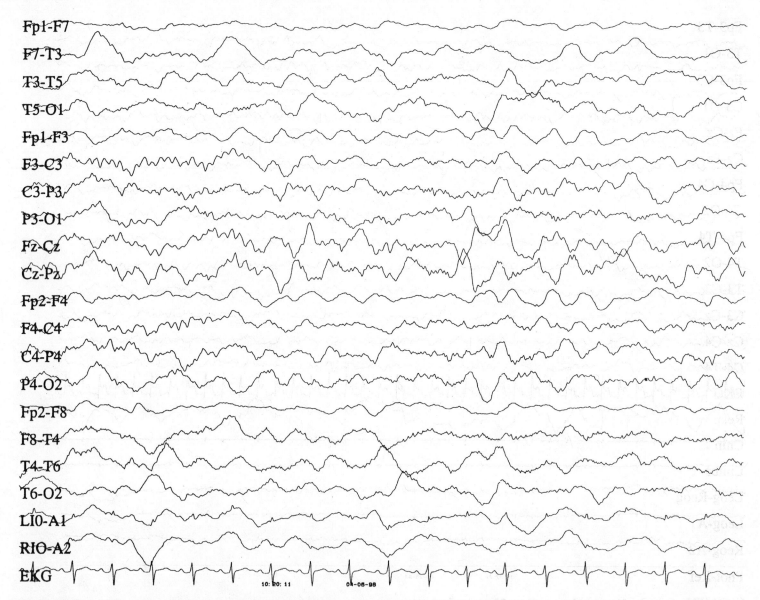

Fp1-F7

F7-T3

T3-T5

T5-O1

Fp1-F3

F3-C3

C3-P3

P3-O1

Fz-Cz

Cz-Pz

Fp2-F4

F4-C4

C4-P4

P4-O2

Fp2-F8

F8-T4

T4-T6

T6-O2

LIO-A1

RIO-A2

EKG

10: 20: 11   04-06-98

FIGURE 2-61   **Infant recording; 15 second page.**
Clinical: 4-month-old patient in NREM sleep.
EEG: Symmetric sleep spindles and vertex waves.

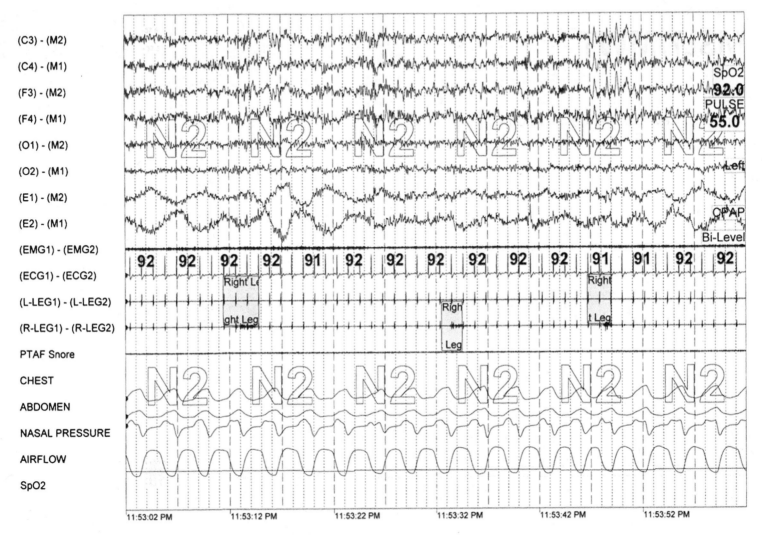

FIGURE 2-62 **Polysomnogram: Standard montage; 60 second page.**
Clinical: 49-year-old man with some snoring and excessive daytime sleepiness. Also just recently started an SSRI for depression and has developed restless sleep. Discontinuation of the SSRI and switching to another antidepressant dramatically improved the restless sleep and daytime sleepiness.
Staging: Awakening with a position change.
Eye leads: Slow eye movements on eye channels.
Leg leads: PLMs. The PLM index was 63.7.

MSLT/MWT

James D. Geyer, MD and Paul R. Carney, MD

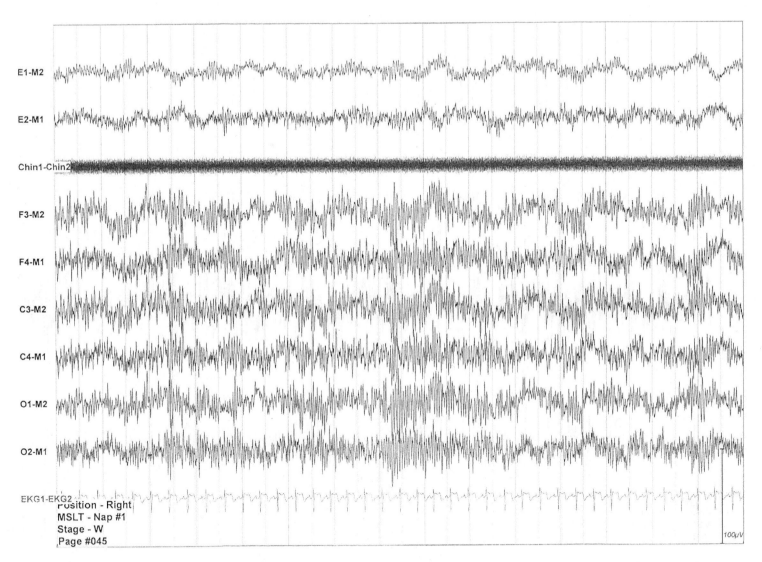

E1-M2

E2-M1

Chin1-Chin2

F3-M2

F4-M1

C3-M2

C4-M1

O1-M2

O2-M1

EKG1-EKG2

Position - Right
MSLT - Nap #1
Stage - W
Page #045

100µV

FIGURE 3-1 **Multiple Sleep Latency Test; 30 second page.**
Clinical: 32-year-old man with excessive daytime sleepiness.
Staging: Stage W—Wakefulness. There is prominent alpha activity.

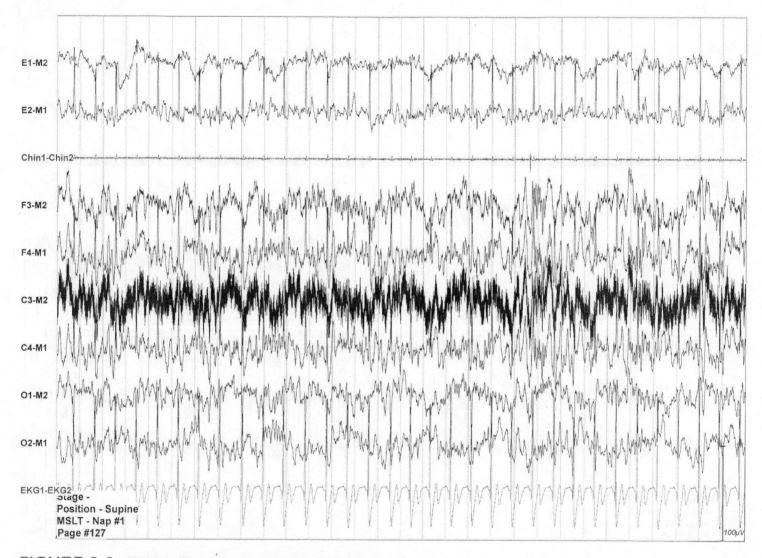

E1-M2

E2-M1

Chin1-Chin2

F3-M2

F4-M1

C3-M2

C4-M1

O1-M2

O2-M1

EKG1-EKG2

Stage -
Position - Supine
MSLT - Nap #1
Page #127

100µV

FIGURE 3-2 **Multiple Sleep Latency Test; 30 second page.**
Clinical: 32-year-old man with excessive daytime sleepiness.
Staging: Stage W—Wakefulness. There is prominent EKG artifact. The alpha activity is attenuated with eye
opening. There is artifact secondary to a loose C3 electrode.

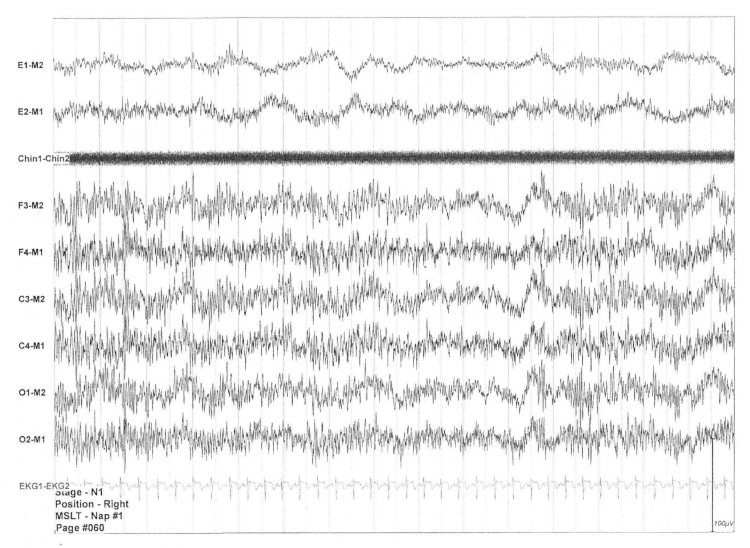

E1-M2

E2-M1

Chin1-Chin2

F3-M2

F4-M1

C3-M2

C4-M1

O1-M2

O2-M1

EKG1-EKG2

Stage - N1
Position - Right
MSLT - Nap #1
Page #060

100µV

FIGURE 3-3 **Multiple Sleep Latency Test; 30 second page.**
Clinical: 32-year-old man with excessive daytime sleepiness.
Staging: Stage N1. There is slowing of the eye movements. There is an increase in the theta activity. The patient had alpha intrusion throughout the prior nocturnal polysomnogram.

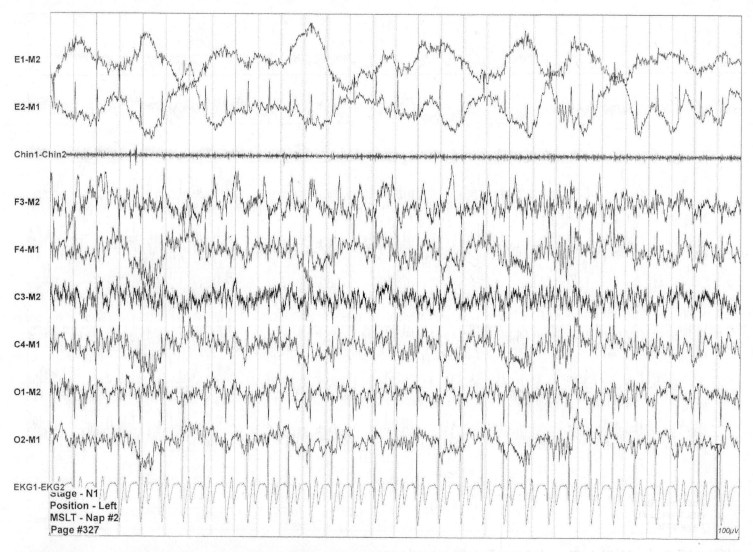

Stage - N1
Position - Left
MSLT - Nap #2
Page #327

100µV

FIGURE 3-4   Multiple Sleep Latency Test; 30 second page.
Clinical: 24-year-old woman with excessive daytime sleepiness.
Staging: Stage N1 sleep with slow eye movements and attenuation of the alpha rhythm. Theta activity is evident present. There is prominent EKG artifact.

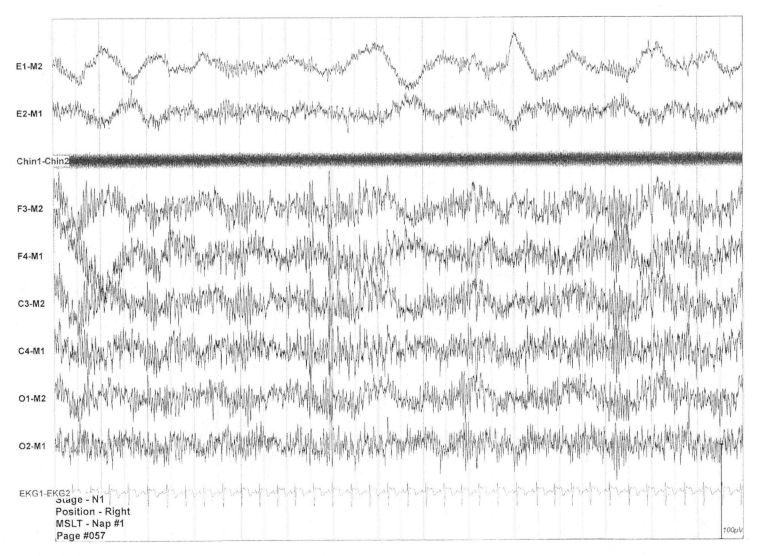

FIGURE 3-5 **Multiple Sleep Latency Test; 30 second page**.
Clinical: 48-year-old man with excessive daytime sleepiness.
Staging: Stage N1. The transition from wakefulness to stage 1 sleep often entails a decrease in the alpha rhythm and the appearance of central theta activity. Slow eye movements are prominent throughout the epoch.

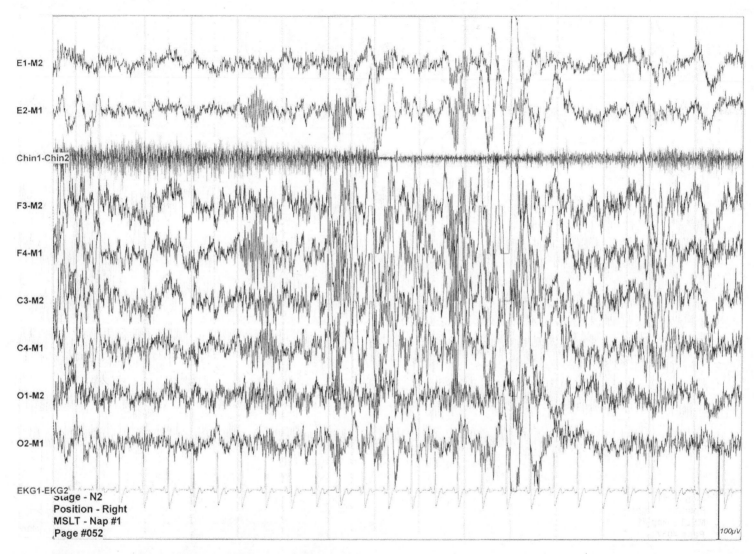

E1-M2

E2-M1

Chin1-Chin2

F3-M2

F4-M1

C3-M2

C4-M1

O1-M2

O2-M1

EKG1-EKG2

Stage - N2
Position - Right
MSLT - Nap #1
Page #052

100µV

FIGURE 3-6   **Multiple Sleep Latency Test; 30 second page.**
Clinical: 27-year-old man with excessive daytime sleepiness.
Staging: Stage N2 sleep with a K-complex and sleep spindles.

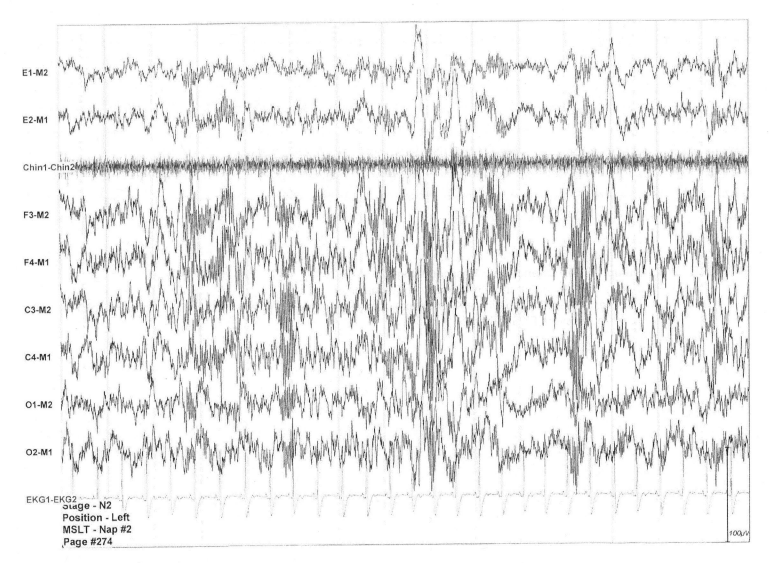

E1-M2

E2-M1

Chin1-Chin2

F3-M2

F4-M1

C3-M2

C4-M1

O1-M2

O2-M1

EKG1-EKG2

Stage - N2
Position - Left
MSLT - Nap #2
Page #274

100μV

FIGURE 3-7 **Multiple Sleep Latency Test; 30 second page.**
Clinical: 27-year-old man with excessive daytime sleepiness.
Staging: Stage N2 sleep with a K-complex and sleep spindles.

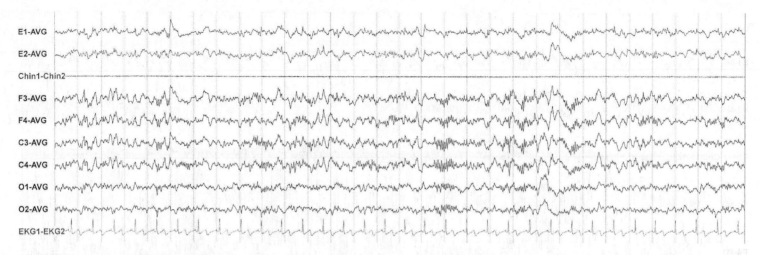

FIGURE 3-8   **Multiple Sleep Latency Test; 30 second page.**
Clinical: 32-year-old man with excessive daytime sleepiness.
Staging: Stage N2 sleep with a K-complex and sleep spindles. The average (AVG) reference was used because of severe EKG artifact.

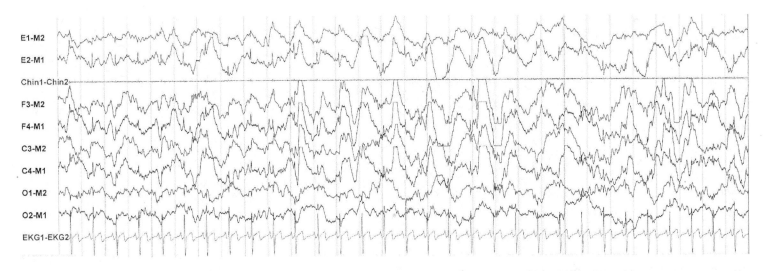

FIGURE 3-9 **Multiple Sleep Latency Test; 30 second page.**

Clinical: 28-year-old man with excessive daytime sleepiness and sleep attacks.

Staging: Stage 3 sleep. Delta activity is evident in the EOG derivations.

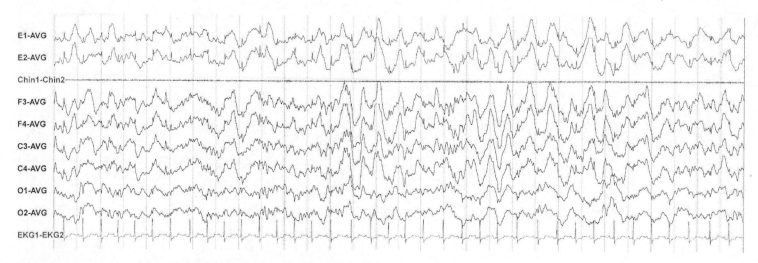

FIGURE 3-10   **Multiple Sleep Latency Test; 30 second page.**
Clinical: 30-year-old woman with excessive sleepiness.
Staging: Stage 3 sleep. Delta activity is evident in the EOG derivations. There is some admixed alpha activity. The average (AVG) reference was used because of severe EKG artifact.

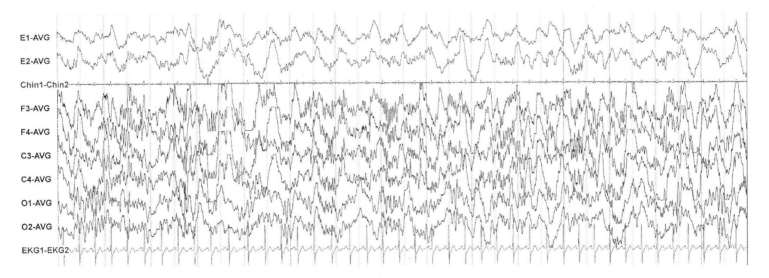

FIGURE 3-11   **Multiple Sleep Latency Test; 30 second page.**

Clinical: 32-year-old man with excessive daytime sleepiness.

Staging: Stage 3 sleep. Delta activity is evident in the EOG derivations. There is prominent admixed alpha activity. The average (AVG) reference was used because of severe EKG artifact.

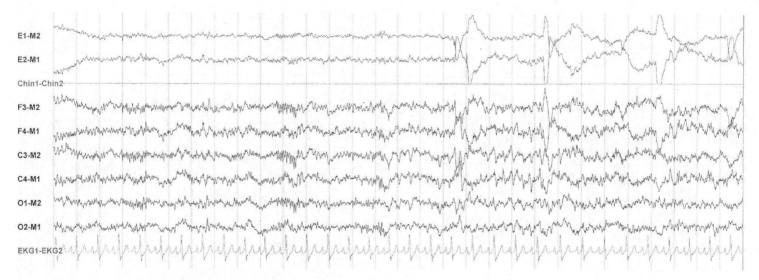

E1-M2

E2-M1

Chin1-Chin2

F3-M2

F4-M1

C3-M2

C4-M1

O1-M2

O2-M1

EKG1-EKG2

FIGURE 3-12   **Multiple Sleep Latency Test; 30 second page.**
Clinical: 22-year-old man with excessive daytime sleepiness and episodes of cataplexy.
Staging: Stage REM sleep with alpha activity posteriorly. There is a transition from tonic REM sleep (without eye movements) to phasic REM sleep (with rapid eye movements). Some sawtooth waves are present.

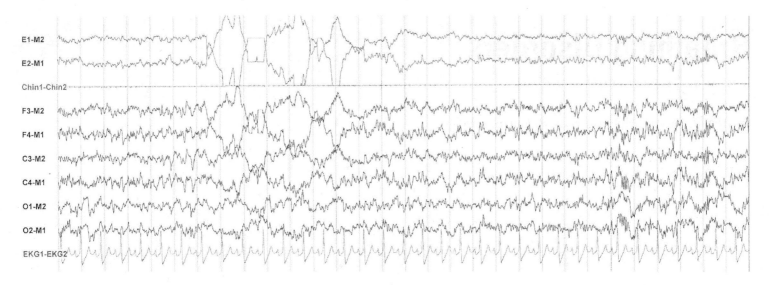

FIGURE 3-13   **Multiple Sleep Latency Test; 30 second page.**
Clinical: 30-year-old woman with excessive sleepiness.
Staging: Stage REM sleep. There is a burst of phasic REM activity.

Breathing Disorders

James D. Geyer, MD and Paul R. Carney, MD

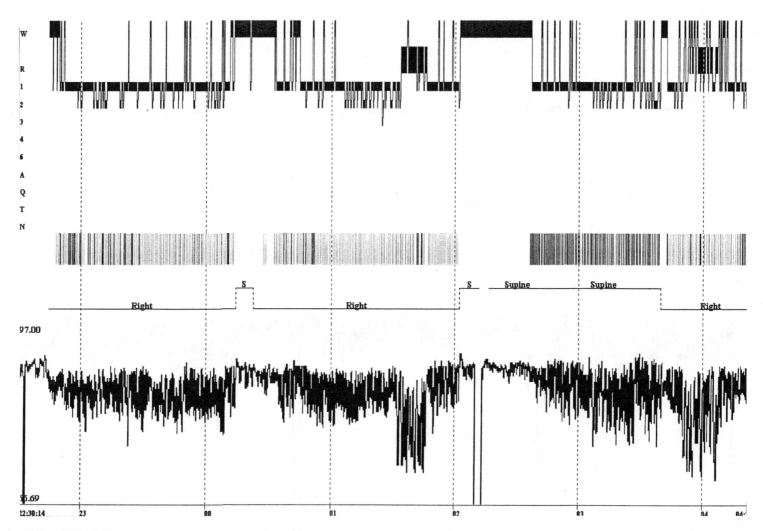

FIGURE 4-1 **Strip chart: Position chart and pulse oximetry.**
Clinical: 46-year-old obese man with severe obstructive sleep apnea.
Pulse oximetry: Frequent oxygen desaturations, which are most prominent during REM sleep. Apneas occurred repeatedly while the patient was supine and in the right lateral decubitus position.

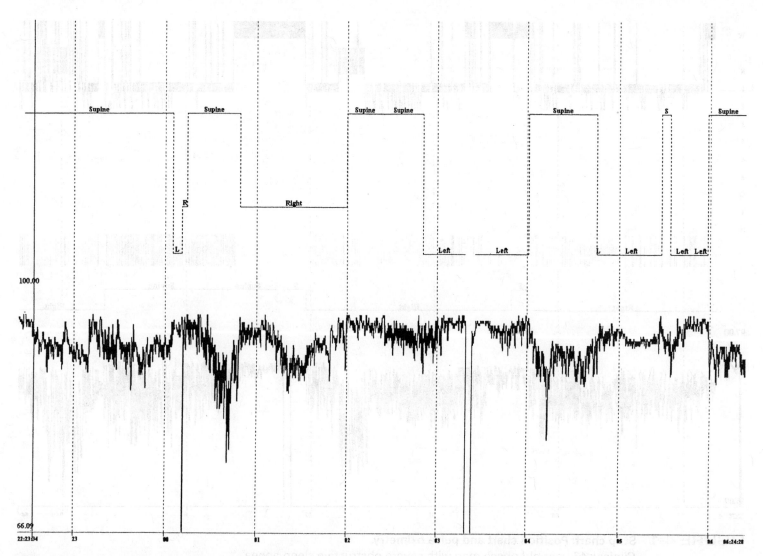

FIGURE 4-2   Strip chart: Pulse oximetry and position.

Pulse oximetry: Obstructive sleep apnea with prolonged oxygen desaturations when supine. This finding can be seen with hypoventilation or with conditions associated with ventilation–perfusion mismatch.

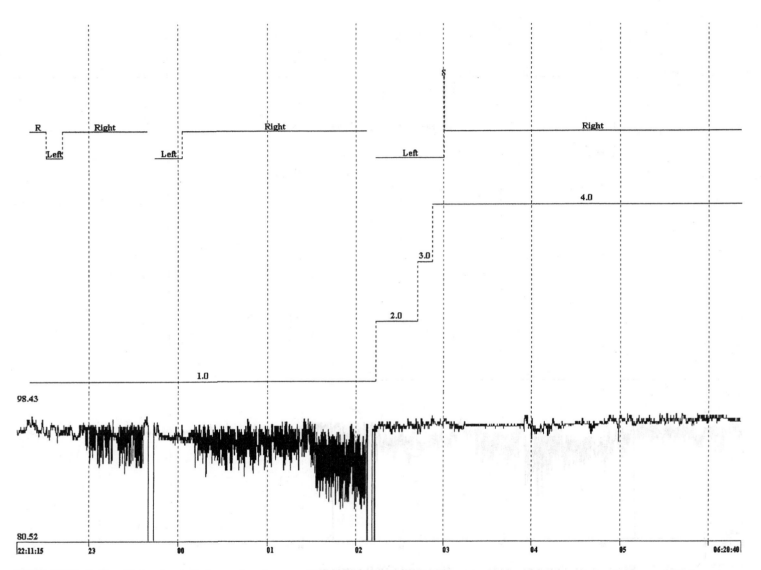

FIGURE 4-3   **Strip chart: Pulse oximetry, position, and CPAP settings.**
Pulse oximetry: Severe obstructive sleep apnea. The initial half of the night (labeled CPAP setting 1.0) is the baseline portion of the recording with no CPAP. CPAP is applied at four different settings, ranging from 5 cm of water (setting 2.0) to 11 cm of water (setting 5.0). Continued moderate obstructive sleep apnea is present with CPAP at levels 2.0 and 3.0. Further improvement of the obstructive sleep apnea is evident at CPAP levels 4.0 and 5.0.

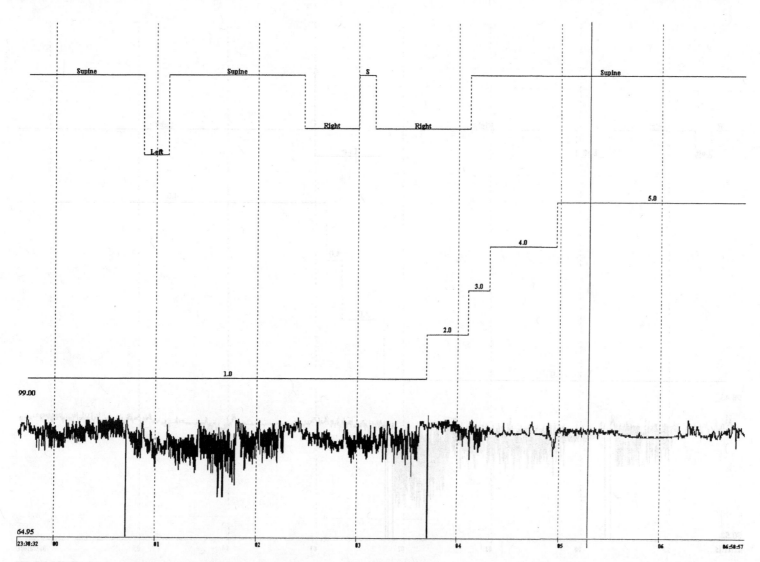

FIGURE 4-4   **Strip chart: Pulse oximetry, position, and CPAP settings.**
Pulse oximetry: Severe obstructive sleep apnea. The initial half of the night (labeled CPAP setting 1.0) is the baseline portion of the recording with no CPAP. CPAP is applied at three different settings, ranging from 5 cm of water (setting 2.0) to 9 cm of water (setting 4.0). Continued moderate obstructive sleep apnea is present with CPAP at levels 2.0 and 3.0. Further improvement of the obstructive sleep apnea is evident at CPAP level 4.0.

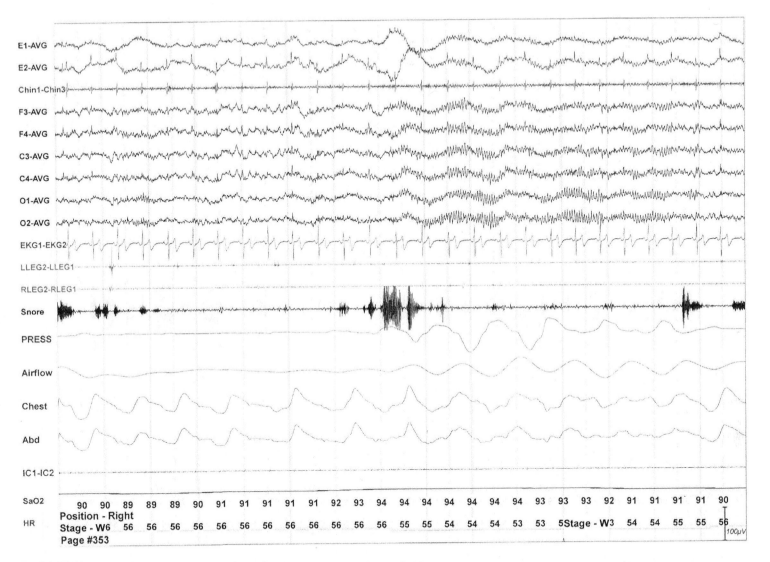

FIGURE 4-5   **Polysomnogram: Standard montage; 30 second page.**
Clinical: 32-year-old man with retrognathia and suspected obstructive sleep apnea.
Staging: Stage W in this epoch because of the timing of the event.
Respiratory: Obstructive apnea followed by a snort, arousal, and an oxygen desaturation.
(Copyright NeuroTexion, 2017.)

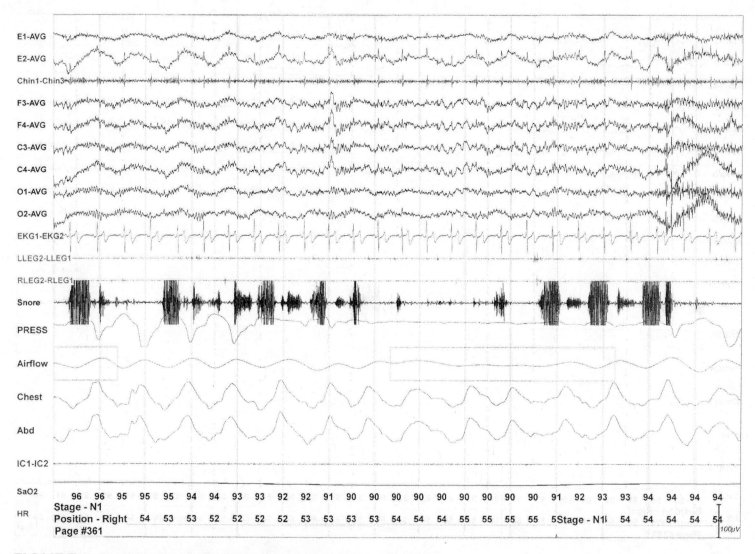

FIGURE 4-6   **Polysomnogram: Standard montage; 30 second page.**
Clinical: 36-year-old woman with retrognathia and suspected obstructive sleep apnea.
Staging: Stage N1 with an arousal.
Respiratory: Obstructive apnea followed by a snort, arousal, and oxygen desaturation.
(Copyright NeuroTexion, 2017.)

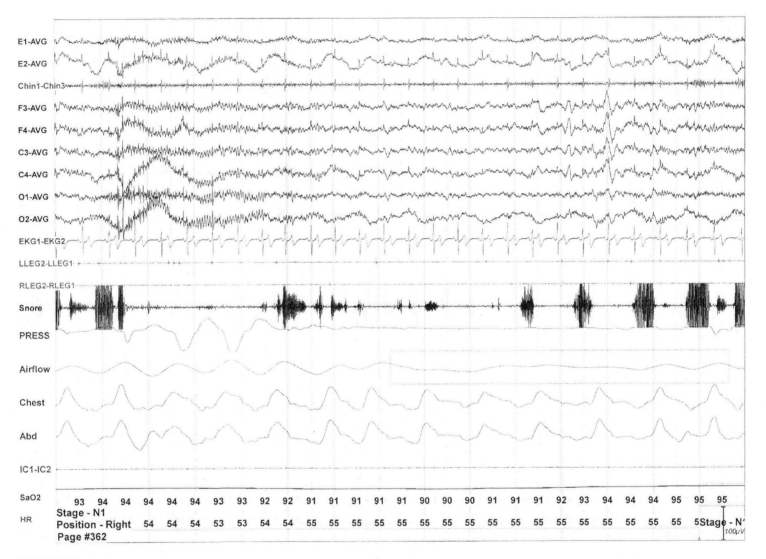

FIGURE 4-7 **Polysomnogram: Standard montage; 30 second page.**
Clinical: 36-year-old woman with retrognathia and suspected obstructive sleep apnea.
Staging: Stage N1 with an arousal.
Respiratory: Obstructive apnea followed by a snort, arousal, and oxygen desaturation on the following page. (Copyright NeuroTexion, 2017.)

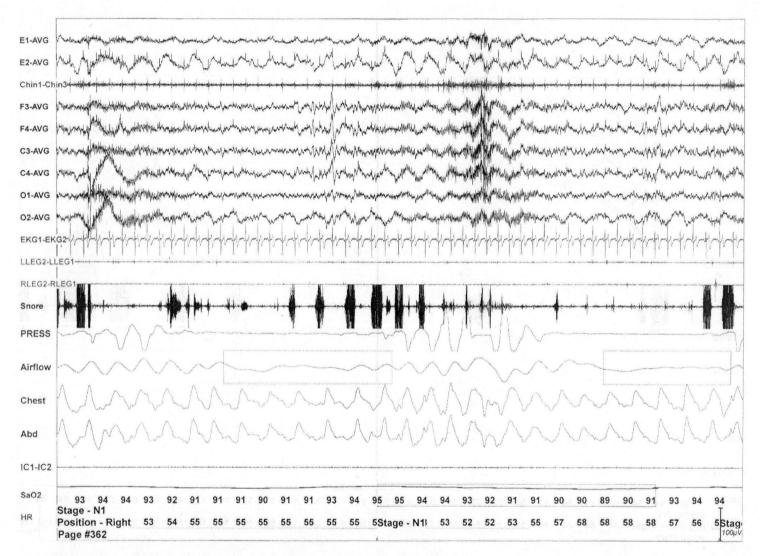

FIGURE 4-8 **Polysomnogram: Standard montage; 60 second page.**
Clinical: 36-year-old woman with retrognathia and suspected obstructive sleep apnea.
Staging: Stage N1 with arousals.
Respiratory: Obstructive apnea followed by snorts, arousals, and oxygen desaturations. (Copyright NeuroTexion, 2017.)

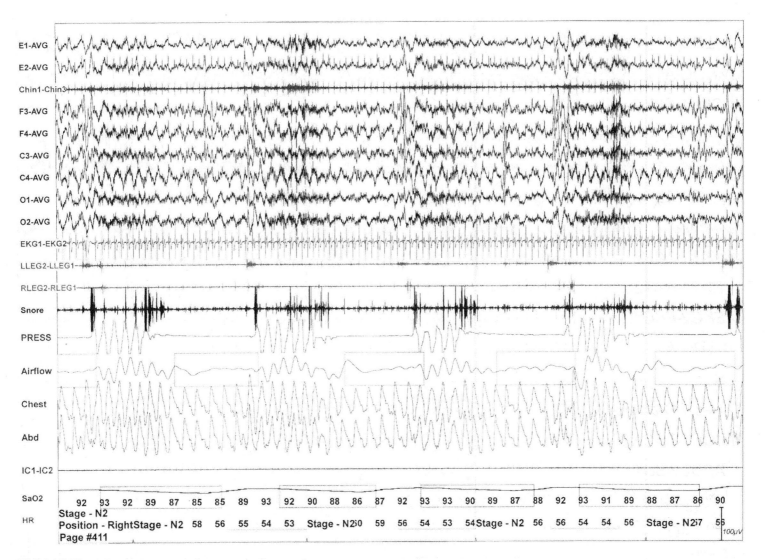

FIGURE 4-9 **Polysomnogram: Standard montage; 120 second page.**
Clinical: 36-year-old woman with retrognathia and suspected obstructive sleep apnea.
Staging: Stage N2 with arousals.
Respiratory: Obstructive apnea followed by snorts, arousals, and oxygen desaturations. (Copyright NeuroTexion, 2017.)

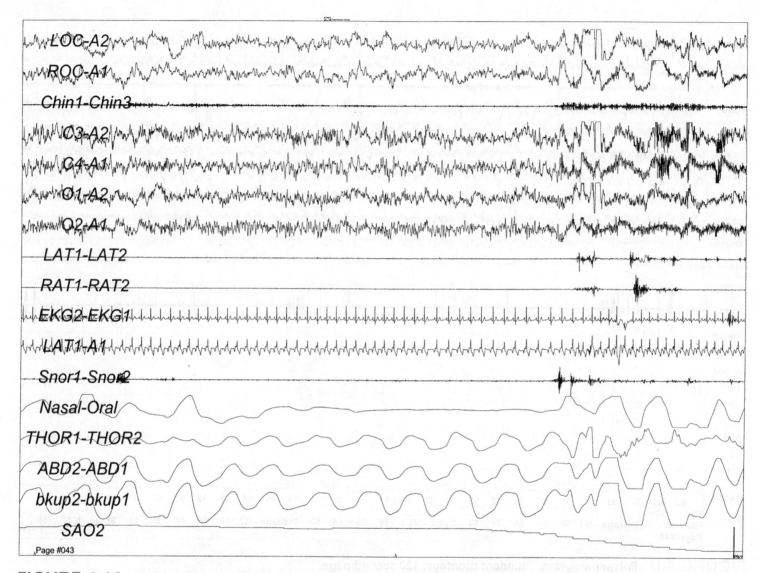

FIGURE 4-10 **Polysomnogram: Standard montage (prior recording/display montage); 60 second page.**

Clinical: 29-year-old obese woman with a thick neck and suspected obstructive sleep apnea.

Staging: Stage N2 sleep with an arousal.

Respiratory: Obstructive apnea with inphase respiratory effort in the thoracic and abdominal channels followed by an arousal, a snort, and an oxygen desaturation.

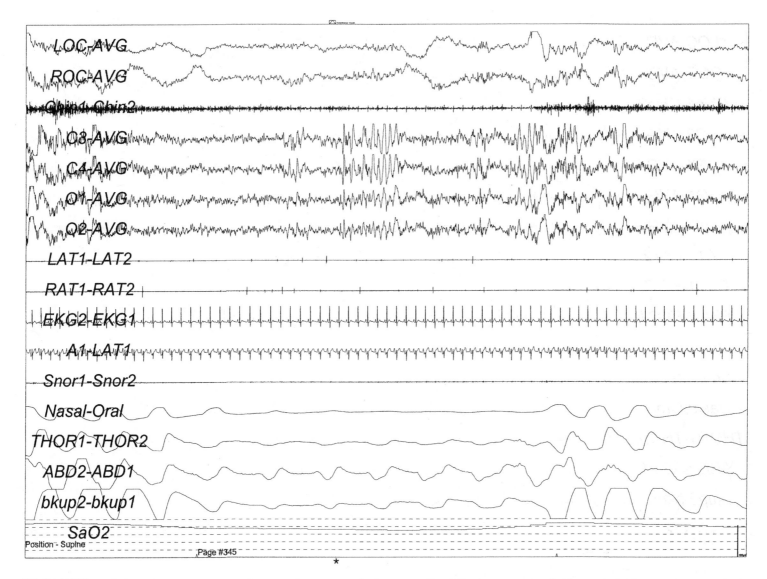

FIGURE 4-11   **Polysomnogram: Standard montage (prior recording/display montage); 60 second page.**

Clinical: 42-year-old man with a low-lying soft palate and suspected obstructive sleep apnea.

Staging: Stage N2 sleep with transition into REM sleep. Although the epoch does not meet scoring criteria for REM sleep due to the absence of rapid eye movements, the reduction in chin EMG activity and the occurrence of sawtooth waves (*) are consistent with REM sleep.

Respiratory: Obstructive apnea with decreased but inphase respiratory effort followed by an arousal and an oxygen desaturation.

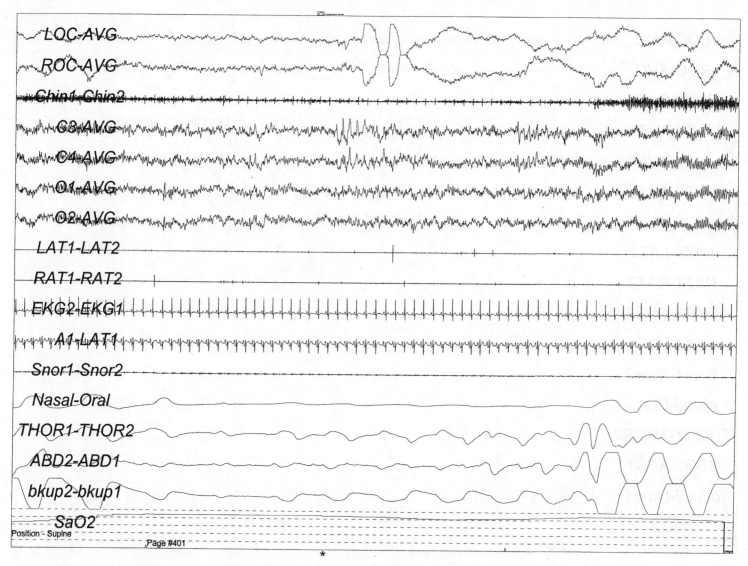

FIGURE 4-12 **Polysomnogram: Standard montage (prior recording/display montage); 60 second page.**
Clinical: 42-year-old man with a low-lying soft palate and suspected obstructive sleep apnea.
Staging: Stage R sleep with rapid eye movements and arousals.
Respiratory: Obstructive apnea with increasing respiratory effort followed by an arousal.
EEG: Sawtooth waves (*) in REM sleep.

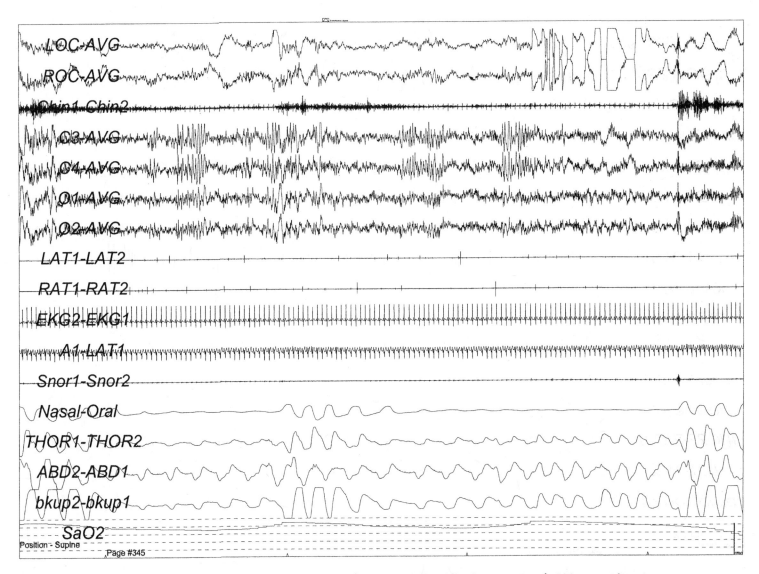

FIGURE 4-13 **Polysomnogram: Standard montage (prior recording/display montage); 120 second page.**
Clinical: 42-year-old man with a low-lying soft palate and suspected obstructive sleep apnea.
Staging: Stage R sleep with rapid eye movements and arousals.
Respiratory: Obstructive apneas with increasing respiratory effort followed by arousals, snorts, and oxygen desaturations.
EEG: Sawtooth waves in REM sleep.

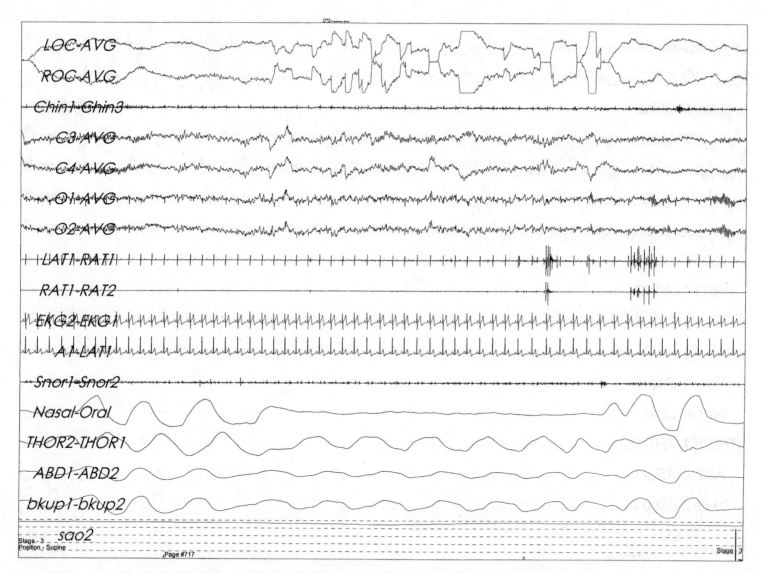

FIGURE 4-14   **Polysomnogram: Standard montage (prior recording/display montage); 30 second page.**
Clinical: 12-year-old with large tonsils and suspected obstructive sleep apnea.
Staging: Stage R sleep with rapid eye movements and bursts of leg EMG activity.
Respiratory: Obstructive apnea with decreased but inphase respiratory effort followed by an arousal.

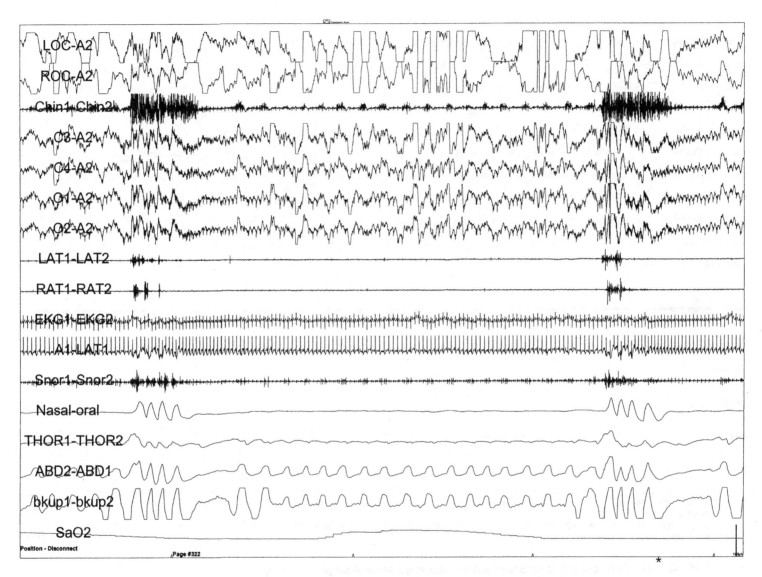

FIGURE 4-15 **Polysomnogram: Standard montage (prior recording/display montage); 120 second page.**
Clinical: 12-year-old with large tonsils and suspected obstructive sleep apnea.
Staging: Stage R sleep with rapid eye movements.
Respiratory: Prolonged obstructive apnea with decreased but inphase respiratory effort followed by an arousal and an oxygen desaturation. There is also a brief postarousal central apnea (*). The oxygen desaturation at the beginning of this page was caused by an apnea from the preceding page of the record.

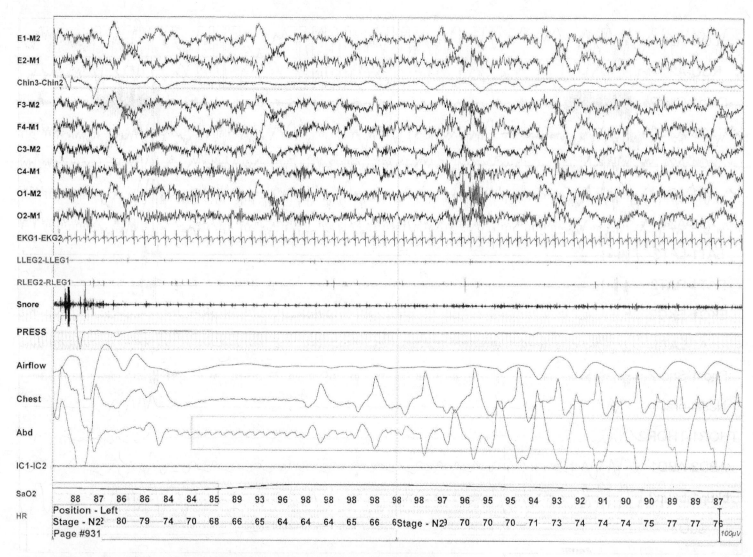

FIGURE 4-16   Polysomnogram: Standard montage; 60 second page.

Clinical: 29-year-old moderately obese woman with excessive daytime sleepiness and suspected obstructive sleep apnea.

Staging: Stage N2.

Respiratory: prolonged mixed apnea.

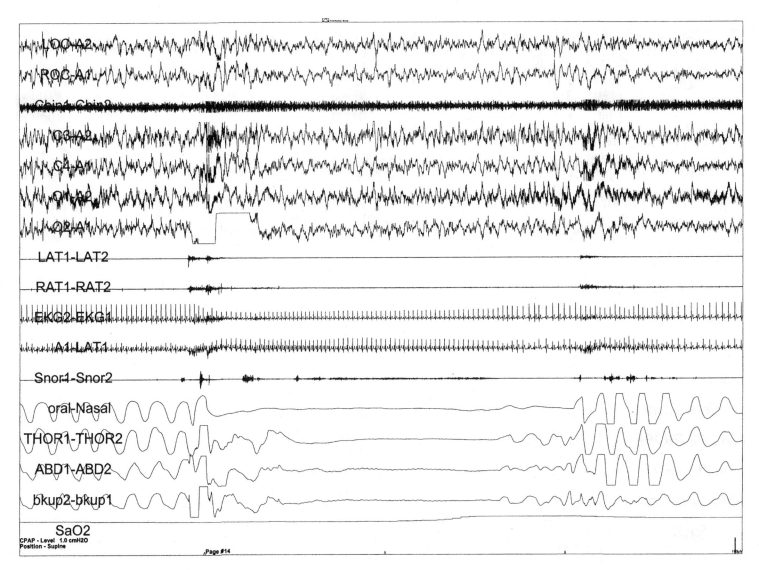

FIGURE 4-17 **Polysomnogram: Standard montage (prior recording/display montage); 120 second page.**
Clinical: 22-year-old obese man with marked retrognathia.
Staging: Stage N3 sleep with arousals.
Respiratory: Mixed apnea with inphase respiratory effort at the beginning and end of the apnea followed by an arousal and an oxygen desaturation. The oxygen desaturation at the beginning of this page is a result of an apnea from the preceding page of the record.

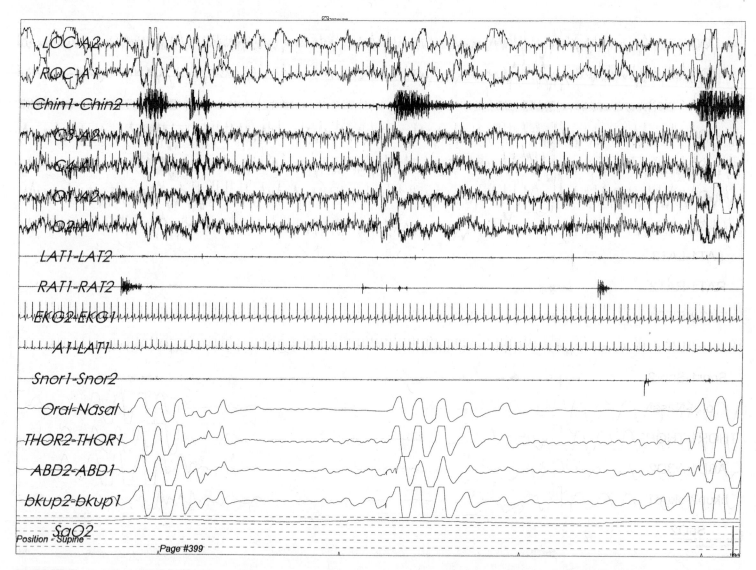

FIGURE 4-18 **Polysomnogram: Standard montage (prior recording/display montage); 120 second page.**
Clinical: 42-year-old woman with multiple sclerosis, restless legs syndrome and suspected obstructive sleep apnea.
Staging: Stage N1 sleep with arousals.
Respiratory: Repeated mixed apneas with arousals and minimal oxygen desaturations.

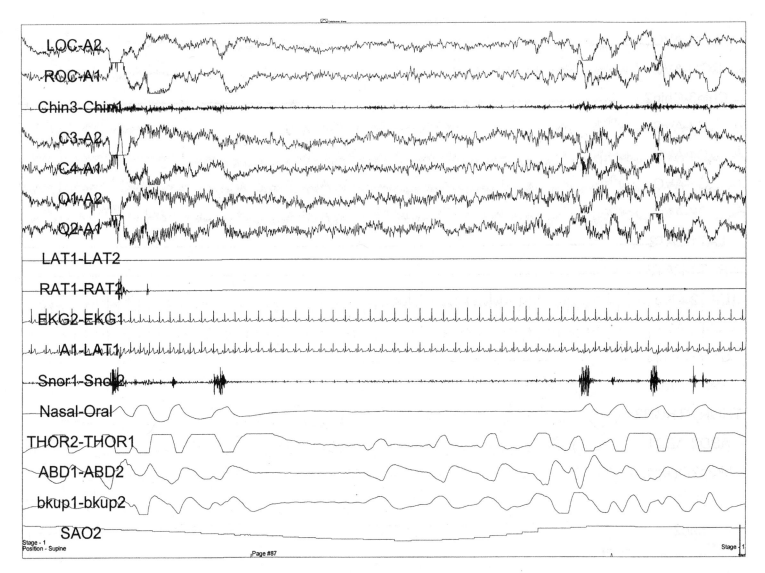

FIGURE 4-19　**Polysomnogram: Standard montage (prior recording/display montage); 60 second page.**

Clinical: 52-year-old man with snoring and excessive daytime sleepiness.

Staging: Stage N1 sleep with arousals.

Respiratory: Mixed apnea with increasing effort and paradoxical respirations followed by a snort, an arousal, an oxygen desaturation, and snoring. The oxygen desaturation on this page was caused by an apnea from the preceding page of the record.

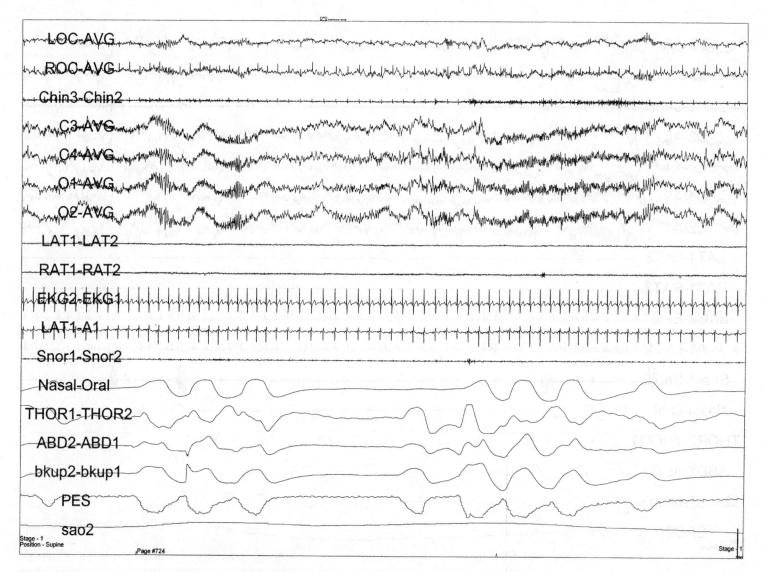

FIGURE 4-20   **Polysomnogram: Standard montage with intrathoracic pressure monitoring (prior recording/display montage); 30 second page.**

Clinical: 44-year-old woman with snoring and excessive daytime sleepiness.

Staging: Stage N1 sleep with arousals.

Respiratory: Mixed apnea with an initial portion without respiratory effort followed by two obstructed breaths. Respiratory effort, as measured by the esophageal pressure monitor (PES), increases with the second obstructed breath and then decreases after the arousal and resumption of breathing. There is minimal oxygen desaturation from 94% to 91%.

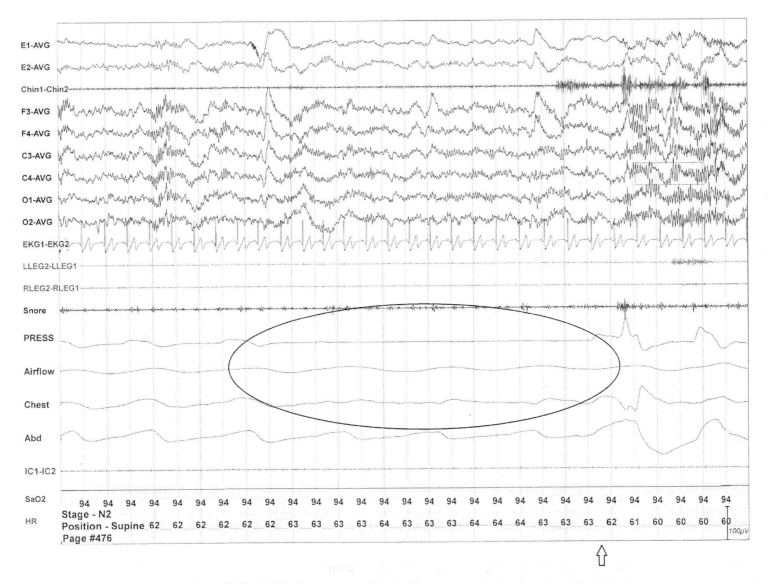

FIGURE 4-21   **Polysomnogram: Standard montage; 30 second page.**
Clinical: 77-year-old thin man with severe peripheral polyneuropathy and excessive daytime sleepiness.
Staging: Stage N2 sleep with an arousal.
Respiratory: Hypopnea (*oval*) with decreased airflow and respiratory effort followed by an arousal
(*arrow*). (Copyright JNP Enterprises, 2017.)

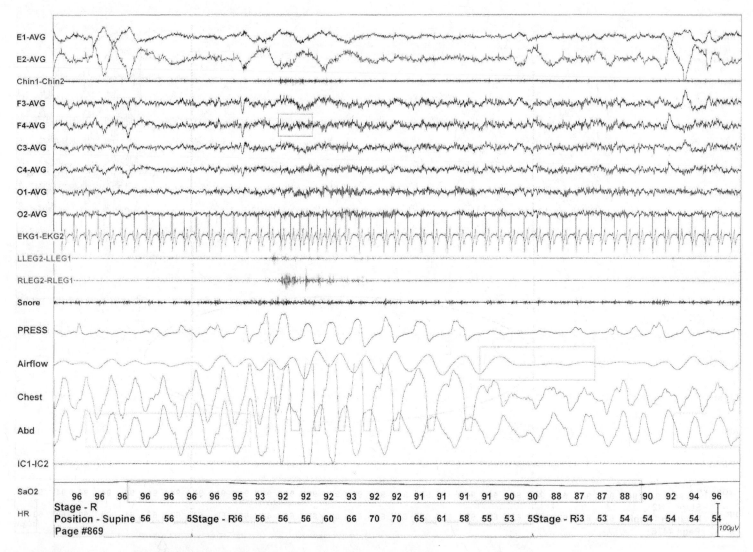

FIGURE 4-22   **Polysomnogram: Standard montage; 60 second page.**

Clinical: 64-year-old obese woman with daytime sleepiness and loud snoring.

Staging: Stage R.

Respiratory: Recurrent hypopneas with arousals and oxygen desaturations.

EKG: Tachycardia–bradycardia with events. (Copyright JNP Enterprises, 2017.)

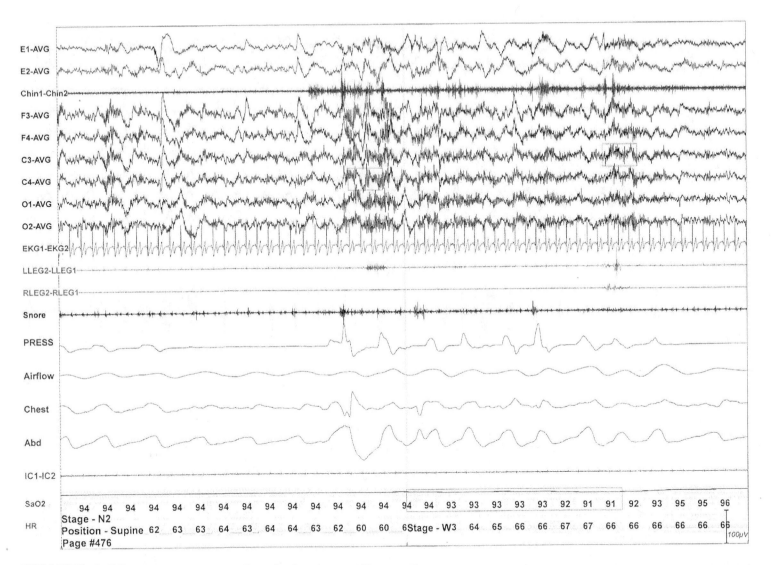

FIGURE 4-23　**Polysomnogram: Standard montage; 60 second page.**
Clinical: 41-year-old woman with excessive daytime sleepiness and intractable headaches.
Staging: Stage N2 sleep.
Respiratory: Repeated hypopneas followed by arousals and oxygen desaturations. The pressure transducer is flat during the event. (Copyright JNP Enterprises, 2017.)

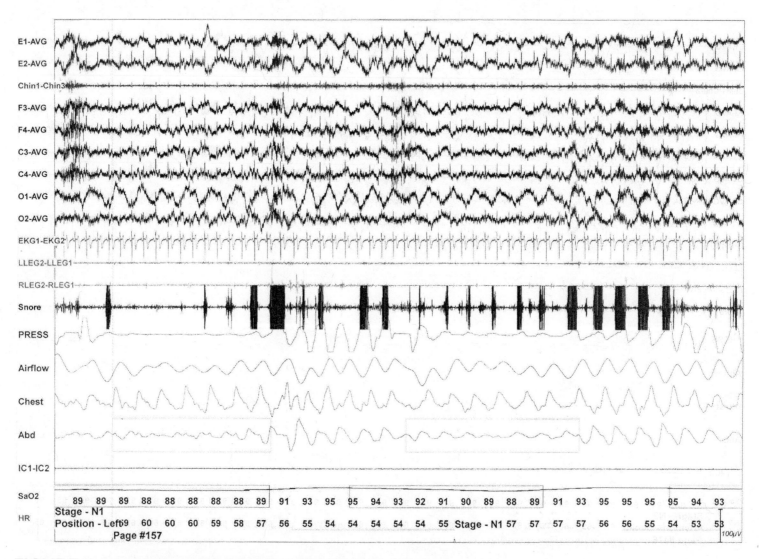

FIGURE 4-24   **Polysomnogram: Standard montage; 60 second page.**
Clinical: 51-year-old man with excessive daytime sleepiness and hypertension.
Staging: Stage N1 sleep with arousals.
Respiratory: Repeated hypopneas followed by arousals and oxygen desaturations. The pressure transducer is flat during the first event, but there are low-amplitude deflections during the second event.
(Copyright JNP Enterprises, 2017.)

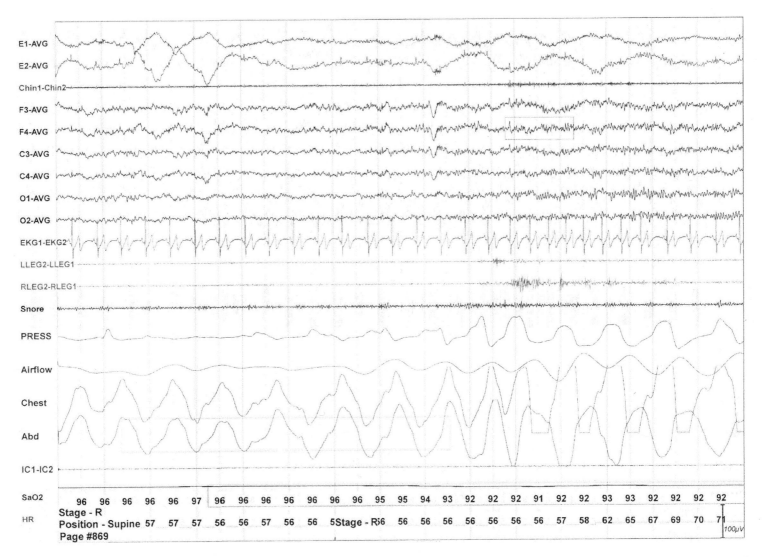

FIGURE 4-25   **Polysomnogram: Standard montage; 30 second page.**
Clinical: 64-year-old obese woman with daytime sleepiness and loud snoring.
Staging: Stage R.
Respiratory: Recurrent hypopneas with arousals and oxygen desaturations.
EKG: Tachycardia–bradycardia with events. (Copyright JNP Enterprises, 2017.)

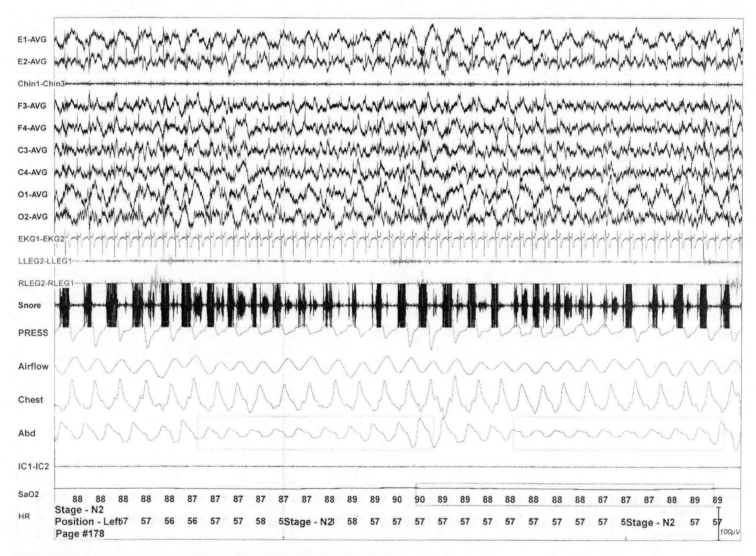

FIGURE 4-26   **Polysomnogram: Standard montage; 60 second page.**
Clinical: 37-year-old man with fatigue and loud snoring.
Staging: Stage N2 sleep.
Respiratory: Hypopnea with increasing respiratory effort followed by an oxygen desaturation. (Copyright JNP Enterprises, 2017.)

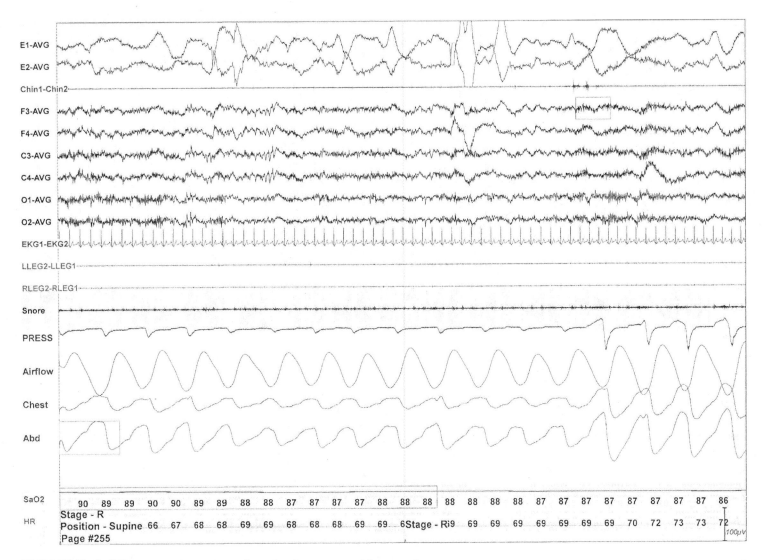

FIGURE 4-27   **Polysomnogram: Standard montage; 60 second page.**
Clinical: 29-year-old obese woman with excessive daytime sleepiness.
Staging: Stage R sleep.
Respiratory: Prolonged hypopnea with an associated oxygen desaturation during phasic REM
sleep. There is an arousal and increased respiratory effort at the end of the page. (Copyright JNP
Enterprises, 2017.)

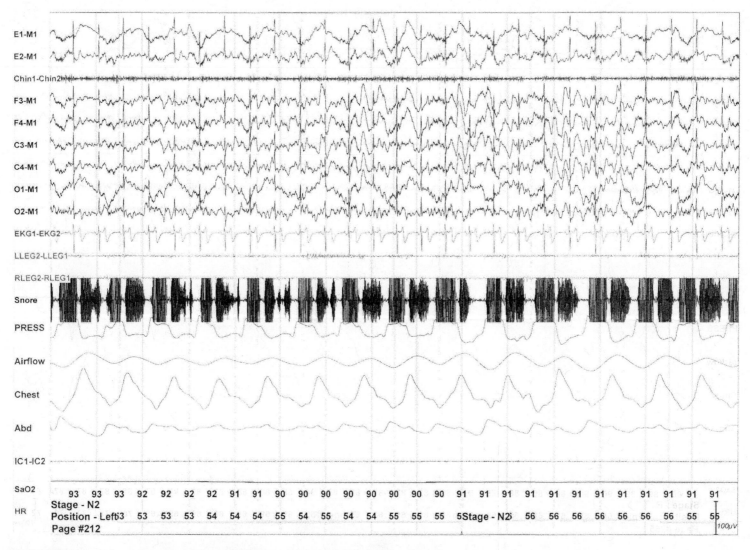

FIGURE 4-28   **Polysomnogram: Standard montage; 30 second page.**
Clinical: 33-year-old woman with excessive daytime sleepiness.
Staging: Stage N2 sleep with an arousal.
Respiratory: There are paradoxical respirations with flattening of the nasal pressure transducer waveform. This suggests resistance in the upper airway. There is loud snoring. (Copyright JNP Enterprises, 2017.)

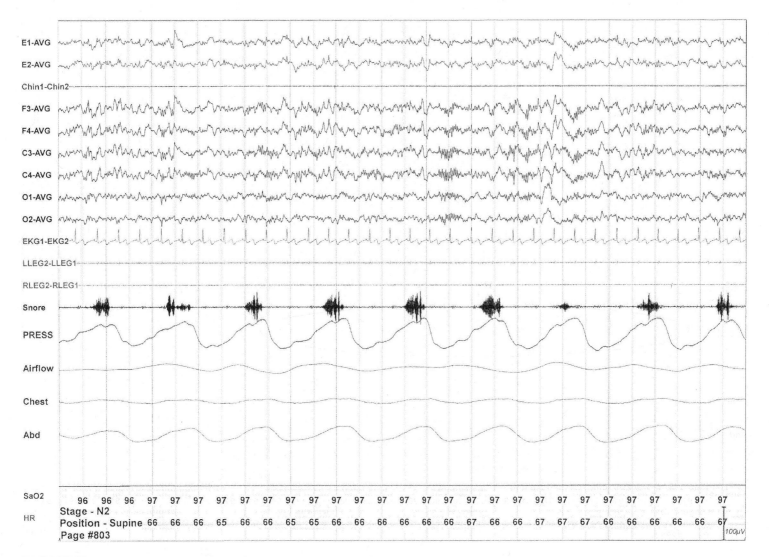

FIGURE 4-29 **Polysomnogram: Standard montage; 30 second page.**
Clinical: 36-year-old man with snoring and coronary artery disease.
Staging: Stage N2 sleep.
Respiratory: Snoring is present. Normal respirations. (Copyright JNP Enterprises, 2017.)

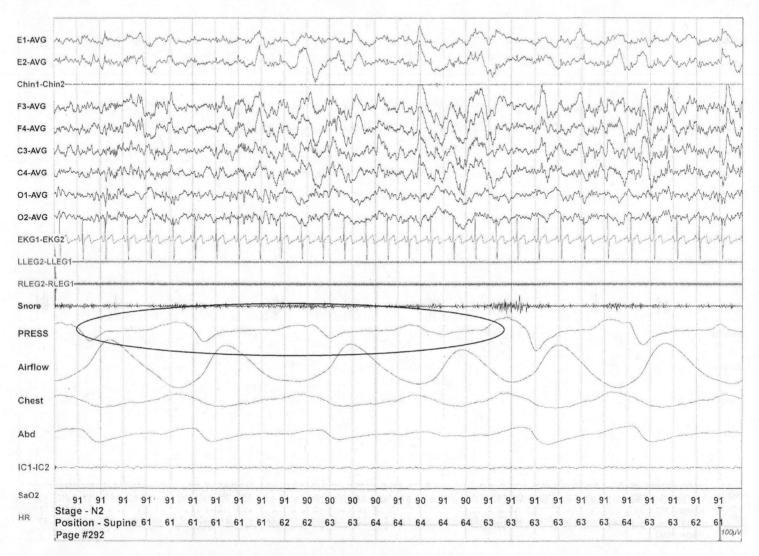

FIGURE 4-30 **Polysomnogram: Standard montage; 30 second page.**
Clinical: 49-year-old man with unrefreshing sleep.
Staging: Stage N2 sleep transitioning toward N3.
Respiratory: Decreased nasal pressure waveform amplitude (*oval*) followed by a small snort. There is no significant associated change in the airflow or effort channels. Furthermore, there is no arousal or associated oxygen desaturation. (Copyright JNP Enterprises, 2017.)

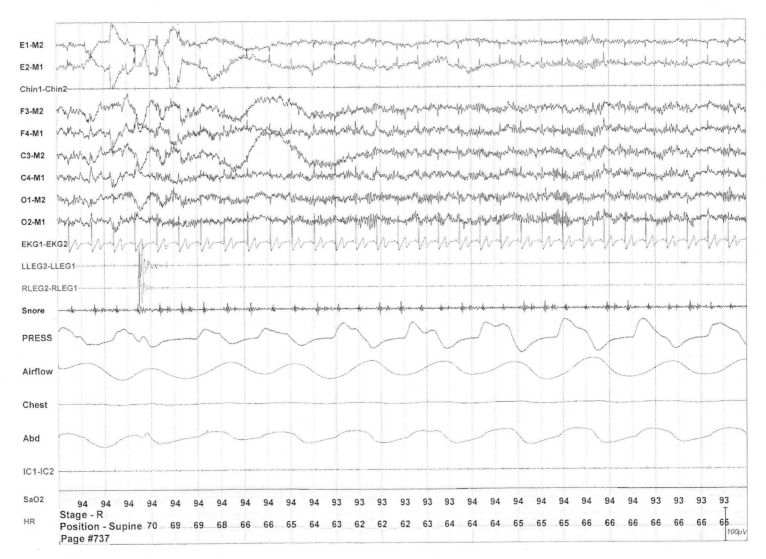

FIGURE 4-31   **Polysomnogram: Standard montage; 30 second page.**
Clinical: 34-year-old man with daytime sleepiness and irritability.
Staging: Stage R sleep.
Respiratory: There is some respiratory irregularity, which is a normal component of REM sleep, especially phasic REM sleep. (Copyright JNP Enterprises, 2017.)

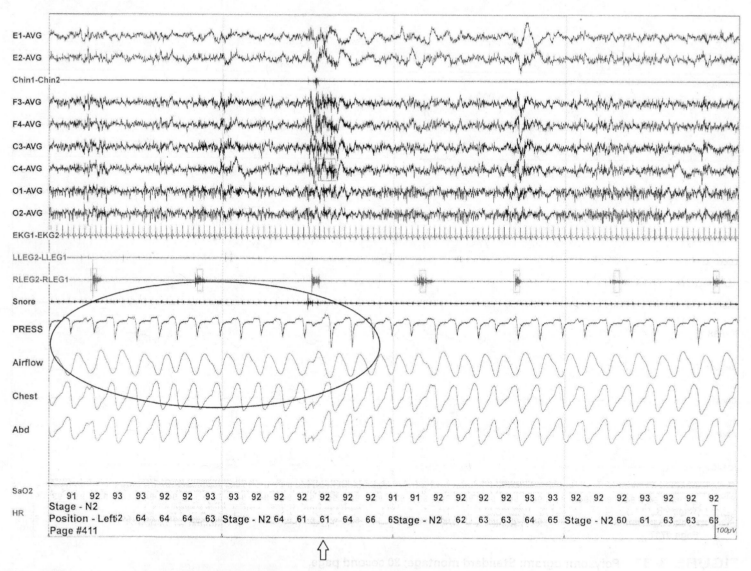

FIGURE 4-32 **Polysomnogram: Standard montage; 120 second page.**
Clinical: 37-year-old woman with excessive fatigue and daily headaches.
Staging: Stage N2 sleep.
Respiratory: There is a respiratory event–related arousal. There is a decrease in the nasal pressure waveform followed by a sudden increase (*oval*) with an associated arousal (*arrow*).
Limb movements: There are periodic limb movements involving the right leg. (Copyright JNP Enterprises, 2017.)

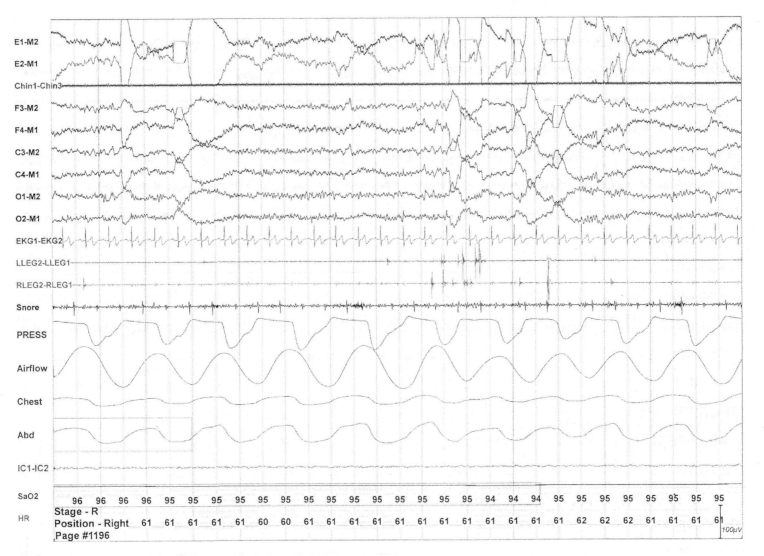

FIGURE 4-33 **Polysomnogram: Standard montage; 30 second page.**
Clinical: 50-year-old man with snoring and fatigue.
Staging: Stage R sleep.
Respiratory: There is flattening of the nasal pressure transducer waveform. (Copyright JNP Enterprises, 2017.)

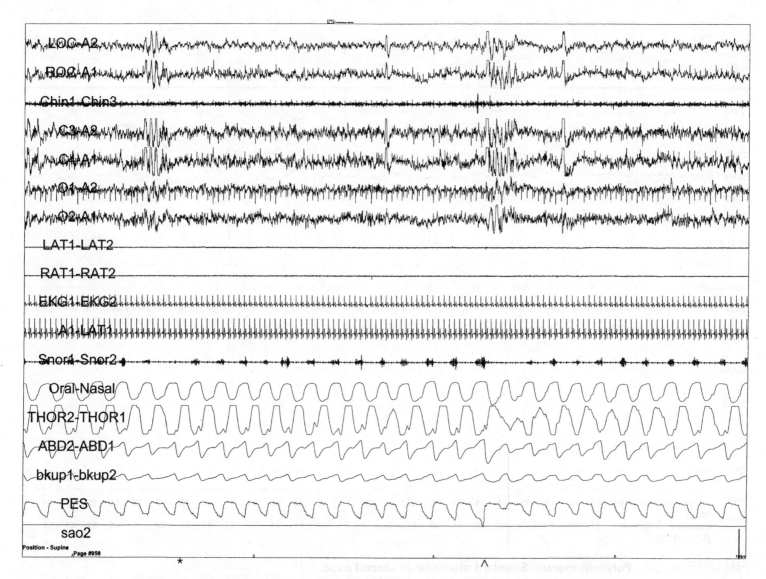

FIGURE 4-34   **Polysomnogram: Standard montage with intrathoracic pressure (Pes) monitoring (prior recording/display montage); 120 second page.**

Clinical: 49-year-old man with upper airway resistance syndrome.

Staging: Stage N2 sleep with an arousal.

Respiratory: Negative intrathoracic pressure increases gradually from −12 (*) to 19 (^) cm of water. There is a subsequent arousal but no oxygen desaturation.

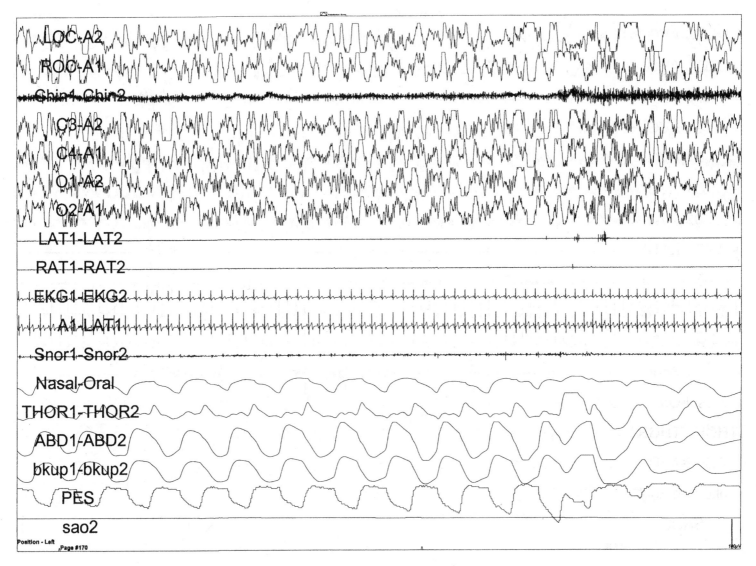

FIGURE 4-35   **Polysomnogram: Standard montage with intrathoracic pressure monitoring (prior recording/display montage); 30 second page.**

Clinical: 17-year-old woman with mild retrognathia, excessive daytime sleepiness associated with recent weight gain.

Staging: Stage N3 sleep with alpha intrusion and an arousal.

Respiratory: Negative intrathoracic pressure increases gradually over several breaths followed by an arousal but no oxygen desaturation. Snoring is minimal. The increased respiratory effort preceding the arousal would be more difficult to appreciate without the Pes monitoring.

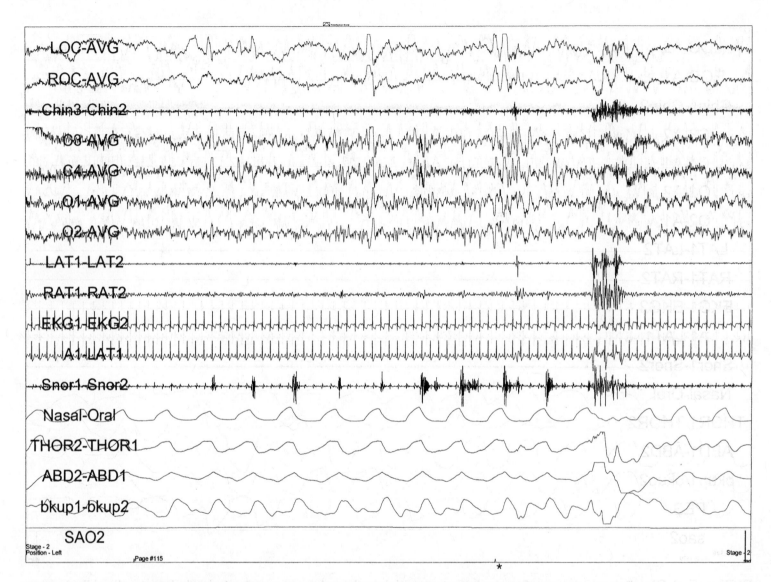

FIGURE 4-36 **Polysomnogram: Standard montage (prior recording/display montage); 60 second page.**
Clinical: 39-year-old man with snoring, unrefreshing sleep and headaches.
Staging: Stage N2 sleep with an arousal.
Respiratory: Snoring increases in amplitude for several breaths and then is followed by an arousal (*).
The increase in snoring is inferential evidence of increased respiratory effort, which is difficult to detect in
the thoracic and abdominal channels.

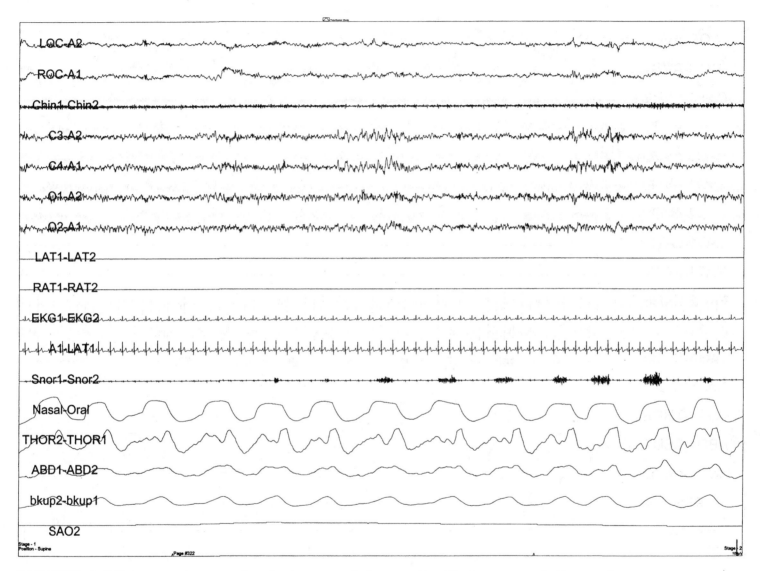

FIGURE 4-37   **Polysomnogram: Standard montage (prior recording/display montage); 30 second page.**

Clinical: 24-year-old man with snoring and hypertension.

Staging: Stage N1 sleep.

Respiratory: Snoring increases in amplitude over several breaths accompanied by subtle evidence of increased respiratory effort in the thoracic and abdominal channels.

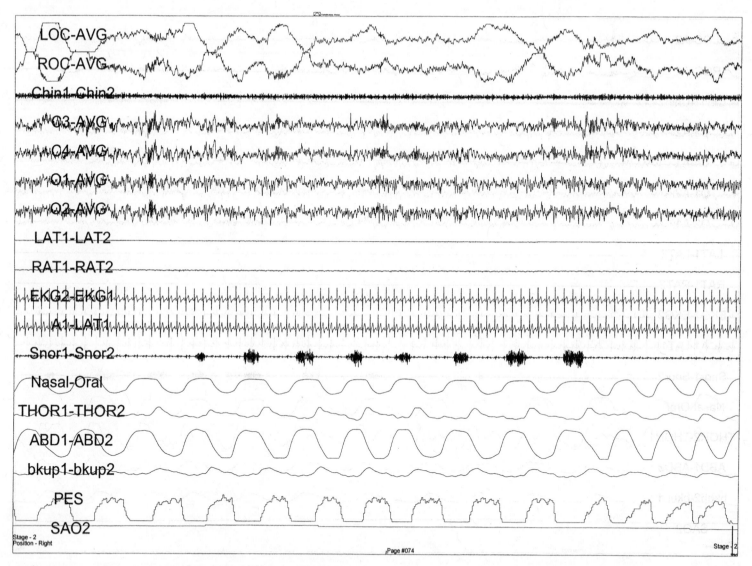

FIGURE 4-38   **Polysomnogram: Standard montage (prior recording/display montage); 60 second page.**
Clinical: 24-year-old man with snoring and hypertension.
Staging: Stage N2 sleep.
Respiratory: Snoring increases over several breaths without a subsequent arousal. Blocking of the intra-thoracic pressure signal does not allow quantitation of inspiratory force.

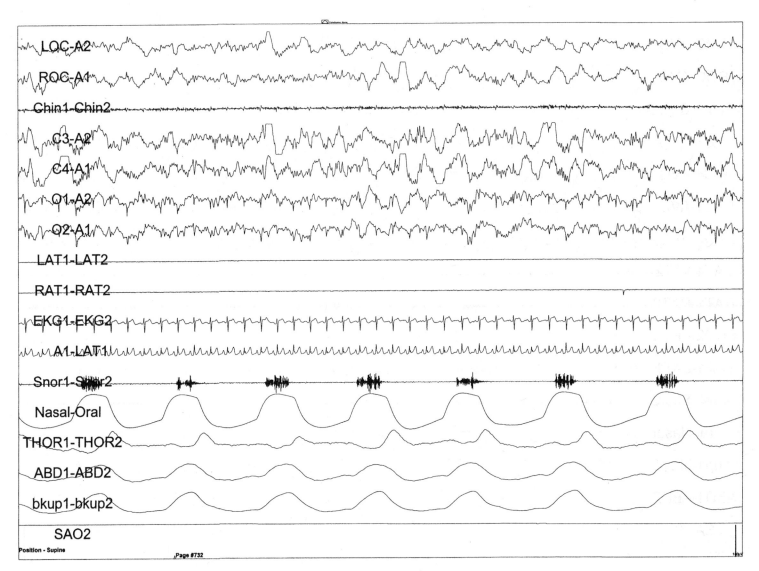

FIGURE 4-39   **Polysomnogram: Standard montage (prior recording/display montage); 30 second page.**
Clinical: 39-year-old man with loud snoring and excessive daytime sleepiness.
Staging: Stage N2 sleep.
Respiratory: Snoring with otherwise normal respirations.

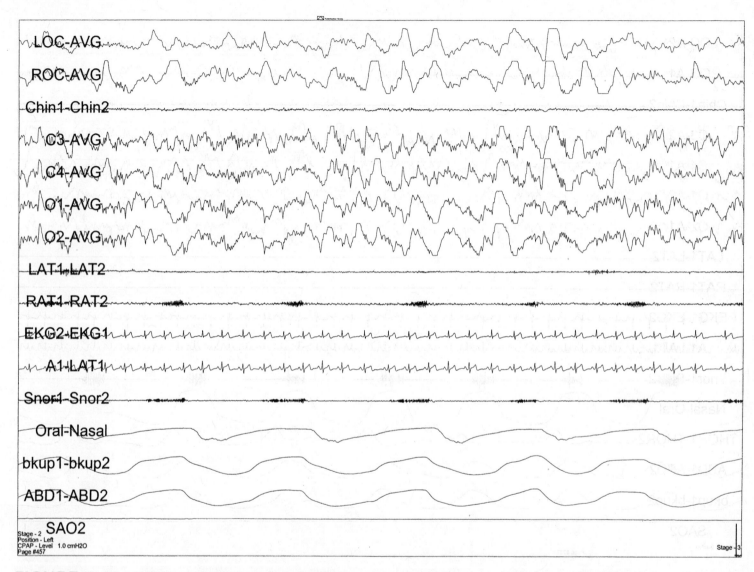

LOC-AVG
ROC-AVG
Chin1-Chin2
C3-AVG
C4-AVG
O1-AVG
O2-AVG
LAT1-LAT2
RAT1-RAT2
EKG2-EKG1
A1-LAT1
Snor1-Snor2
Oral-Nasal
bkup1-bkup2
ABD1-ABD2
SAO2

Stage - 2
Position - Left
CPAP - Level 1.0 cmH2O
Page #457

Stage - 3

FIGURE 4-40 **Polysomnogram: Standard montage (prior recording/display montage); 30 second page.**
Clinical: 47-year-old woman with fatigue and snoring.
Staging: Stage N3 sleep.
Respiratory: Snoring with otherwise normal respirations.

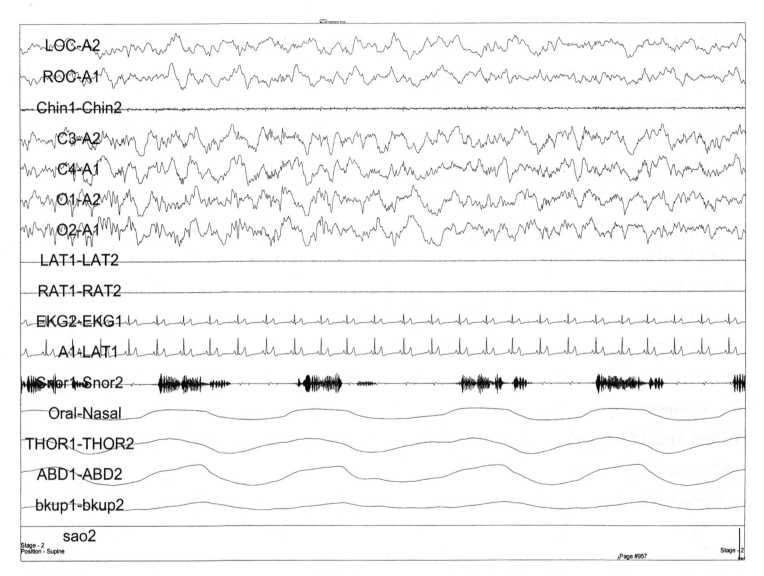

FIGURE 4-41   **Polysomnogram: Standard montage (prior recording/display montage); 30 second page.**
Clinical: 45-year-old man with snoring and hypertension.
Staging: Stage N3 sleep.
Respiratory: Normal respirations except for pronounced snoring.

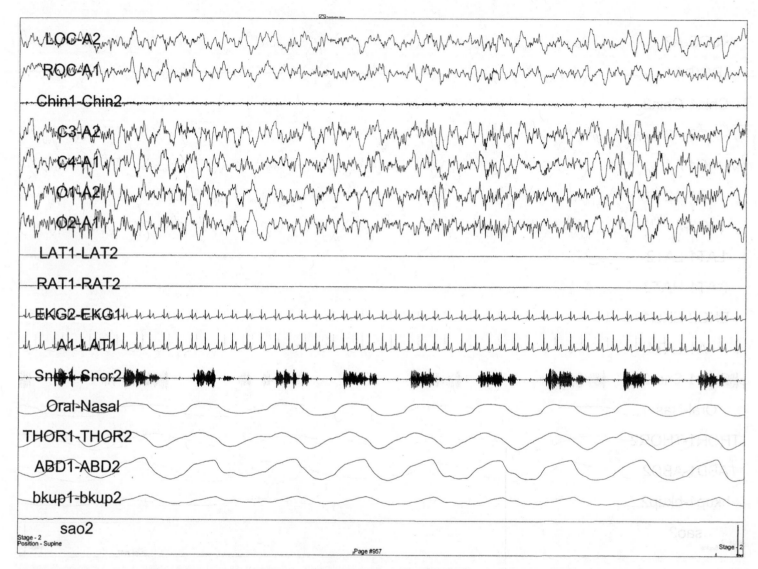

LOC-A2

ROC-A1

Chin1-Chin2

C3-A2

C4-A1

O1-A2

O2-A1

LAT1-LAT2

RAT1-RAT2

EKG2-EKG1

A1-LAT1

Snor1-Snor2

Oral-Nasal

THOR1-THOR2

ABD1-ABD2

bkup1-bkup2

sao2

Stage - 2
Position - Supine

Page #957

Stage - 2

FIGURE 4-42   **Polysomnogram: Standard montage (prior recording/display montage); 60 second page.**
Clinical: 45-year-old man with snoring and hypertension.
Staging: Stage N3 sleep.
Respiratory: Normal respirations except for loud snoring.

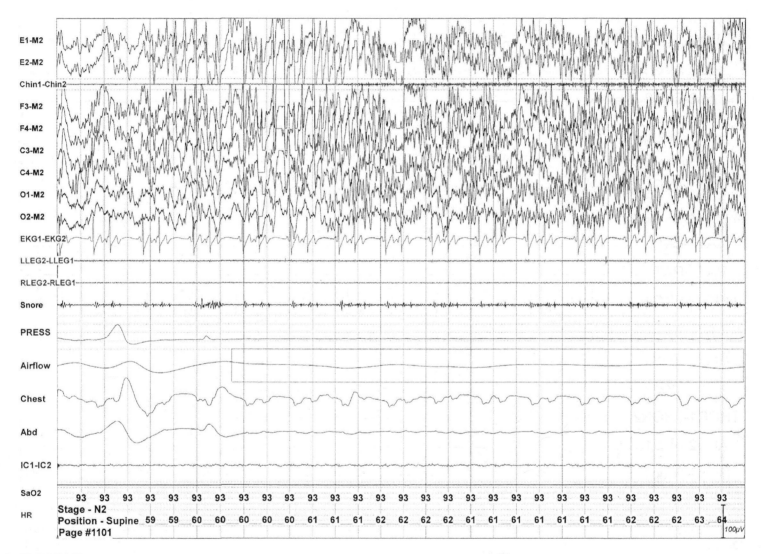

FIGURE 4-43 **Polysomnogram: Standard montage; 30 second page.**
Clinical: 44-year-old man with excessive daytime sleepiness and witnessed apneas.
Staging: Stage N2 sleep with an electrographic seizure.
Respiratory: Central apnea. There is cardioballistic artifact in the chest effort channel.
EKG: Premature atrial contractions. (Copyright JNP Enterprises, 2017.)

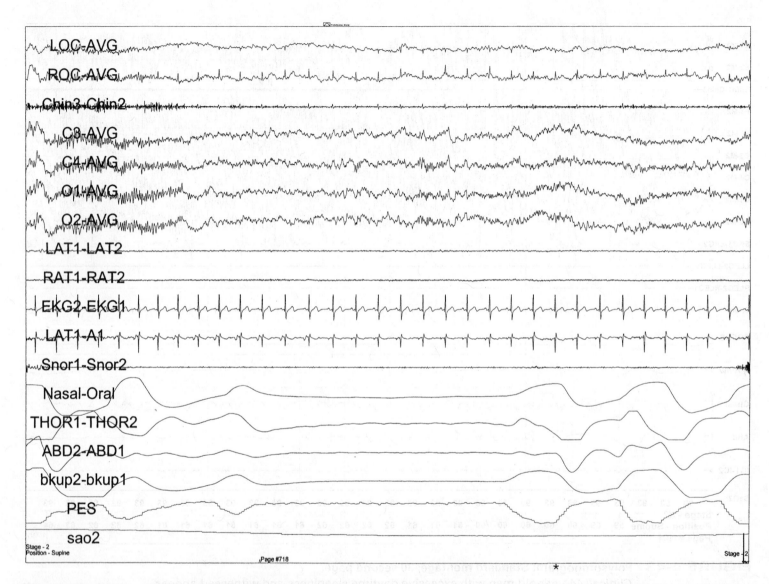

FIGURE 4-44 **Polysomnogram: Standard montage with intrathoracic pressure monitoring (prior recording/display montage); 30 second page.**

Clinical: 33-year-old man with witnessed episodes of apnea.

Staging: Stage N2 sleep with an arousal (*).

Respiratory: Central apnea with no effort on intrathoracic pressure monitoring.

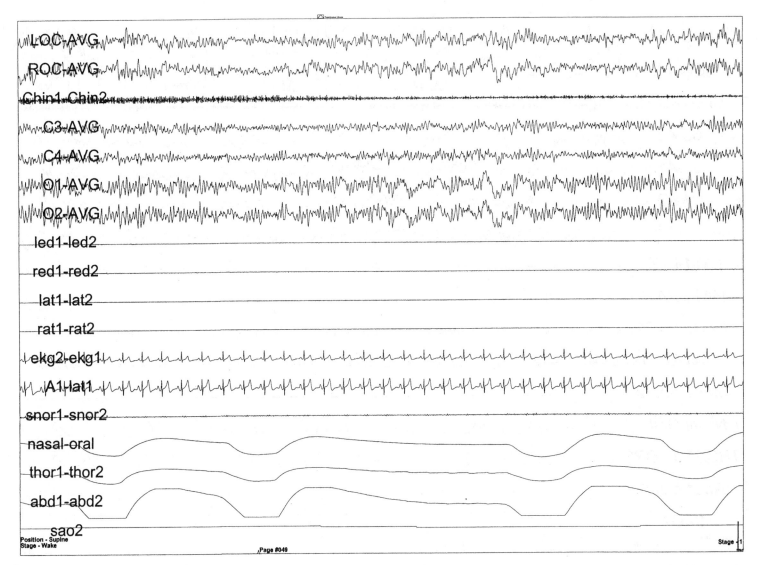

FIGURE 4-45   **Polysomnogram: Periodic limb movements montage (prior recording/display montage); 30 second page.**
Clinical: 41-year-old man with frequent nocturnal movements.
Staging: Transition from wake to stage N1 sleep.
Respiratory: Sleep onset central apnea. Brief central apneas that occur in the transition from wakefulness to sleep are common in normal persons.

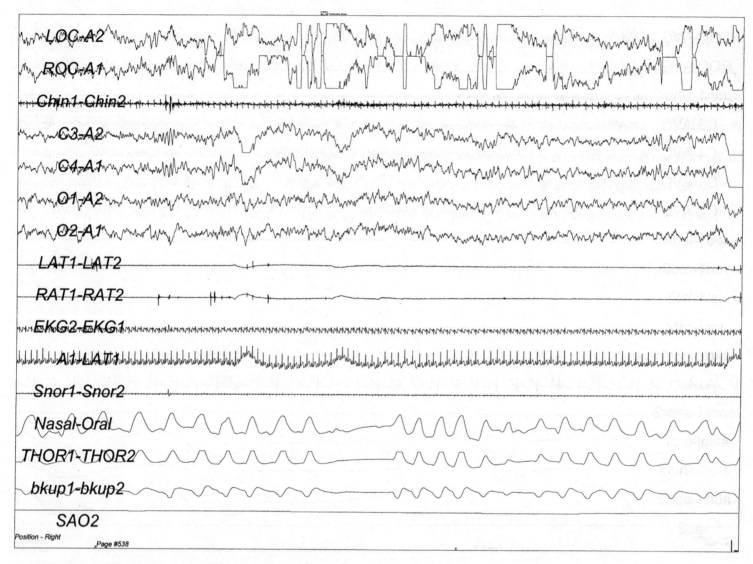

LOC-A2

ROC-A1

Chin1-Chin2

C3-A2

C4-A1

O1-A2

O2-A1

LAT1-LAT2

RAT1-RAT2

EKG2-EKG1

A1-LAT1

Snor1-Snor2

Nasal-Oral

THOR1-THOR2

bkup1-bkup2

SAO2

Position - Right

Page #538

FIGURE 4-46   **Polysomnogram: Standard montage (prior recording/display montage); 120 second page.**
Clinical: 46-year-old woman with excessive daytime sleepiness.
Staging: Stage R sleep.
Respiratory: Central apnea with no associated arousal or oxygen desaturation. Brief central apneas are common during REM sleep in normal individuals.

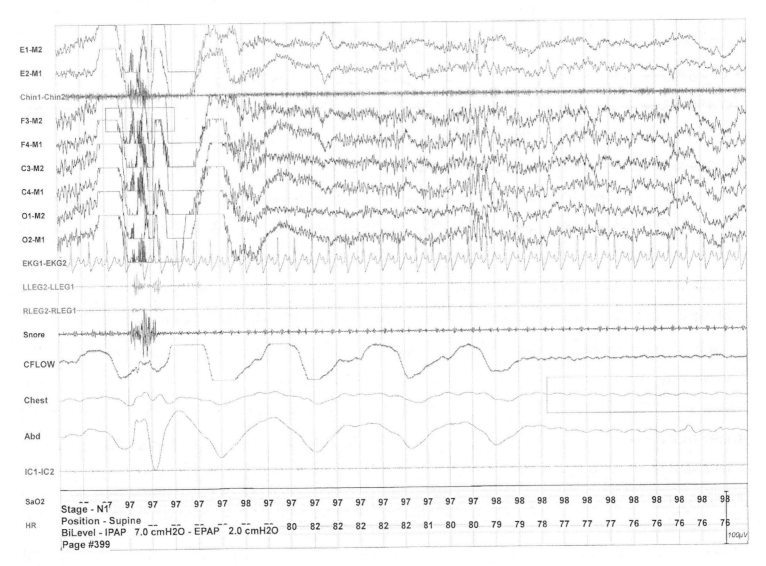

FIGURE 4-47   **Polysomnogram: CPAP monitoring; 30 second page.**

Clinical: 38-year-old man with obstructive sleep apnea.

Staging: Stage N1 sleep.

Respiratory: Sleep onset central apnea followed by an arousal on the following page. (Copyright JNP Enterprises, 2017.)

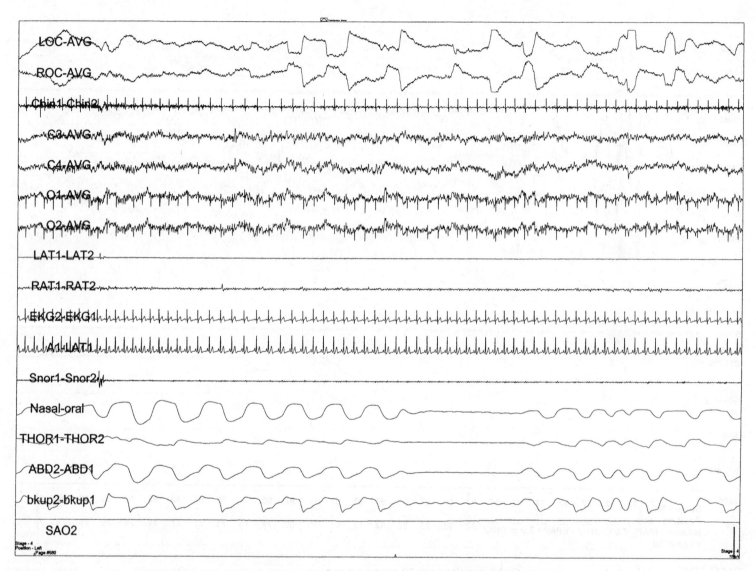

FIGURE 4-48   **Polysomnogram: Standard montage (prior recording/display montage); 60 second page.**
Clinical: 51-year-old man with snoring and witnessed apneas.
Staging: Stage R sleep.
Respiratory: Central apnea during phasic REM sleep without associated arousal or oxygen desaturation.
Brief central apneas are common during REM sleep in normal individuals.

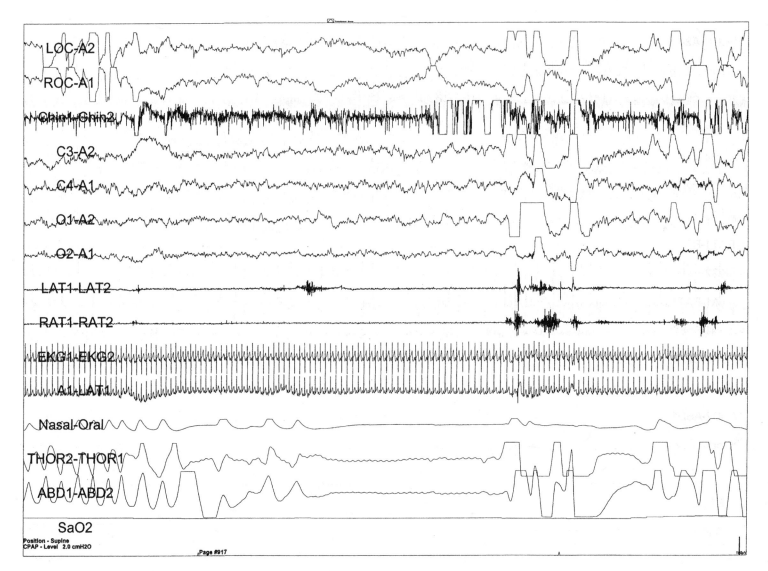

FIGURE 4-49 **Polysomnogram: Standard montage (prior recording/display montage); 60 second page.**
Clinical: 5-week-old infant girl with frequent witnessed apneas.
Staging: Stage R sleep with an arousal.
Respiratory: Central apnea followed by an arousal.

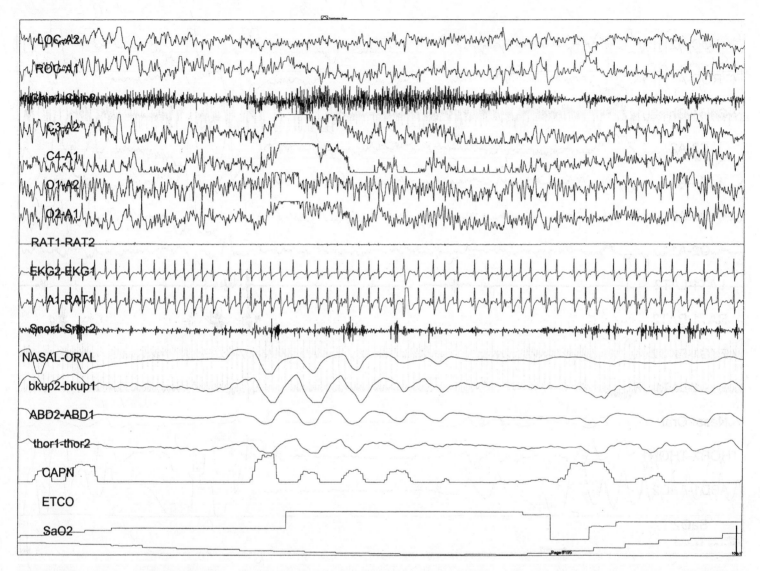

FIGURE 4-50   **Polysomnogram: Standard montage with CO$_2$ monitoring (prior recording/display montage); 60 second page.**

Clinical: 52-year-old obese man with witnessed apneas.

Staging: Stage N2 sleep with arousals.

Respiratory: Central apnea. The capnogram indicates that CO$_2$ is highest with the first breath following the apnea and then rapidly returns to normal (60 to 41 torr).

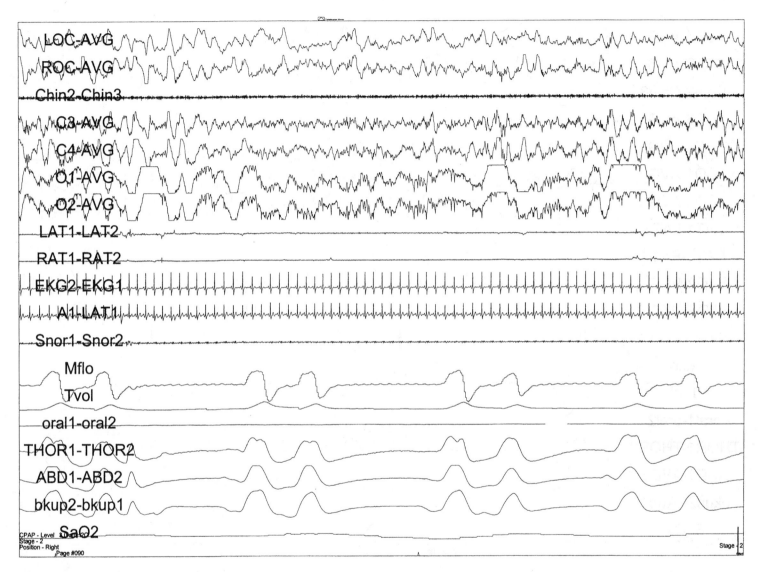

FIGURE 4-51   **Polysomnogram: CPAP montage (prior recording/display montage); 60 second page.**

Clinical: 55-year-old man with snoring and frequent pauses in breathing.

Staging: Stage N2 sleep.

Respiratory: Periodic breathing with two normal breaths followed by a central apnea. The central apneas are followed by oxygen desaturations from 95% to 88%.

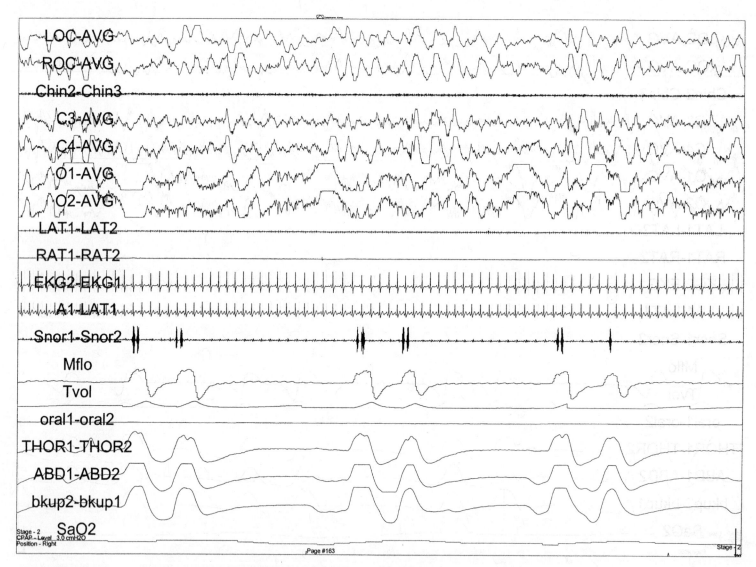

FIGURE 4-52 **Polysomnogram: CPAP montage (prior recording/display montage); 60 second page.**

Clinical: 55-year-old man with snoring and frequent pauses in breathing.

Staging: Stage N2 sleep.

Respiratory: Periodic breathing consisting of 2 normal breaths with snoring followed by a central apnea. The central apneas are followed by oxygen desaturations from 95% to 88%.

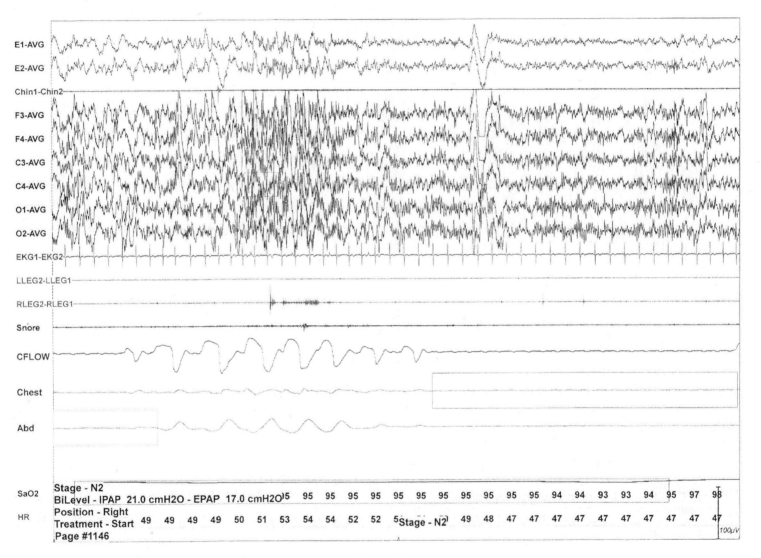

FIGURE 4-53   **Polysomnogram: CPAP montage; 60 second page.**
Clinical: 59-year-old man with congestive heart failure and excessive daytime sleepiness.
Staging: Stage N2 sleep with an arousal at maximum effort.
Respiratory: Central apnea and Cheyne-Stokes respirations with an EEG arousal occurring at the apex of the respiratory cycle. (Copyright JNP Enterprises, 2017.)

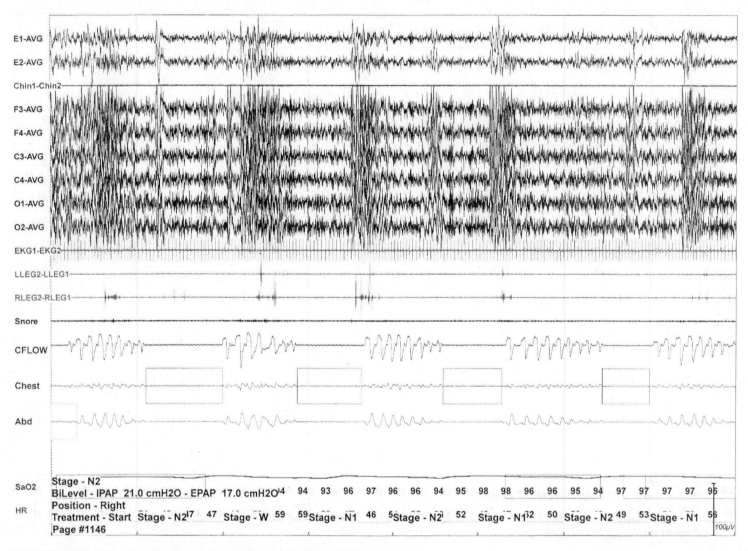

FIGURE 4-54 **Polysomnogram: CPAP montage; 240 second page.**
Clinical: 59-year-old man with congestive heart failure and excessive daytime sleepiness.
Staging: Stage N2 and N1 sleep with arousals.
Respiratory: Central apnea and Cheyne-Stokes respirations with an EEG arousal occurring both at the
onset of the respiratory cycle and at the apex of the respiratory cycle. (Copyright JNP Enterprises, 2017.)

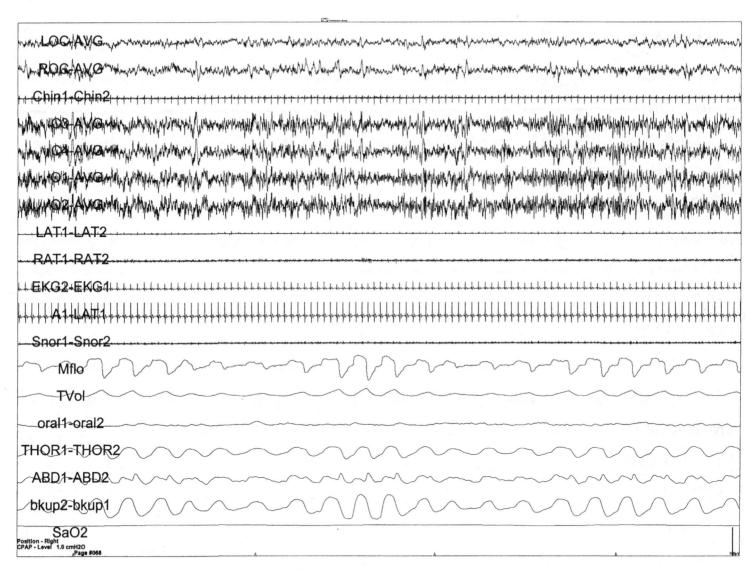

FIGURE 4-55 **Polysomnogram: CPAP montage (prior recording/display montage); 120 second page.**
Clinical: 64-year-old woman with a recent myocardial infarction and excessive daytime sleepiness.
Staging: Stage R sleep.
Respiratory: Cyclic variation in respiratory effort and airflow without arousals or oxygen desaturations.
Patients with Cheyne-Stokes respirations and central apneas in NREM sleep may show this pattern in
REM sleep and wakefulness.

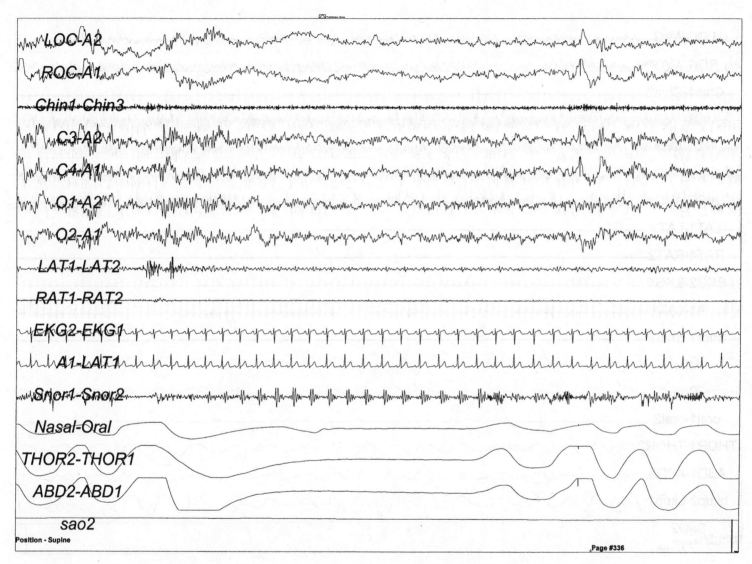

FIGURE 4-56 **Polysomnogram: Standard montage (prior recording/display montage); 30 second page.**
Clinical: 44-year-old man with recent weight gain and excessive daytime sleepiness.
Staging: Stage N1 sleep.
Respiratory: Postarousal central apnea.

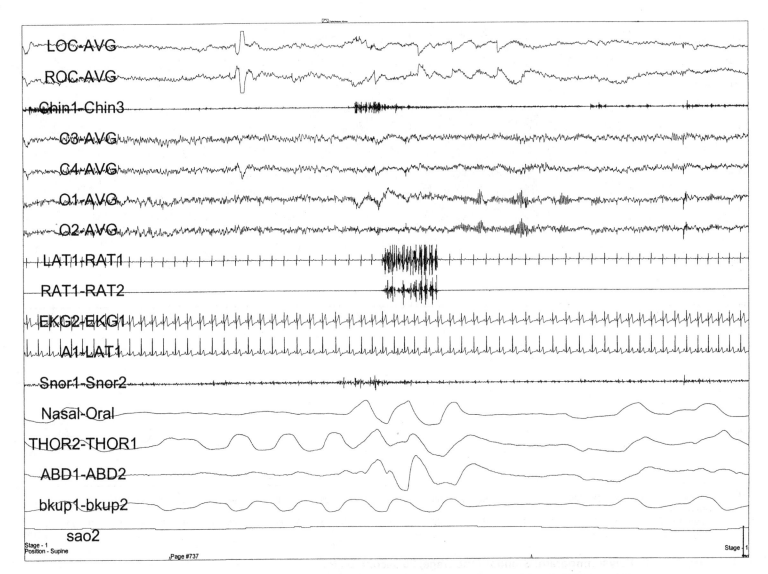

LOC-AVG

ROC-AVG

Chin1-Chin3

C3-AVG

C4-AVG

O1-AVG

O2-AVG

LAT1-RAT1

RAT1-RAT2

EKG2-EKG1

A1-LAT1

Snor1-Snor2

Nasal-Oral

THOR2-THOR1

ABD1-ABD2

bkup1-bkup2

sao2

Stage - 1
Position - Supine

Page #737

Stage - 1

FIGURE 4-57   **Polysomnogram: Standard montage (prior recording/display montage); 60 second page.**
Clinical: 44-year-old man with recent weight gain and excessive daytime sleepiness.
Staging: Stage R with an arousal.
Respiratory: Obstructive apnea followed by an arousal and then a postarousal central apnea. The oxygen desaturation at the beginning of this page is a result of an apnea from the preceding page of the record.

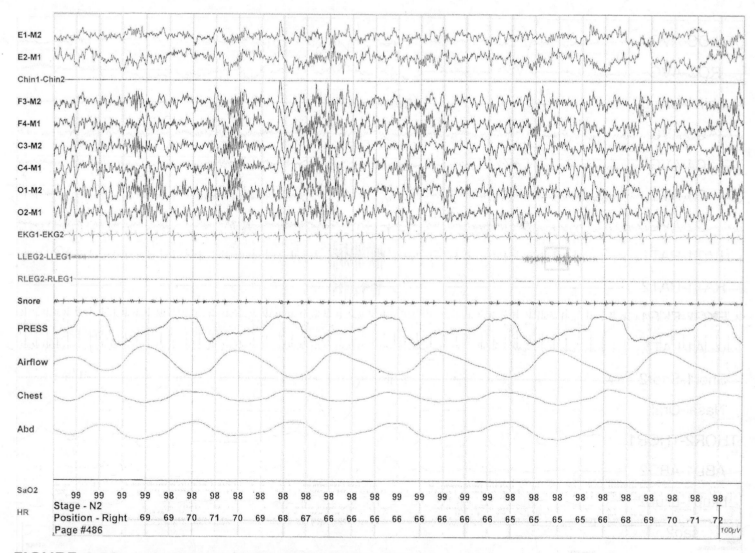

FIGURE 4-58   **Polysomnogram: Standard montage; 30 second page.**
Clinical: 55-year-old man with disturbed, unrefreshing sleep.
Staging: Stage N2 sleep.
Respiratory: Normal respirations. (Copyright JNP Enterprises, 2017.)

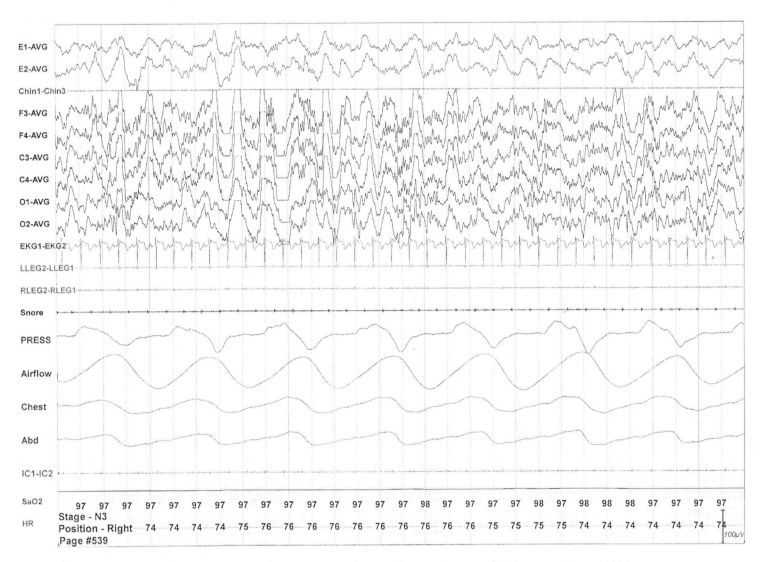

FIGURE 4-59 **Polysomnogram: Standard montage; 30 second page.**
Clinical: 24-year-old man with severe fatigue.
Staging: Stage N3 sleep.
Respiratory: Normal respirations. (Copyright JNP Enterprises, 2017.)

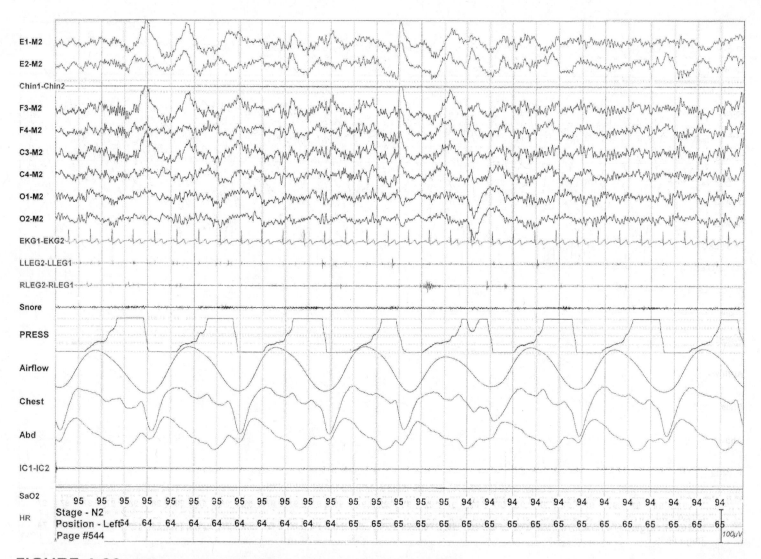

FIGURE 4-60   **Polysomnogram: Standard montage; 30 second page.**
Clinical: 40-year-old man with headaches upon awakening.
Staging: Stage N2 sleep.
Respiratory: Normal respirations. There is clipping of the pressure transducer signal, which could obscure mild respiratory events. (Copyright JNP Enterprises, 2017.)

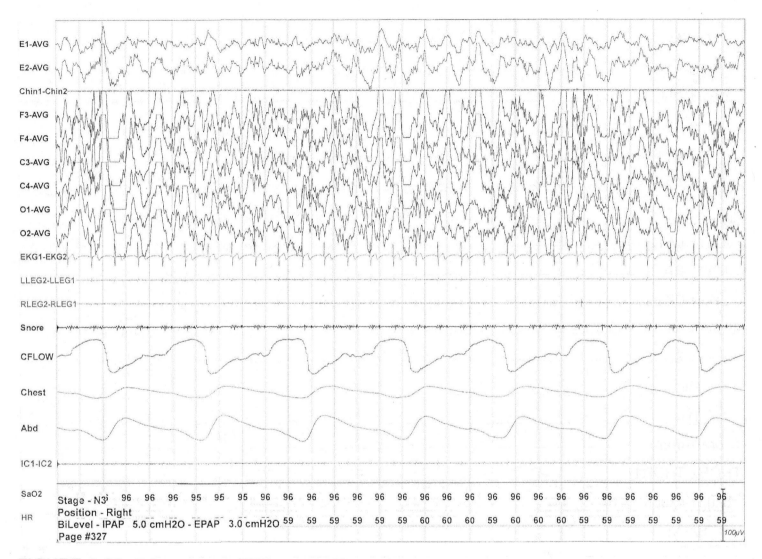

FIGURE 4-61   **Polysomnogram: CPAP montage; 30 second page.**
Clinical: 66-year-old man with obstructive sleep apnea.
Staging: Stage N3 sleep.
Respiratory: Normal respirations. (Copyright JNP Enterprises, 2017.)

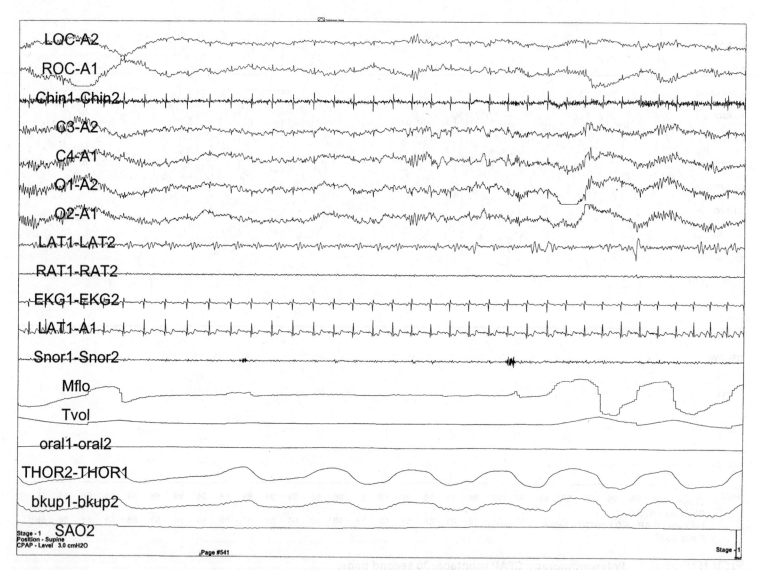

Stage - 1
Position - Supine
CPAP - Level 3.0 cmH2O

Page #541

Stage - 1

FIGURE 4-62 **Polysomnogram: CPAP montage (prior recording/display montage); 30 second page.**
Clinical: 42-year-old woman with obstructive sleep apnea.
Staging: Stage N1 sleep with an arousal.
Respiratory: Obstructive apnea followed by a snort and an arousal. The oxygen desaturation at the beginning of this page was caused by an apnea from the preceding page of the record. Nasal CPAP was set at 7 cm of water for this portion of the recording. Obstructive apneas were eliminated with higher levels of CPAP.

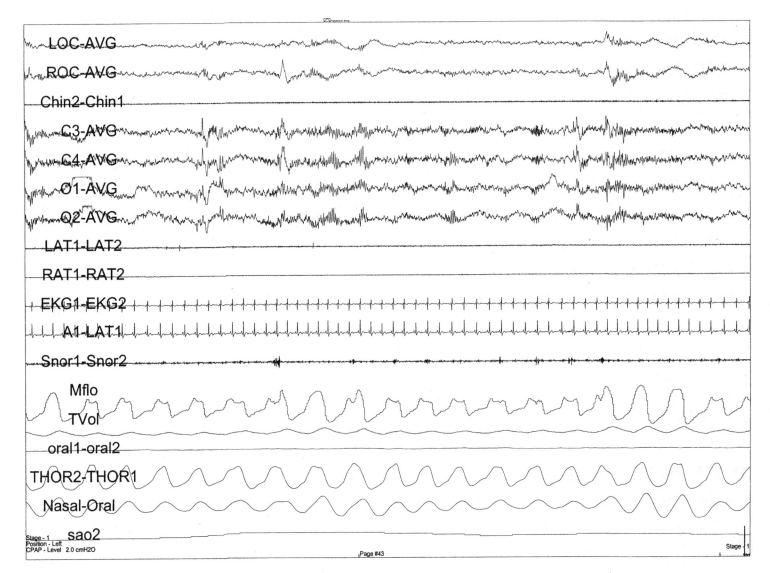

FIGURE 4-63   **Polysomnogram: CPAP montage (prior recording/display montage); 60 second page.**

Clinical: 53-year-old man with obstructive sleep apnea.

Staging: Stage N1 sleep with arousals.

Respiratory: Two hypopneas are followed by snorts, arousals, and oxygen desaturations. Hypopneas resolved at higher levels of CPAP. The oxygen desaturation at the beginning of this page was caused by an apnea from the preceding page of the record.

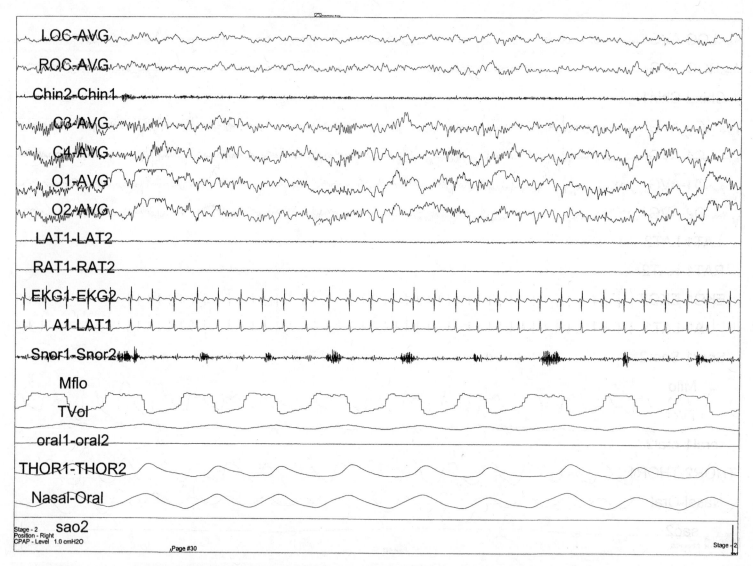

FIGURE 4-64   **Polysomnogram: CPAP montage (prior recording/display montage); 30 second page.**
Clinical: 28-year-old man with obstructive sleep apnea.
Staging: Stage N2 sleep.
Respiratory: Snoring with no associated hypopneas or apneas with CPAP at 5 cm of water. The snoring resolved with higher levels of CPAP.

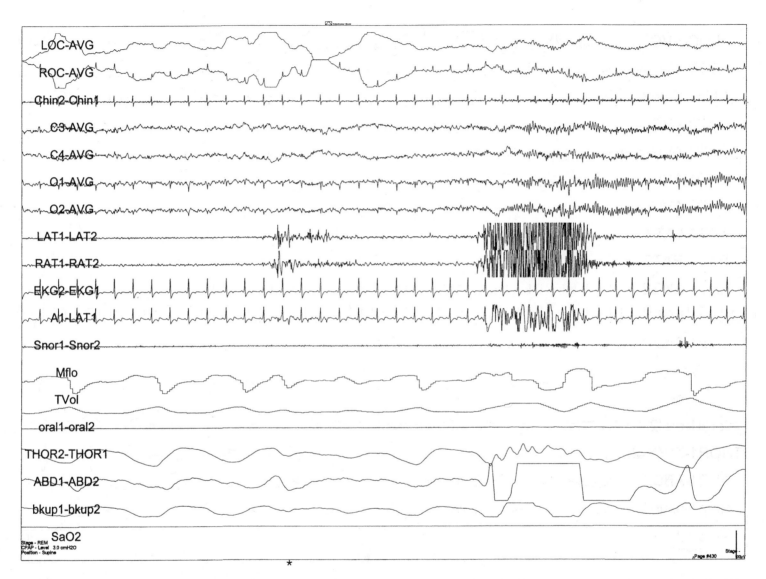

FIGURE 4-65   **Polysomnogram: CPAP montage (prior recording/display montage); 60 second page.**
Clinical: 28-year-old man with obstructive sleep apnea.
Staging: Stage R sleep with an arousal.
Respiratory: Hypopnea followed by an arousal and movement. The beginning of the hypopnea is marked (*).

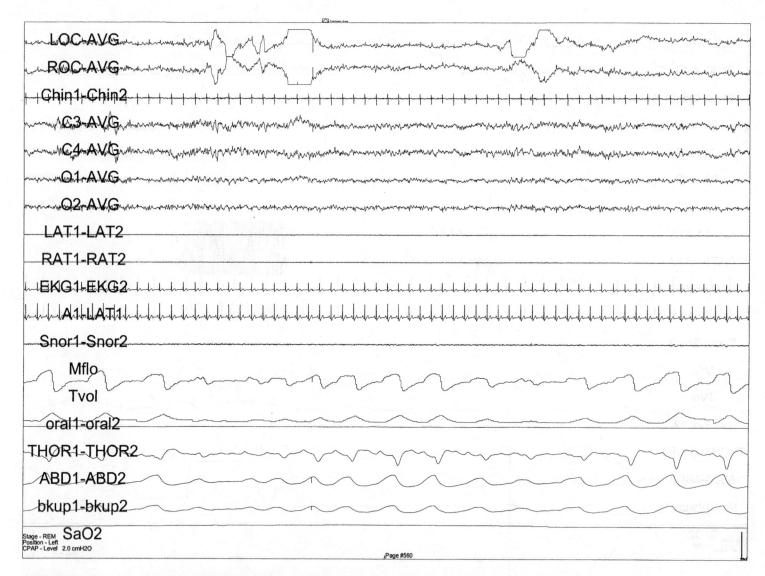

LOC-AVG

ROC-AVG

Chin1-Chin2

C3-AVG

C4-AVG

O1-AVG

O2-AVG

LAT1-LAT2

RAT1-RAT2

EKG1-EKG2

A1-LAT1

Snor1-Snor2

Mflo

Tvol

oral1-oral2

THOR1-THOR2

ABD1-ABD2

bkup1-bkup2

Stage - REM
Position - Left
CPAP - Level 2.0 cmH2O

SaO2

Page #560

FIGURE 4-66   **Polysomnogram: CPAP montage (prior recording/display montage); 60 second page.**
Clinical: 35-year-old man with obstructive sleep apnea.
Staging: Stage R sleep.
Respiratory: Decreased respiratory effort and airflow without an arousal or an oxygen desaturation during phasic REM sleep. Brief reductions in ventilation often accompany phasic REM sleep in normal persons.

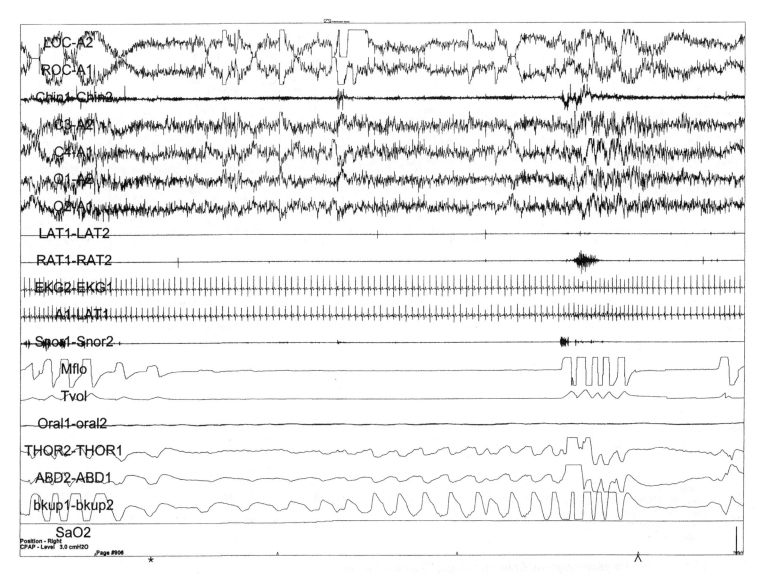

FIGURE 4-67 **Polysomnogram: CPAP montage (prior recording/display montage); 120 second page.**
Clinical: 49-year-old morbidly obese man with obstructive sleep apnea and poorly controlled hypertension.
Staging: Stage R sleep.
Respiratory: Prolonged obstructive apnea (*) followed by an arousal, a snort, right leg movement, and a brief postarousal central apnea (^).

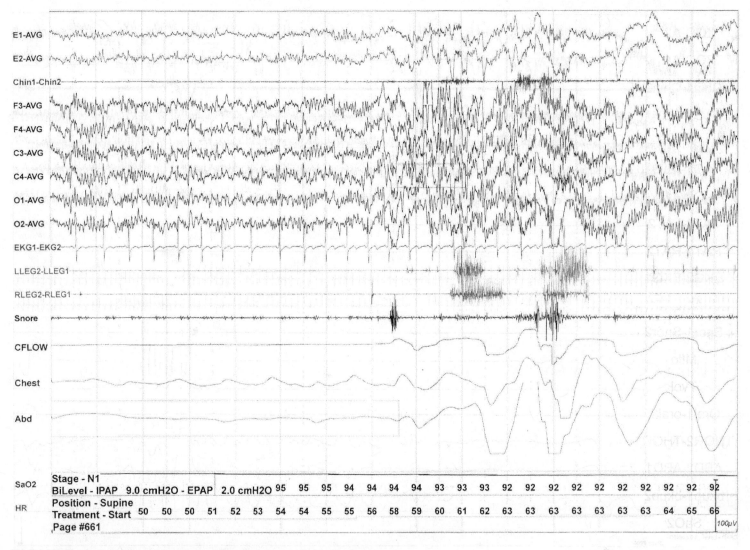

FIGURE 4-68 **Polysomnogram: CPAP montage; 30 second page.**
Clinical: 53-year-old thin woman with obstructive sleep apnea.
Staging: Stage N1 sleep with an arousal.
Respiratory: Central apnea with an associated arousal and oxygen desaturation. Cardioballistic artifact is present in the chest effort channel. (Copyright JNP Enterprises, 2017.)

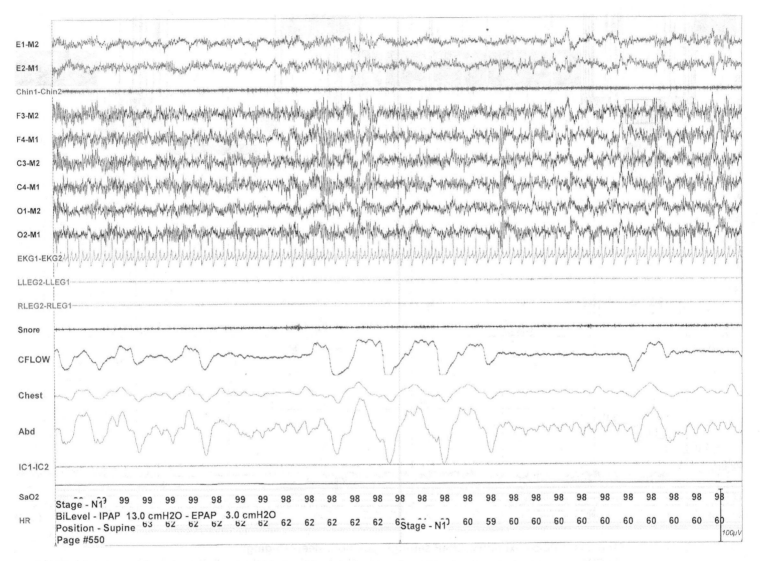

FIGURE 4-69 **Polysomnogram: CPAP montage; 60 second page.**

Clinical: 58-year-old man with obstructive sleep apnea.

Staging: Stage N1 sleep.

Respiratory: Central apneas with no associated oxygen desaturation. Cardioballistic artifact is present in the chest and abdominal effort channels. (Copyright JNP Enterprises, 2017.)

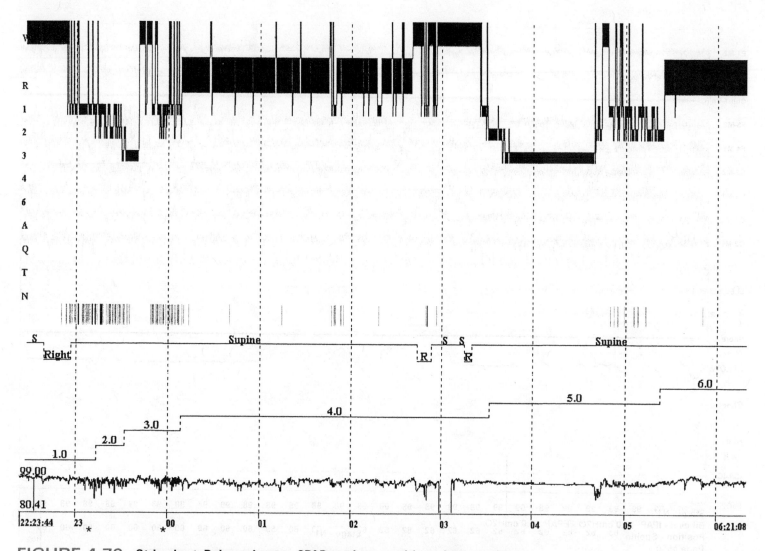

FIGURE 4-70   **Strip chart: Pulse oximetry, CPAP settings, position, sleep staging.**
Six CPAP settings were used during the study. The first three settings (5, 7, and 9 cm) were inadequate and apneas continued to occur (*). At the fourth CPAP setting (11 cm), apneas became much less frequent, and there was marked REM sleep rebound (increased amounts of REM sleep).

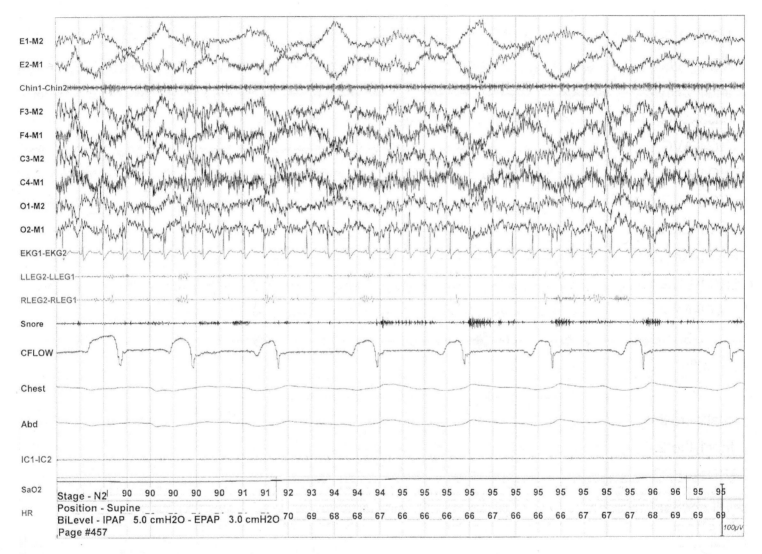

| | Stage - N2 | 90 | 90 | 90 | 90 | 90 | 91 | 91 | 92 | 93 | 94 | 94 | 94 | 95 | 95 | 95 | 95 | 95 | 95 | 95 | 95 | 95 | 95 | 95 | 96 | 96 | 95 | 95 |

Position - Supine
BiLevel - IPAP 5.0 cmH2O - EPAP 3.0 cmH2O
Page #457

HR: 70 69 68 68 67 66 66 66 66 67 66 66 66 67 67 67 68 69 69 69

SaO2

100µV

FIGURE 4-71 **Polysomnogram: CPAP montage; 30 second page.**
Clinical: 65-year-old man with obstructive sleep apnea and continued excessive daytime sleepiness despite nasal CPAP.
Staging: Stage N2 sleep.
Respiratory: CPAP mask leak seen as a sharp dip below the baseline at the end of breaths on the mask flow channel. (Copyright JNP Enterprises, 2017.)

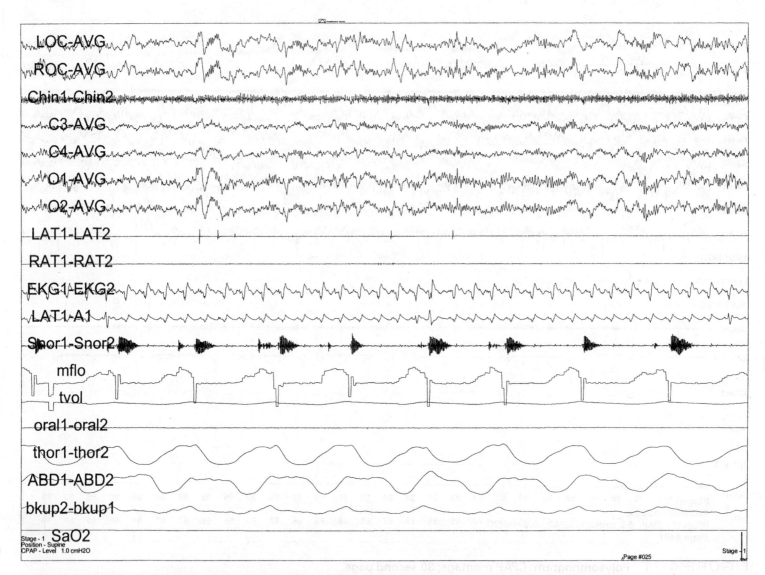

FIGURE 4-72 **Polysomnogram: CPAP montage (prior recording/display montage); 30 second page.**
Clinical: 27-year-old man with obstructive sleep apnea.
Staging: Stage N1 sleep.
Respiratory: CPAP mask leak seen as a sharp dip below the baseline at the end of breaths on the mask flow channel. Lip quiver recorded in the snore channel coincides with the mask leak.

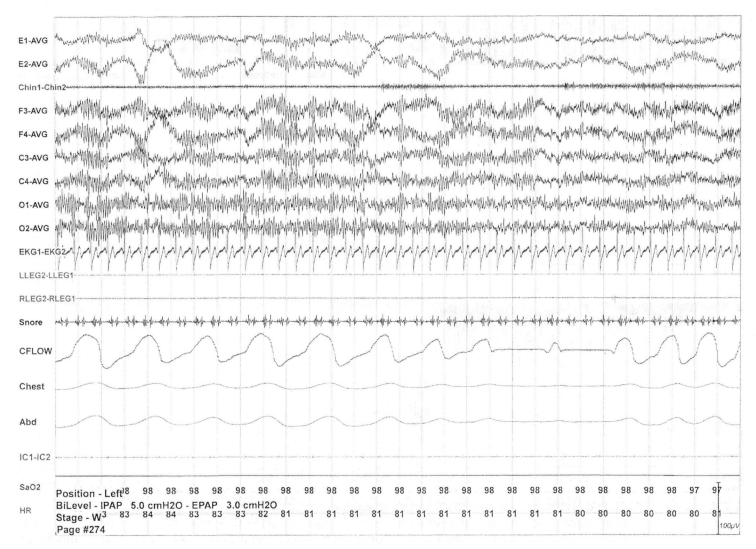

FIGURE 4-73   **Polysomnogram: CPAP montage; 30 second page.**

Clinical: 27-year-old man with obstructive sleep apnea.

Staging: Stage W.

Respiratory: There is a brief breath hold during wakefulness. (Copyright JNP Enterprises, 2017.)

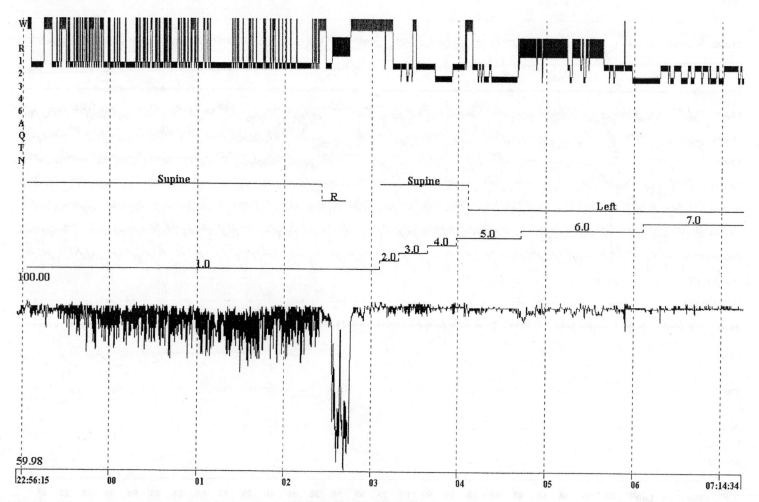

FIGURE 4-74   **Strip chart: Pulse oximetry, CPAP settings, position.**
Obstructive sleep apnea with severe oxygen desaturations during REM sleep. The initial half of the night (labeled CPAP setting 1.0) is the baseline portion of the recording with no CPAP. When CPAP is applied, at six different settings, ranging from 5 cm of water (setting 2.0) to 15 cm of water (setting 7.0), apneas and associated hypoxemia were almost completely eliminated.

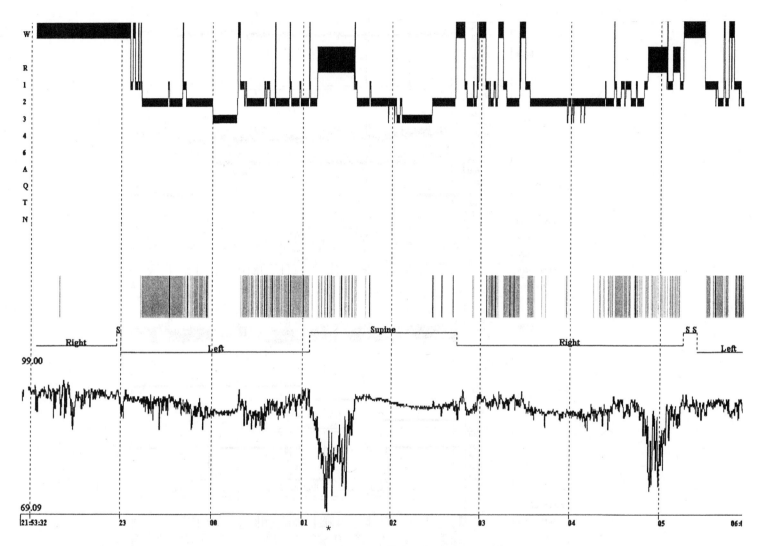

FIGURE 4-75 **Strip chart: Pulse oximetry, CPAP settings, position, sleep staging.**
Prolonged oxygen desaturation during REM sleep (*) in a patient with obesity hypoventilation syndrome. There are also frequent oxygen desaturations caused by obstructive sleep apnea.

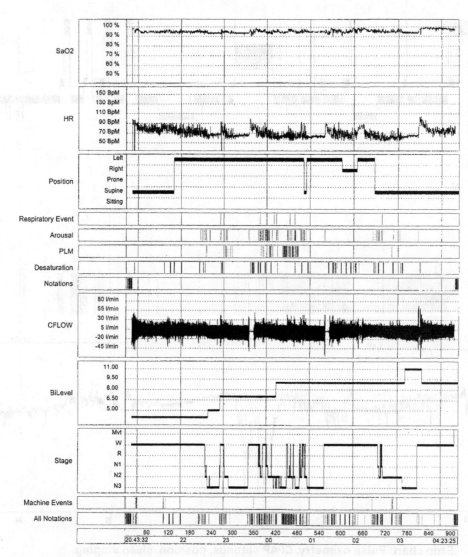

FIGURE 4-76   **Strip chart: Pulse oximetry, PAP settings, position, sleep staging.**
PAP titration in a patient with obstructive sleep apnea.

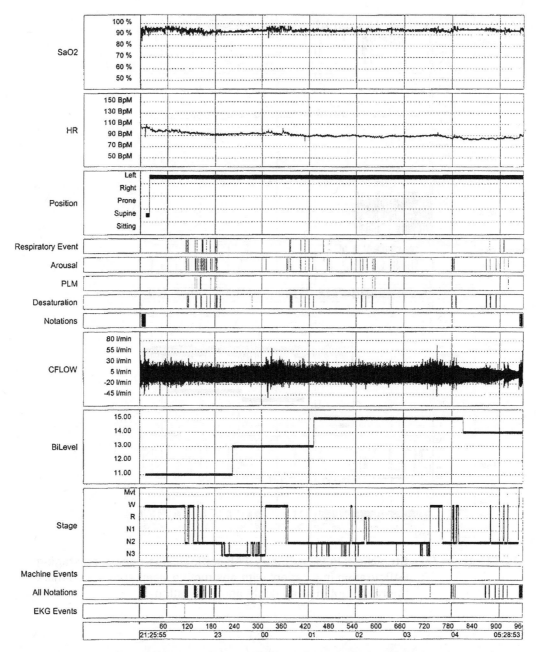

FIGURE 4-77   **Strip chart: Pulse oximetry, PAP settings, position, sleep staging.**
PAP titration in a patient with obstructive sleep apnea.

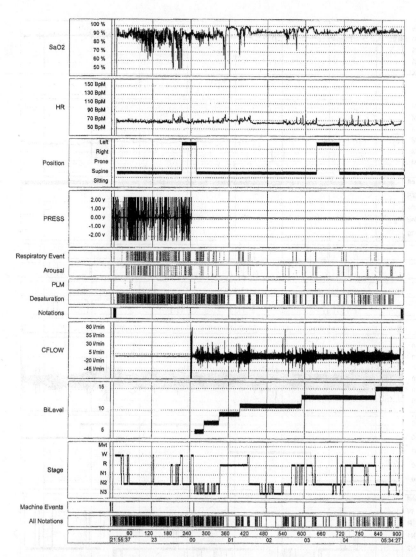

FIGURE 4-78   Strip chart: Pulse oximetry, PAP settings, position, sleep staging. PAP titration in a patient with obstructive sleep apnea with marked improvement in sleep depth and respirations.

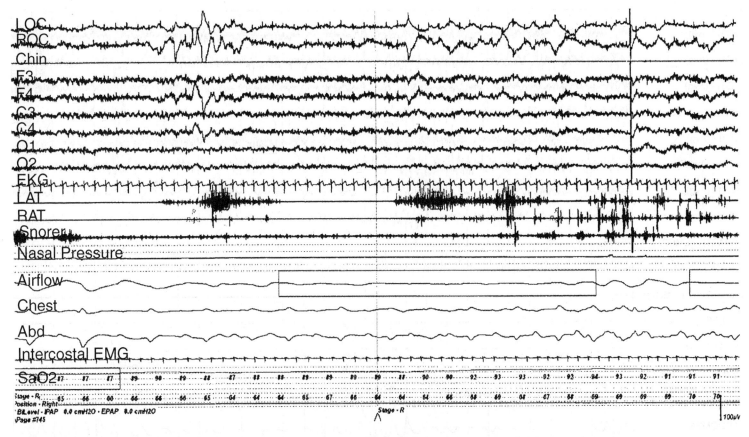

FIGURE 4-79   **Polysomnogram: CPAP montage (prior recording/display montage); 30 second page.**
Clinical: 37-year-old man with obstructive sleep apnea.
Staging: Stage R.
Respiratory: Apnea primarily during phasic REM sleep.

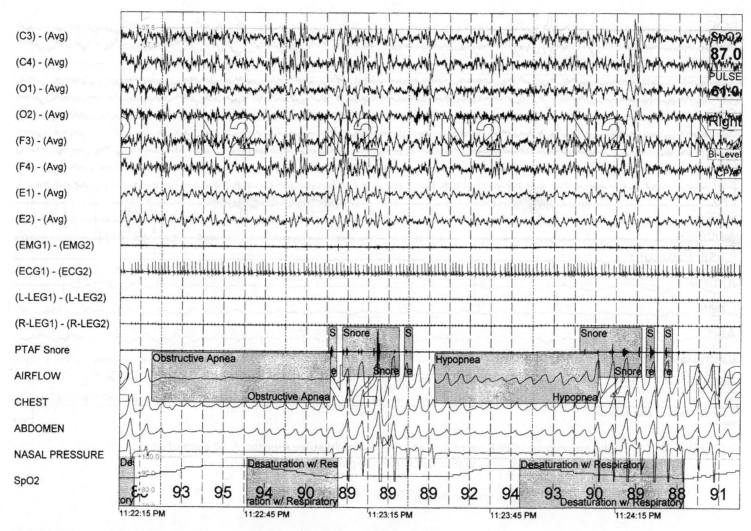

FIGURE 4-80   **Polysomnogram: Standard montage; 120 second page.**
Clinical: 39-year-old man with witnessed apneas and a recent myocardial infarction.
Staging: Stage 2 sleep.
Respiratory: Apneas and hypopneas are seen in this recording made with RIP recording.
Obstructive apnea: There is a drop in the peak thermal sensor excursion by ≥90% of the baseline. The event last at least 10 seconds. At least 90% of the event's duration meets the amplitude reduction criteria for apnea. There is continued or increased effort throughout the entire period of absent airflow. (From The AASM Manual for Scoring Sleep, 2007.)

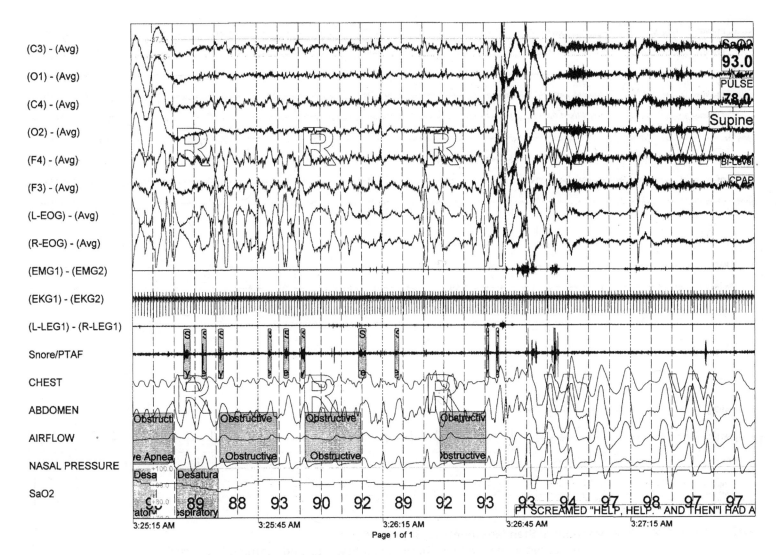

FIGURE 4-81   **Polysomnogram: Standard montage; 150 second page.**

Clinical: 53-year-old female with bad dreams, most in the last half of the night, usually of being smothered or held down. Snoring.

Staging: Stage R.

Respiratory: Obstructive apneas are seen in this recording made with RIP recording. The patient screamed "Help, Help." She then said "I had a terrible dream" and sat up in bed on video monitoring.

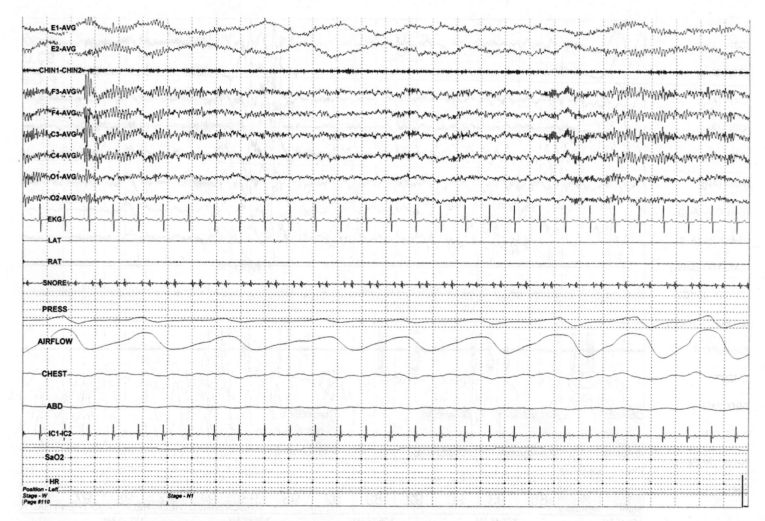

FIGURE 4-82   **Polysomnogram: Standard montage; 30 second page.**

Clinical: 41-year-old man with loud snoring, night sweats, and morning headaches.

Staging: Stage N2 sleep.

Respiratory: The hypopnea is scored by the alternative method.

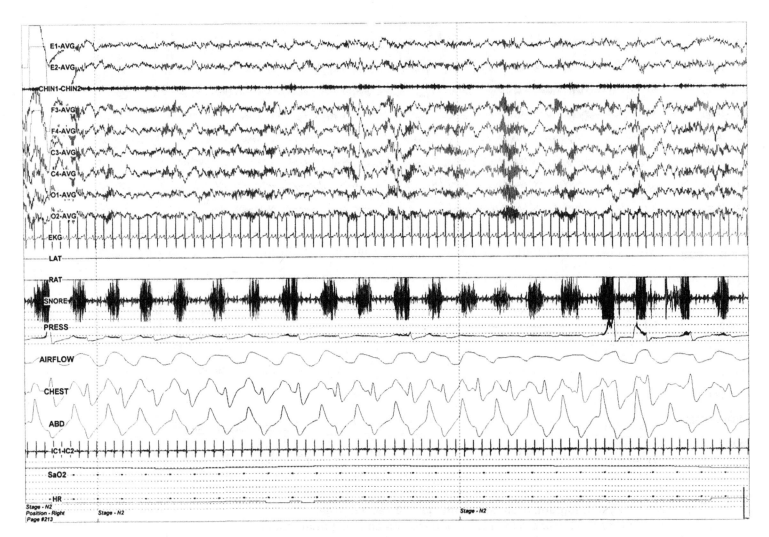

FIGURE 4-83 **Polysomnogram: Standard montage; 30 second page.**

Clinical: 41-year-old man with loud snoring, night sweats, and morning headaches.

Staging: Stage N2 sleep.

Respiratory: The hypopnea is scored by the standard method.

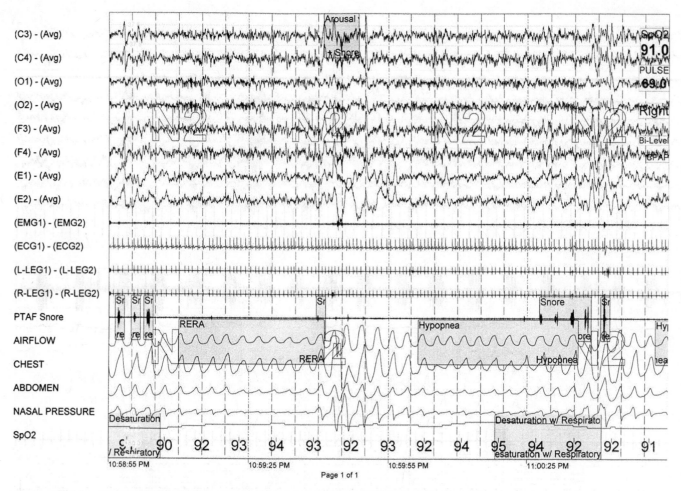

FIGURE 4-84   Polysomnogram: Standard montage; 120 second page.

Clinical: 52-year-old man with loud snoring and nocturnal reflux.

Staging: Stage N2 sleep.

Respiratory: RERA—there is a sequence of breaths lasting at least 10 seconds characterized by increasing respiratory effort or flattening of the nasal pressure waveform leading to an arousal from sleep when the sequence of breaths does not meet criteria for an apnea or hypopnea. (From The ASM Manual for Scoring Sleep, 2007.) In this example, there is no ≥4% desaturation, and therefore, it cannot be a hypopnea. Hypopnea—the nasal pressure signal excursion drops by ≥30% of baseline. The duration of this drop occurs for a period lasting at least 10 seconds. There is a ≥4% desaturation form pre-event baseline. At least 90% of the event's duration meets the amplitude reduction criteria. (From The AASM Manual for Scoring Sleep, 2007.)

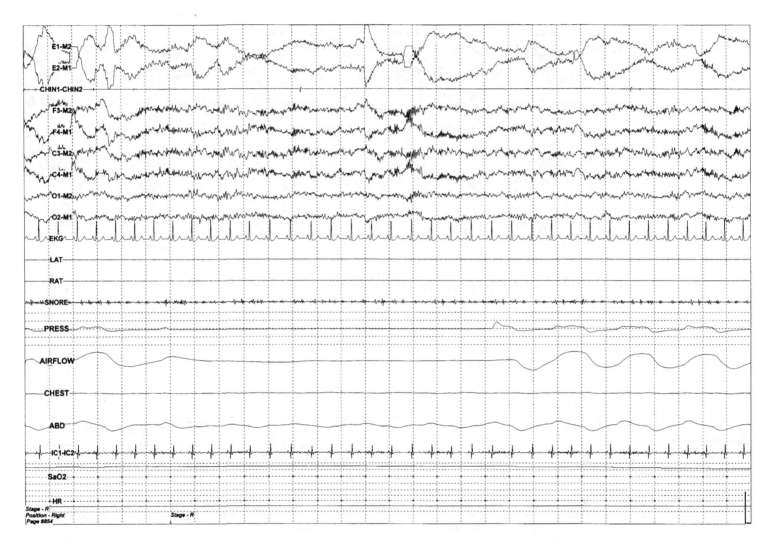

FIGURE 4-85 **Polysomnogram: Standard montage; 120 second page.**
Clinical: 56-year-old woman with fatigue and reported fibromyalgia.
Staging: Stage N2 sleep with an arousal.
Respiratory: Respiratory event related arousal.

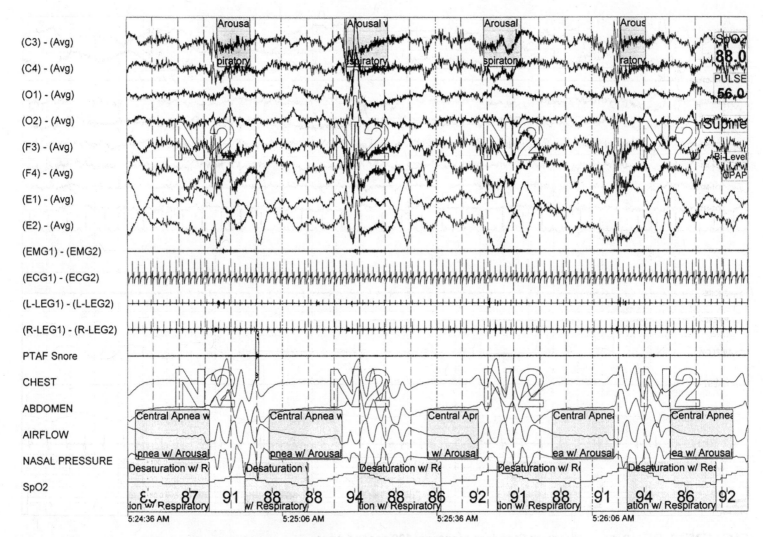

FIGURE 4-86 **Polysomnogram: Standard montage; 120 second page.**
Clinical: 68-year-old man with poor sleep and heart failure.
Staging: Stage N2 sleep with arousals.
Respiratory: Periodic central apneas with oxygen desaturations.

TABLE 4-1 Sample Report: Obstructive Sleep Apnea

Patient:
Account Number:
Medical Records:
Study Number:
Date of Study:
Date of Birth:
Requesting Physician:
Referring Physician:
Indications for Study: Sleep disturbance with hypersomnolence (780.54)
Study Description: Polysomnogram
Equipment: Central, frontal, and occipital EEG, EOG, EKG, submentalis EMG, intercostal EMG, airflow, thoracic motion, abdominal motion, snore sensor, anterior tibialis EMG, and pulse oximetry were recorded throughout the study. The tracing was recorded in 30-second epochs.

Sleep Study Summary Report:
Record time: 485.5 minutes; sleep time: 423.5 minutes
Analysis—see detailed analysis tables
EEG/Sleep stage

Stage N1 sleep: 15.7% (4%–8%)	Sleep latency: 43 minutes
Stage N2 sleep: 65.1% (45%–63%)	REM latency: 130.5 minutes
Stage N3 sleep: 0% (4%–20%)	Sleep efficiency: 87.2%
Stage R sleep: 19.2% (23%–31%)	

Respiratory
  AHI: 9.1 NREM AHI: 4.6 REM AHI: 28 Supine AHI: 9.1
  RERA index: 9.8 (69 RERA)
  Total respiratory events: 64 (63 obstructive)
  Arousal index: 19.7
  Minimum oxygen saturation: 90%
Snoring: loud
EKG: PVCs
Limb movement
  PLM index: 0
  PLM arousal index: 0.8
Impression: Obstructive sleep apnea (327.23)

The findings indicate obstructive sleep apnea consisting apneas and hypopneas with associated arousals and oxygen desaturations, which was most prominent during REM sleep. Obstructive sleep apnea may be related to other medical conditions. Clinical correlation is advised.
    Recommendations: The patient will be scheduled for a follow-up visit along with a CPAP titration.

_____, M.D.

The physician reviewed the record in its entirety, including sleep staging, EMG activity, EKG, EEG, respiration, oxygen saturation, body position, and behavior unless otherwise noted. The interpretation is based on this information in addition to the available clinical history and physical examination. This is a summary report. Please see the additional tabular report from this study for more detailed analysis.

TR:
DD:
DT:

TABLE 4-2 Sample Report: Severe Obstructive Sleep Apnea

Patient:
Account Number:
Medical Records:
Study Number:
Date of Study:
Date of Birth:
Requesting Physician:
Referring Physician:
Indications for Study: Sleep disturbance with hypersomnolence (780.54) and witnessed apneas
Study Description: Polysomnogram
Equipment: Central, frontal, and occipital EEG, EOG, EKG, submentalis EMG, intercostal EMG, airflow, thoracic motion, abdominal motion, snore sensor, anterior tibialis EMG, and pulse oximetry were recorded throughout the study. The tracing was recorded in 30-second epochs.

Sleep Study Summary Report:
Record time: 393.5 minutes; sleep time: 355.5 minutes
Analysis—see detailed analysis tables
EEG/Sleep stage

Stage N1 sleep: 11% (2%–9%)	Sleep latency: 25 minutes
Stage N2 sleep: 78.9% (50%–64%)	REM latency: 264.5 minutes
Stage N3 sleep: 0% (7%–18%)	Sleep efficiency: 90.3%
Stage R sleep: 10.1% (20%–27%)	

Respiratory
　AHI: 35.6　　NREM AHI: 32.1　　REM AHI: 66.7　　Supine AHI: 35.6
　RERA index: 0 (0 RERA)
　Total respiratory events: 211 (211 obstructive)
　Arousal index: 35.3
　Minimum oxygen saturation: 80%
Snoring: moderate
EKG: unremarkable
Limb movement
　PLM index: 0.7
　PLM arousal index: 0.8
Impression: Obstructive sleep apnea (327.23)

The findings indicate severe obstructive sleep apnea consisting of apneas and hypopneas with associated arousals and oxygen desaturations. Obstructive sleep apnea may be related to other medical conditions. Clinical correlation is advised.
　　Recommendations: The patient will be scheduled for a follow-up visit along with a CPAP titration.
　　　　　　　　_____, M.D.

The physician reviewed the record in its entirety, including sleep staging, EMG activity, EKG, EEG, respiration, oxygen saturation, body position, and behavior unless otherwise noted. The interpretation is based on this information in addition to the available clinical history and physical examination. This is a summary report. Please see the additional tabular report from this study for more detailed analysis.
TR:
DD:
DT:

TABLE 4-3 Sample Report: Long Form

Diagnostic Polysomnographic Report

Patient:	Date:
DOB:	PSG Study #:
Age:	Referring Physician: Physician:
Sex:	Account #:
PSG Tech:	Medical Record #:
Scored by:	

Sleep Architecture Summary

Lights Out:	11:12:54 PM	**Lights On:**	05:46:24 AM
Total Record Time:	413.0 minutes	**# REM Episodes:**	1
		# of Awakenings[a]**:**	5

	Time (minutes)	% of TST	% of SPT
Time in Bed (TIB):	393.5		
Total Sleep Time (TST):	355.5	100%	96.5%
Total Stage N1:	39	11.0%	10.6%
Total Stage N2:	280.5	78.9%	76.1%
Total Stage N3:	0	0%	0.0%
Total Stage R:	36	10.1%	9.8%
Total Movement Time:	0		0.0%
Total Wake Time:	38		
WASO:	13.0		
Wake Time During SPT:	13.0		3.5%
Latency to Sleep Onset:	25		
Latency to Persistent Sleep:	25		
Latency to Stage N2:	29.5		
Latency to REM Sleep:	264.5		
Latency to Persistent Sleep:	25		
Sleep Efficiency:	90.3%		
Sleep Maintenance:	96.5%		

[a]Sleep efficiency is time asleep as a percentage of time in bed. Sleep maintenance is time asleep as a percentage of sleep period time. Awakenings are defined as 30 seconds or more.

Positional Summary

	Time (minutes)[a]	%TST
Left:	0	0.0%
Right:	0	0.0%
Supine:	355.5	100.0%
Prone:	0	0.0%

[a]Positional times are given for TST.

Arousal Summary

Arousal Caused By:	Number	Index
Respiratory Events:	173	29.2
Snore:	0	0.0
LM:	5	0.8
Spontaneous:	31	5.2
Bruxism:	0	0.0
Other:	0	0.0
Total:	209	35.3

Respiratory Events Summary

Oxygen Saturation Summary

	Wake	NREM	REM	Total Record
Total O$_2$ Desaturations:	13	108	28	149
O$_2$ Desaturation Index:	20.5	20.3	46.7	22.7
Average O$_2$ Saturation (%)	96.4	94.8	92.9	94.8
Min O$_2$ Saturation (%)	88	86	80	80
Max O$_2$ Saturation (%)	99	99	98	99
Time @ 90%–100% (minutes)	36.7	315.2	28.6	380.5
Time @ 80%–89% (minutes)	1.3	4.1	7.4	12.8
Time @ 70%–79% (minutes)	0.0	0.0	0.0	0.0
Time @ 60%–69% (minutes)	0.0	0.0	0.0	0.0
Time @ 50%–59% (minutes)	0.0	0.0	0.0	0.0
Time ≤ 88% (minutes)	0.6	1.8	4.9	7.3

SaO$_2$ < 90% for 3.3% of the total sleep time.

Respiratory Event Durations

	Average (seconds)	Maximum (seconds)
Apnea (NREM):	15.2	21.5
Hypopnea (NREM):	17.7	31.9
RERA (NREM):	0	0
Apnea (REM):	13.0	20.6
Hypopnea (REM):	14.4	28.0
RERA (REM):	0	0

Number of Respiratory Events—Position and Sleep Stage

	NREM		REM		
	Nonsupine	Supine	Nonsupine	Supine	Total
Obstructive Apnea:	0	33	0	21	54
Mixed Apnea:	0	0	0	0	0
Central Apnea:	0	0	0	0	0
All Apneas:	0	33	0	21	54
Hypopneas:	0	138	0	19	157
Apneas + Hypopneas:	0	171	0	40	211
RERA:	0	0	0	0	0
A/H INDEX:	0	32.1	0	66.7	35.6
RDI:	0	32.1	0	66.7	35.6
Sleep Time (minutes):	319.5	36	0	355.5	355.5
Obstructive Apnea:	33	21	0	54	54
Mixed Apnea:	0	0	0	0	0
Central Apnea:	0	0	0	0	0
All Apneas:	33	21	0	54	54
Hypopneas:	138	19	0	157	157
Apneas + Hypopneas:	171	40	0	211	211
RERA:	0	0	0	0	0
Apnea Index:	6.2	35	0	9.1	9.1
Hypopnea Index:	25.9	31.7	0	26.5	26.5
A/H INDEX:	32.1	66.7	0	35.6	35.6
RDI[a]:	32.1	66.7	0	35.6	35.6

[a]RDI denotes the average number of all respiratory events (Apnea + Hypopnea + RERA) per hour of sleep.

Positional RDI

Left:	0
Right:	0
Prone:	0
Supine:	35.6

Other Respiratory Patterns

	Yes	No
Cheyne-Stokes:	☐	☐
Hypoventilation:	☐	☐

Hypopnea Rule Used: Alternative

Limb Movements Summary

	Number	Index[a]
LM Arousals:	5	0.8
Isolated Limb Movements:	2	0.3
Periodic Limb Movements:	4	0.7
Total Limb Movements:	6	1.0

[a]Index is number per hour of sleep.

Heart Rate Summary

	Wake	NREM	REM	Total
Average Heart Rate (bpm)	69	69	70	69
Minimum Heart Rate (bpm)	58	55	55	55
Maximum Heart Rate (bpm)	91	91	90	91

Cardiac Events:

Occurrence of the Following Arrhythmias was Observed:

			BPM
Bradycardia:	N/A	**Lowest heart rate observed:**	55
Asystole:	N/A	**Longest pause observed:**	
Sinus Tachycardia During Sleep:	N/A		
Narrow Complex Tachycardia:	N/A	**Highest heart rate observed:**	91
Wide Complex Tachycardia:	N/A		
Atrial Fibrillation:	N/A		
Other Arrhythmias Observed:			

Technologist Comment Section

Highest heart rate: 91 bpm, during wake time. Lowest heart rate: 55 bpm. No pauses observed.

Limb Movement Disorders

James D. Geyer, MD and Paul R. Carney, MD

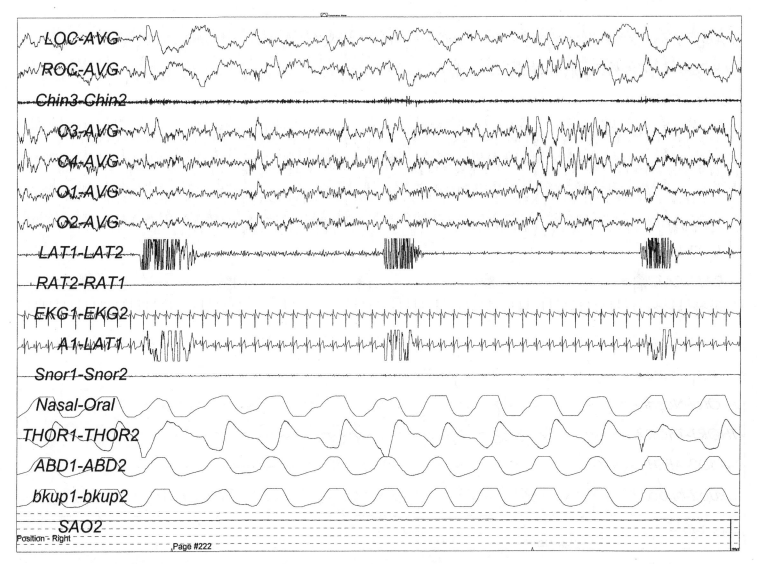

FIGURE 5-1   Polysomnogram: Standard montage (prior display montage); 60 second page.
Clinical: 58-year-old woman with a low back injury and frequent nocturnal leg movements.
Staging: Stage 1 sleep.
EMG: Unilateral (left) periodic leg movements.

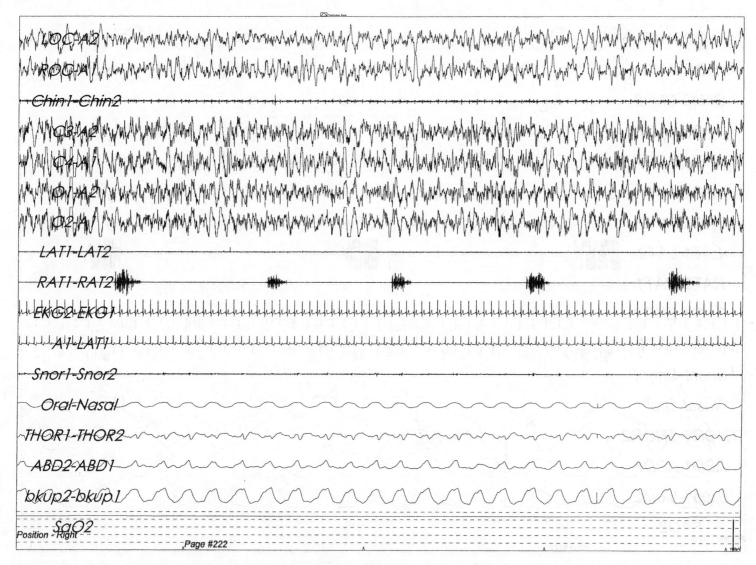

FIGURE 5-2   **Polysomnogram: Standard montage (prior display montage); 60 second page.**
Clinical: 40-year-old woman with restless legs syndrome and a right lumbar radiculopathy.
Staging: Stage 3 sleep.
EMG: Unilateral (right) periodic leg movements.

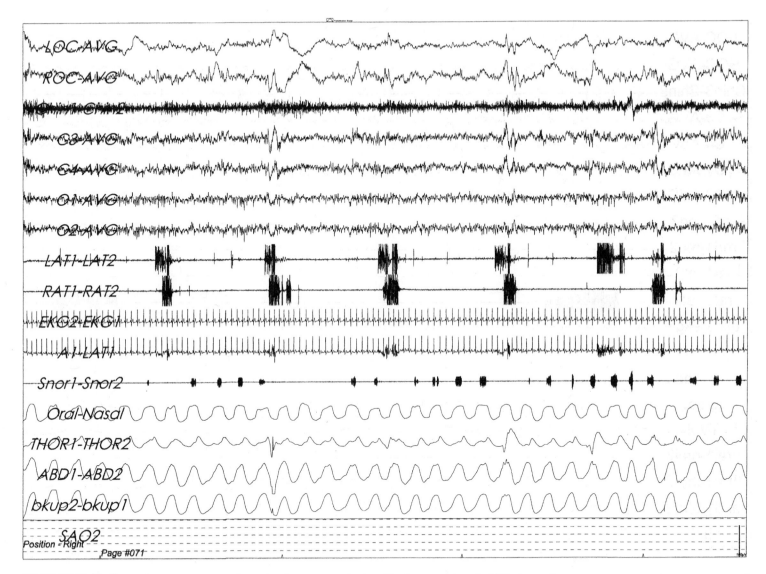

FIGURE 5-3 **Polysomnogram: Standard montage (prior display montage); 120 second page.**

Clinical: 62-year-old man with excessive daytime sleepiness and a history of kicking his wife at night.

Staging: Stage 2 sleep with K-complexes. The K-complexes accompany some but not all of the periodic limb movements.

Respiratory: Snoring with otherwise normal respirations.

EMG: Bilateral periodic leg movements starting slightly earlier on the left side.

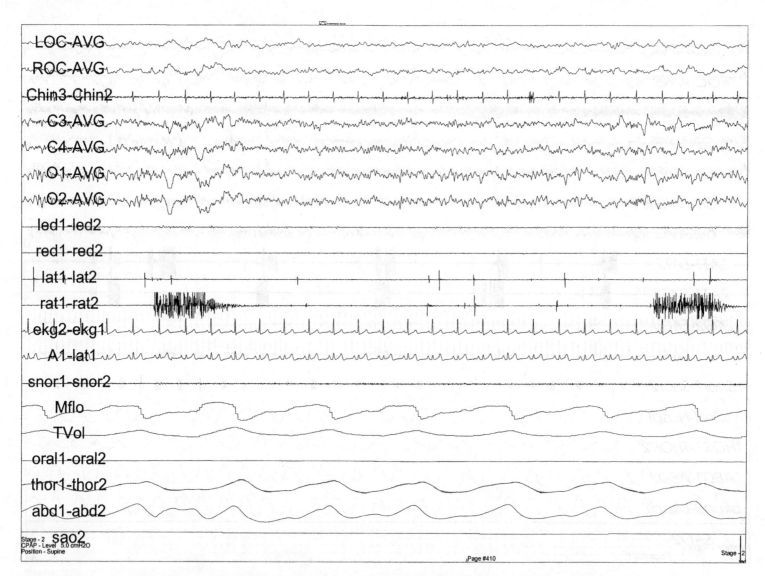

FIGURE 5-4 **Polysomnogram: CPAP and PLM montage (prior display montage); 30 second page.**
Clinical: 68-year-old man with obstructive sleep apnea and peripheral neuropathy.
Staging: Stage 2 sleep.
Respiratory: Normal respirations.
EMG: Right periodic leg movements and fragmentary myoclonus in both right and left leg channels.

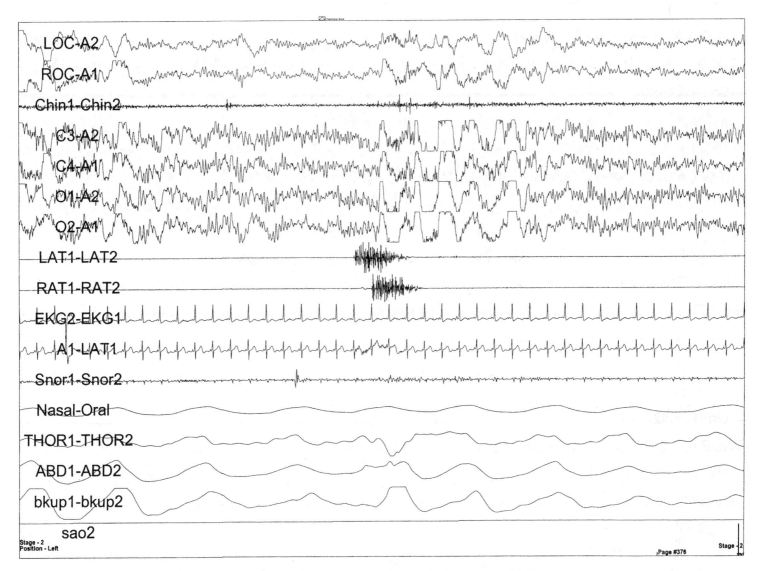

FIGURE 5-5   **Polysomnogram: Standard montage (prior display montage); 30 second page.**

Clinical: 64-year-old man with excessive daytime sleepiness and frequent nocturnal leg movements.

Staging: Stage 2 sleep.

Respiratory: Effort increases with the arousal.

EMG: Bilateral periodic leg movements with an associated arousal.

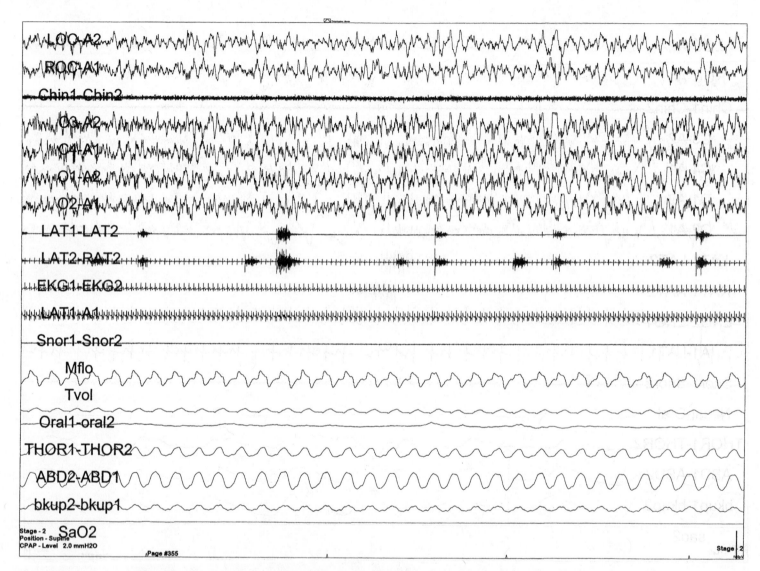

FIGURE 5-6 **Polysomnogram: CPAP montage (prior display montage); 120 second page.**
Clinical: 39-year-old man with obstructive sleep apnea.
Staging: Stage 2 sleep.
Respiratory: Normal respirations while using CPAP.
EMG: Asymmetric periodic leg movements. The compressed time base facilitates identification of the periodicity of the movements.

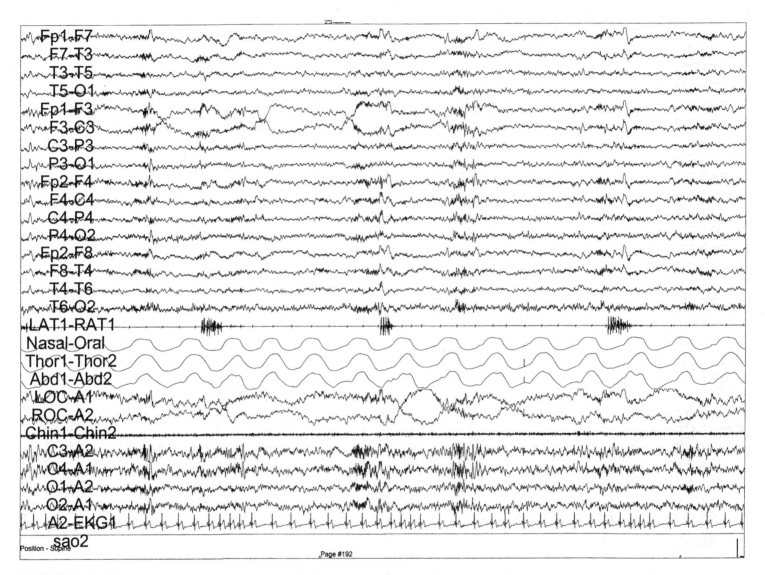

FIGURE 5-7 **Polysomnogram: Expanded EEG montage (prior display montage); 60 second page.**

Clinical: 44-year-old woman with excessive daytime sleepiness and low back pain.

Staging: Stage 2 sleep.

Respiratory: Normal respirations.

EMG: Periodic leg movements with associated tachycardia. The compressed time base facilitates identification of the periodicity of the movements.

EKG: A transient increase in the heart rate accompanies the periodic leg movements, despite no definite EEG evidence of an arousal.

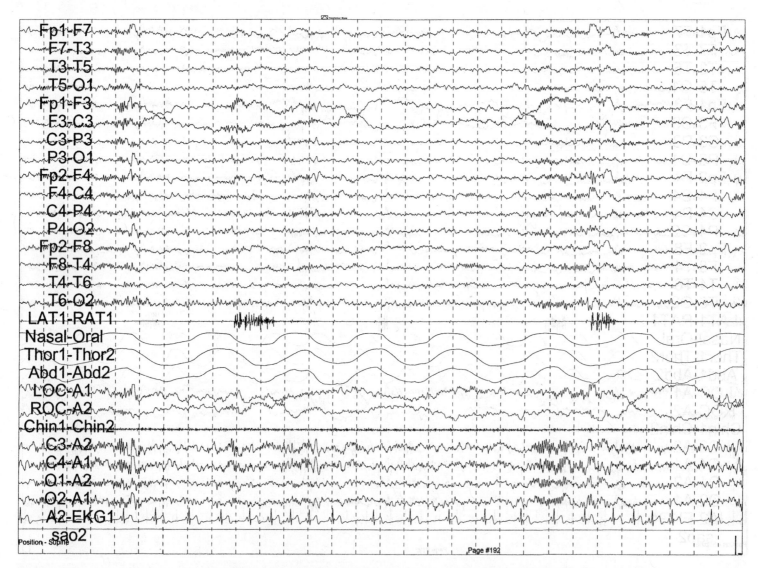

Fp1-F7
F7-T3
T3-T5
T5-O1
Fp1-F3
F3-C3
C3-P3
P3-O1
Fp2-F4
F4-C4
C4-P4
P4-O2
Fp2-F8
F8-T4
T4-T6
T6-O2
LAT1-RAT1
Nasal-Oral
Thor1-Thor2
Abd1-Abd2
LOC-A1
ROC-A2
Chin1-Chin2
C3-A2
C4-A1
O1-A2
O2-A1
A2-EKG1
sao2

Position - Supine

Page #192

FIGURE 5-8   **Polysomnogram: Expanded EEG montage (prior display montage); 30 second page.**
Clinical: 44-year-old woman with excessive daytime sleepiness and low back pain.
Staging: Stage 2 sleep.
Respiratory: Normal respirations.
EMG: Periodic leg movements associated with tachycardia.
EKG: A transient increase in the heart rate accompanies the periodic leg movements, despite no definite
EEG evidence of an arousal.

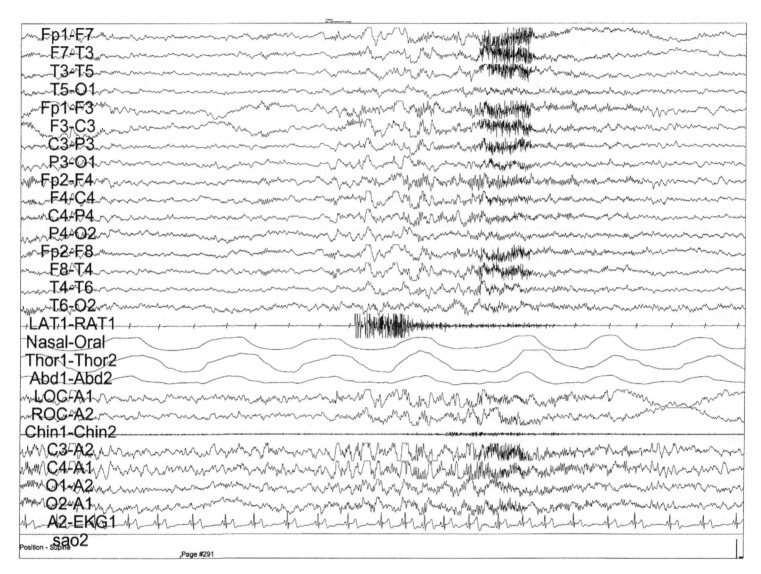

FIGURE 5-9 **Polysomnogram: Expanded EEG montage (prior display montage); 30 second page.**

Clinical: 58-year-old man with excessive daytime sleepiness.

Staging: Stage 2 sleep.

Respiratory: Normal respirations.

EMG: Periodic leg movements with arousals and tachycardia.

EKG: A transient increase in the heart rate occurs with the arousal and periodic leg movement.

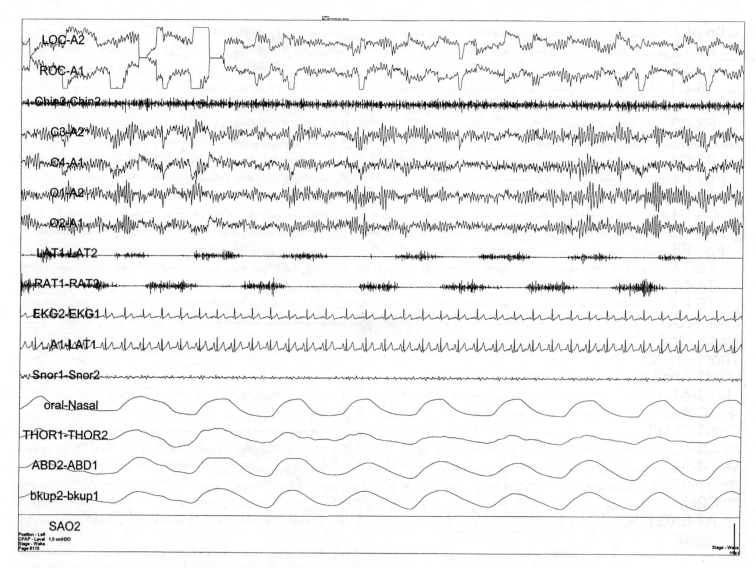

FIGURE 5-10   **Polysomnogram: Standard montage (prior display montage); 30 second page.**
Clinical: 32-year-old woman with restless legs syndrome.
Staging: Stage wake.
Respiratory: Normal respirations.
EMG: Frequent leg movements during wakefulness are typical of restless legs syndrome.

Parasomnias

James D. Geyer, MD and Paul R. Carney, MD

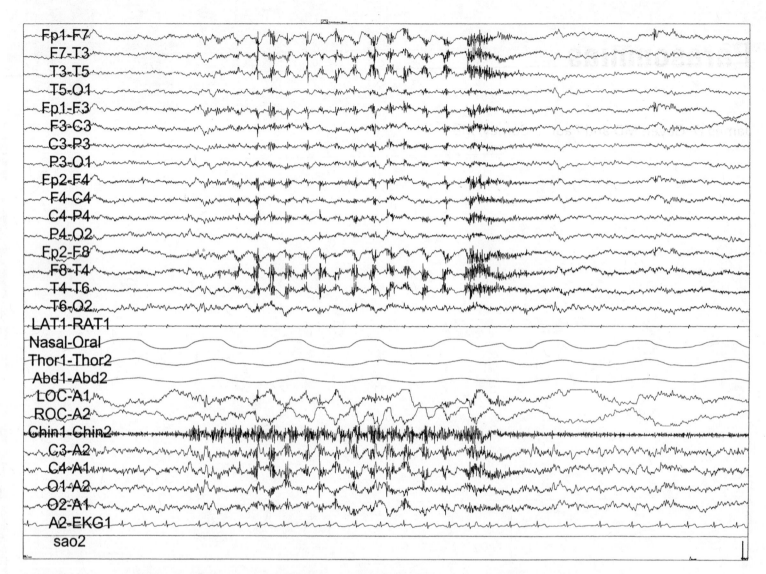

FIGURE 6-1 **Polysomnogram: Expanded EEG montage (prior display montage); 30 second page.**

Clinical: 41-year-old man with witnessed apneas and tooth grinding.

Staging: Stage 1 sleep.

Respiratory: Normal respirations.

Behavior: Bruxism. Bursts of EMG activity occur at a rate of about 1 per second in the EEG, chin EMG, and EOG channels.

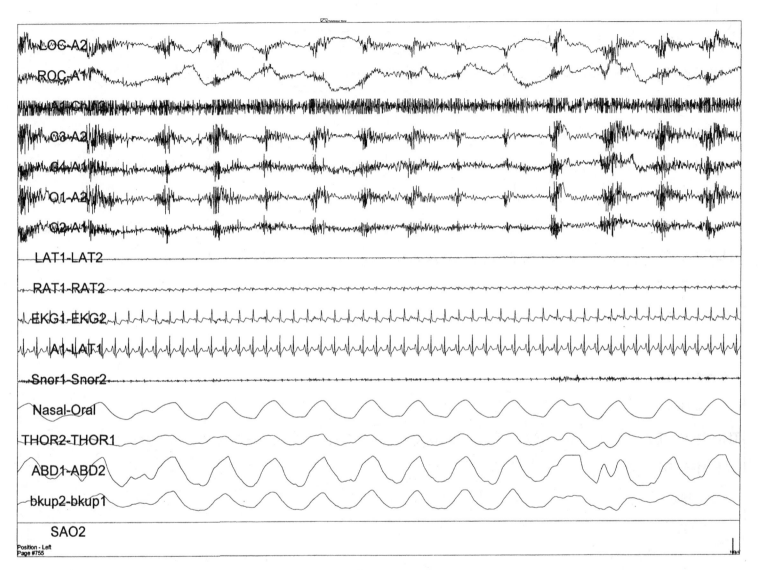

FIGURE 6-2 **Polysomnogram: Standard montage (prior display montage); 60 second page.**

Clinical: 26-year-old woman with excessive daytime sleepiness, tooth grinding, and morning headache.

Staging: Probable stage 1 sleep but difficult to stage because of artifact.

Respiratory: Normal respirations.

Behavior: Bruxism. Rhythmic bursts of EMG activity occur about every 4 seconds.

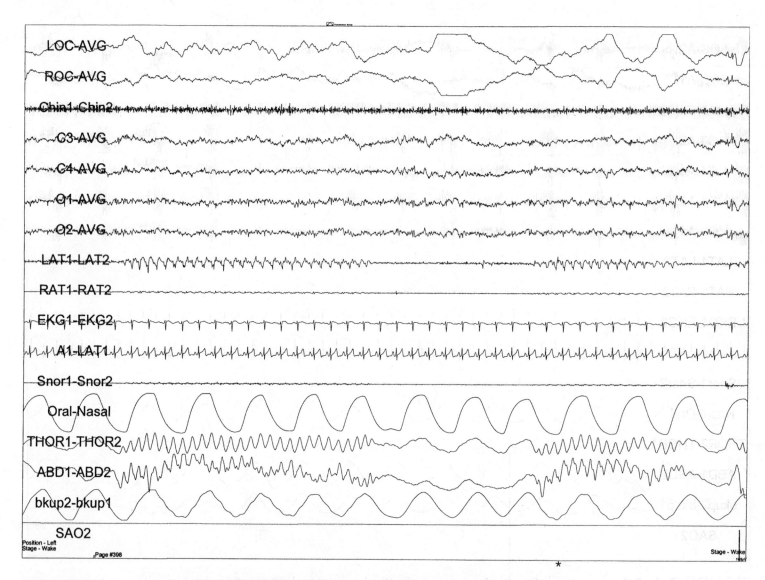

LOC-AVG

ROC-AVG

Chin1-Chin2

C3-AVG

C4-AVG

O1-AVG

O2-AVG

LAT1-LAT2

RAT1-RAT2

EKG1-EKG2

A1-LAT1

Snor1-Snor2

Oral-Nasal

THOR1-THOR2

ABD1-ABD2

bkup2-bkup1

SAO2

Position - Left
Stage - Wake

Page #398

Stage - Wake

*

FIGURE 6-3   **Polysomnogram: Standard montage (prior display montage); 30 second page.**
Clinical: 47-year-old woman with excessive daytime sleepiness.
Staging: Stage 1 sleep.
Respiratory: Normal respirations.
Behavior: Movements of the left leg (*) occur rhythmically at a rate of about 1 per second, characteristic of rhythmic movement disorder. Movement artifact is evident in the thoracic and abdominal channels.

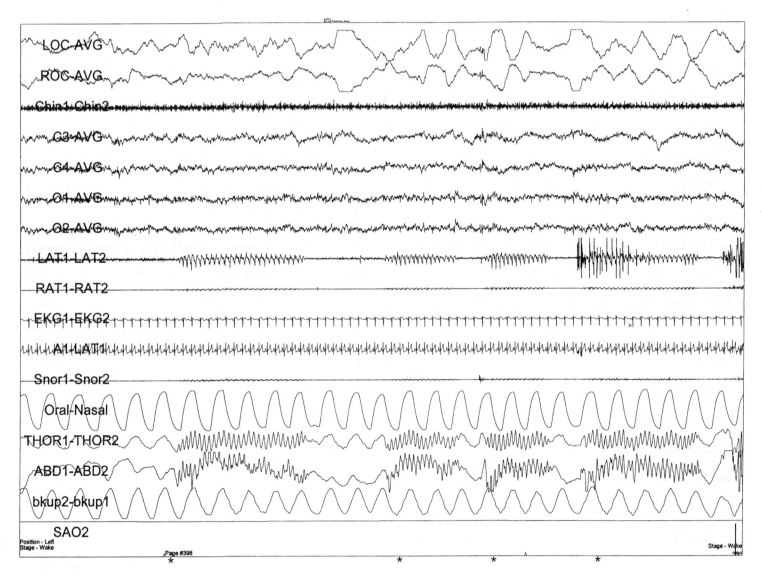

FIGURE 6-4 **Polysomnogram: Standard montage (prior display montage); 120 second page.**

Clinical: 47-year-old woman with excessive daytime sleepiness.

Staging: Stage wake.

Respiratory: Normal respirations.

Behavior: Movements of the left leg (*) occur rhythmically at a rate of about 1 per second, with a brief period of quiescence between the runs of movement. This pattern is characteristic of rhythmic movement disorder. Movement artifact is evident in the thoracic and abdominal channels.

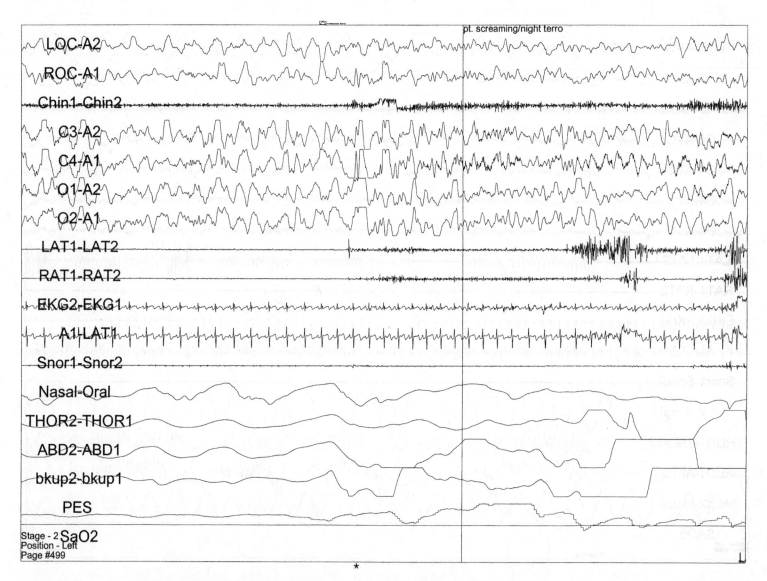

FIGURE 6-5 **Polysomnogram: Standard montage with intrathoracic pressure monitoring (prior display montage); 30 second page.**

Clinical: 7-year-old boy with nocturnal episodes of inconsolable fear.

Staging: Stage 3 sleep with an arousal.

Respiratory: Normal respirations.

EEG: Arousal (*) with delta activity associated with screaming and inconsolable fear, characteristic of sleep terrors. The EEG following the arousal consists of a mixture of delta and faster frequencies. This EEG pattern commonly accompanies arousals from slow-wave sleep in children with arousal disorders.

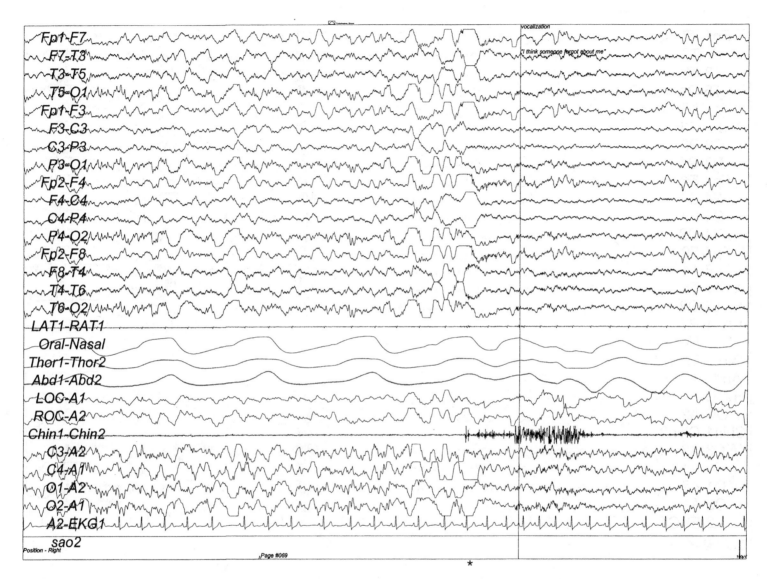

FIGURE 6-6 **Polysomnogram: Expanded EEG montage (prior display montage); 30 second page.**

Clinical: 38-year-old woman with sleep talking.

Staging: Stage 3 sleep.

Respiratory: Normal respirations.

EEG: Spontaneous arousal (*) from stage 3/4 sleep associated with sleep talking. The EEG following the arousal consists of a mixture of theta and delta frequencies.

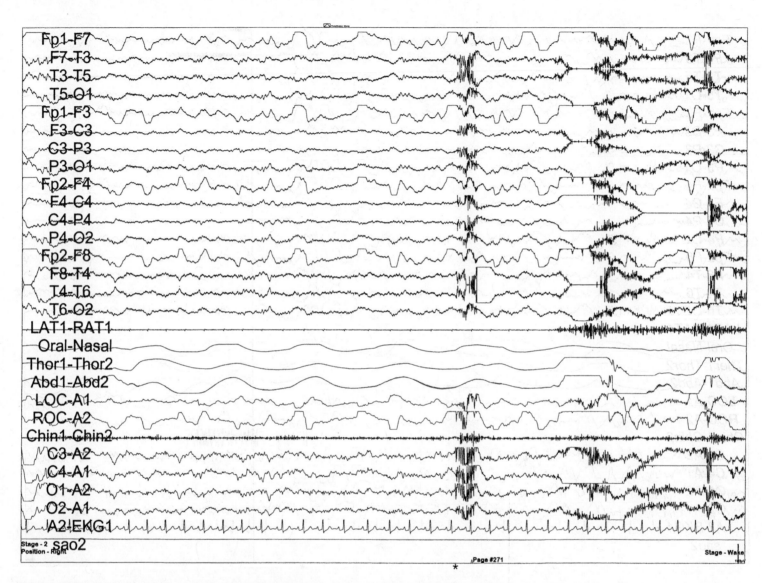

FIGURE 6-7 **Polysomnogram: Expanded EEG montage (prior display montage); 30 second page.**

Clinical: 51-year-old man with frequent nocturnal arousals.

Staging: Stage 2 sleep.

Respiratory: Normal respirations.

EEG: An arousal (*) is followed a few seconds later by a full awakening and sleep talking. Sleep talking can occur with arousals from any stage of sleep.

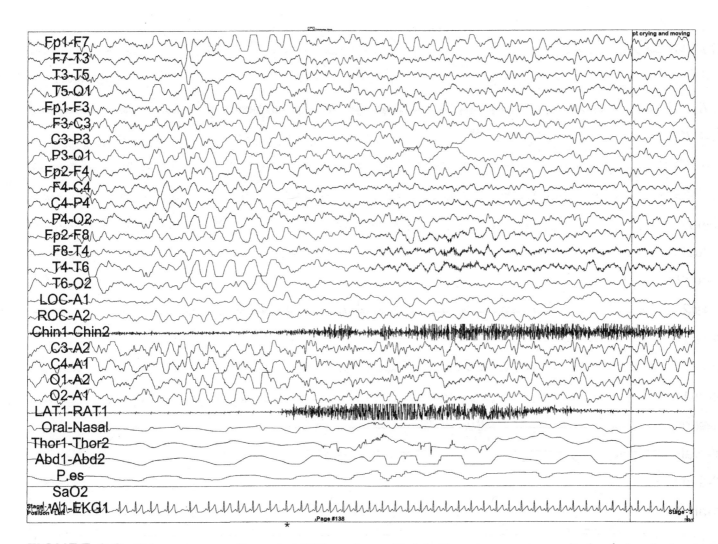

FIGURE 6-8   **Polysomnogram: Expanded EEG montage with intrathoracic pressure monitoring (prior display montage); 30 second page.**

Clinical: 53-year-old man with confusional arousals.

Staging: Stage 3 sleep.

Respiratory: Normal respirations.

EEG: Following the arousal (*), the EEG shows continued delta activity intermixed with faster frequencies, associated with moving and crying. The observed behavior was typical of a confusional arousal. In the 5 to 6 seconds preceding the arousal, the EEG shows delta activity that is more rhythmic and synchronous than the delta activity that usually occurs in slow-wave sleep. Rhythmic, synchronous delta activity sometimes precedes or accompanies arousals from slow-wave sleep in patients with arousal disorders.

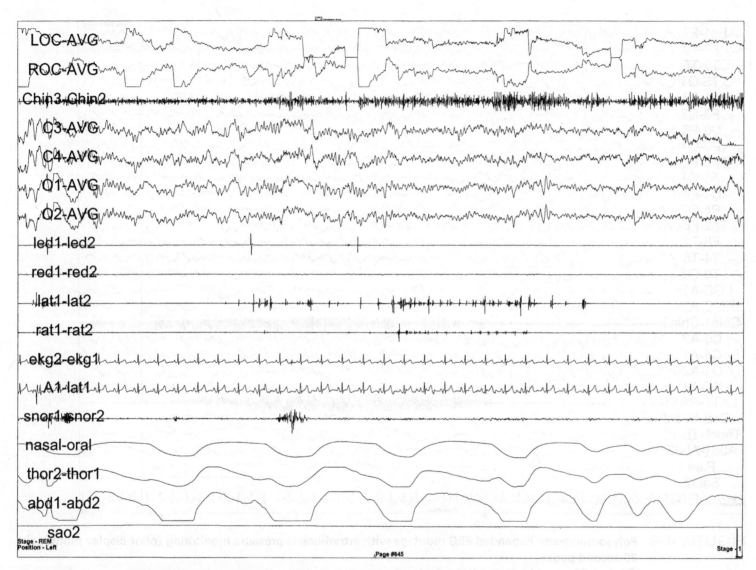

LOC-AVG

ROC-AVG

Chin3-Chin2

C3-AVG

C4-AVG

O1-AVG

O2-AVG

led1-led2

red1-red2

lat1-lat2

rat1-rat2

ekg2-ekg1

A1-lat1

snor1-snor2

nasal-oral

thor2-thor1

abd1-abd2

sao2

Stage - REM
Position - Left

Page #645

Stage - 1

FIGURE 6-9   **Polysomnogram: RLS montage (prior display montage); 30 second page.**

Clinical: 45-year-old with excessive daytime sleepiness.

Staging: Stage REM sleep.

Respiratory: Normal respirations with occasional snoring.

EMG: Increased phasic EMG activity is most prominent in the LAT1-LAT2 derivation. Chin EMG activity is tonically increased. Increased phasic and tonic EMG activity during REM sleep is characteristic of patients with REM sleep behavior disorder.

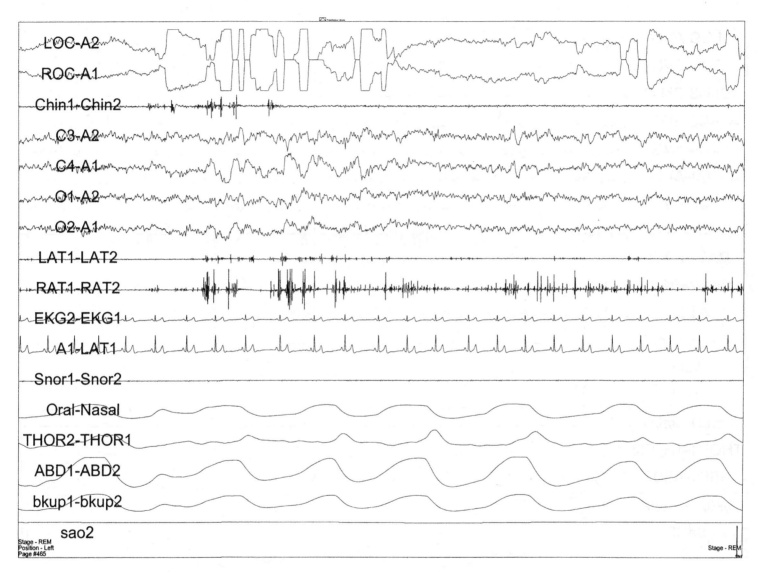

FIGURE 6-10 **Polysomnogram: Standard montage (prior display montage); 30 second page.**

Clinical: 63-year-old man with excessive daytime sleepiness and mild parkinsonism.

Staging: Stage REM sleep with bursts of rapid eye movements.

Respiratory: Mildly irregular breathing accompanying the bursts of rapid eye movements.

EMG: Phasic EMG activity which is most prominent in the right leg. The amount of activity is excessive for an adult. Epochs of REM sleep with excessive phasic EMG activity are common in patients with REM sleep behavior disorder.

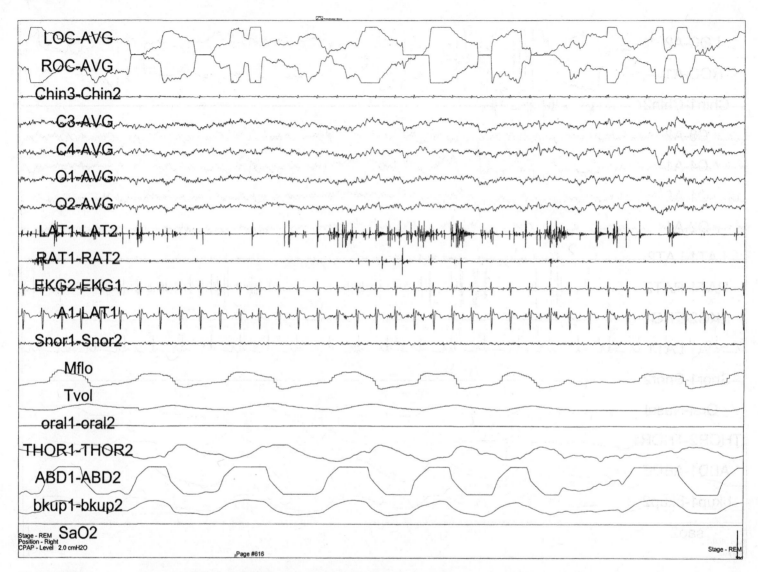

LOC-AVG
ROC-AVG
Chin3-Chin2
C3-AVG
C4-AVG
O1-AVG
O2-AVG
LAT1-LAT2
RAT1-RAT2
EKG2-EKG1
A1-LAT1
Snor1-Snor2
Mflo
Tvol
oral1-oral2
THOR1-THOR2
ABD1-ABD2
bkup1-bkup2
SaO2

Stage - REM
Position - Right
CPAP - Level 2.0 cmH2O

Page #616

Stage - REM

FIGURE 6-11 **Polysomnogram: CPAP montage (prior display montage); 30 second page.**
Clinical: 42-year-old man with a history of poliomyelitis.
Staging: Stage REM sleep with rapid eye movements.
Respiratory: Normal breathing.
EMG: Excessive phasic EMG activity, which is most prominent in the left leg. The amount of activity is excessive for an adult. Epochs of REM sleep with excessive phasic EMG activity are common in patients with REM sleep behavior disorder.

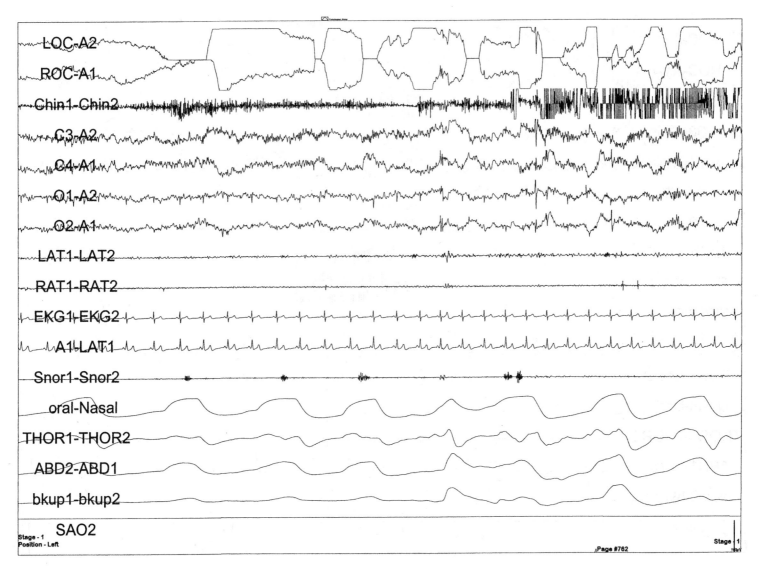

FIGURE 6-12 **Polysomnogram: Standard montage (prior display montage); 30 second page.**
Clinical: 62-year-old man with a history of fighting behavior in his sleep.
Staging: Stage REM sleep with rapid eye movements.
Respiratory: Normal respirations.
EMG: Markedly increased chin EMG tone during REM sleep. Tonic increases in chin EMG activity, with or without excess phasic EMG activity in the limbs, are common during epochs of REM sleep in patients with REM sleep behavior disorder.

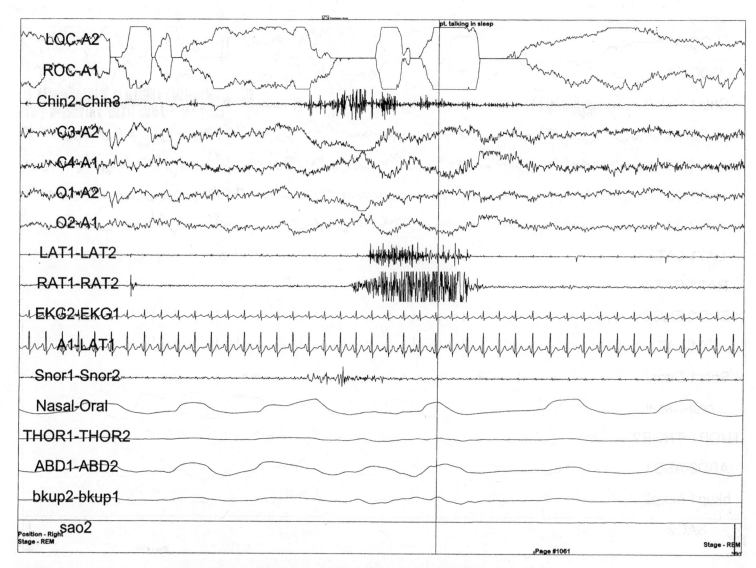

FIGURE 6-13   **Polysomnogram: Standard montage (prior display montage); 30 second page.**
Clinical: 62-year-old man with a history of fighting behavior in his sleep.
Staging: Stage REM sleep with rapid eye movements.
Respiratory: Normal respirations.
EMG: Transiently increased chin EMG tone with leg movements and talking during REM sleep. The behaviors and polysomnographic features are typical of REM sleep behavior disorder.

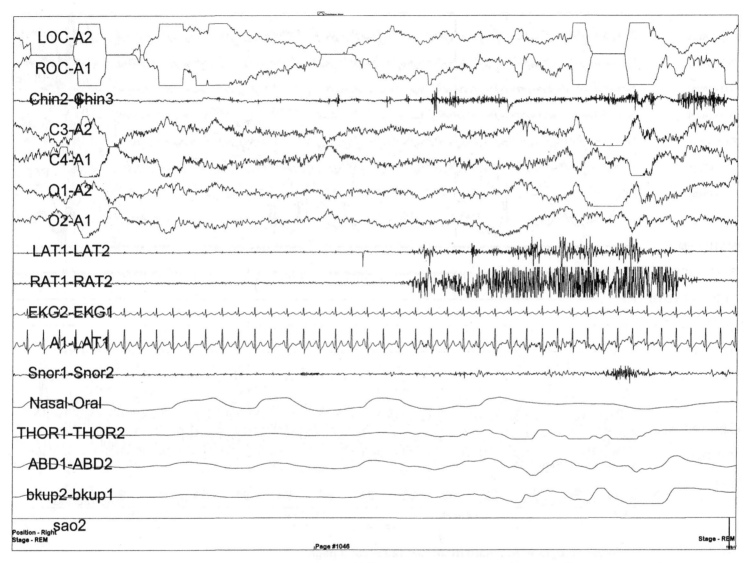

FIGURE 6-14   **Polysomnogram: Standard montage (prior display montage); 30 second page.**
Clinical: 62-year-old man with a history of fighting behavior in his sleep.
Staging: Stage REM sleep with rapid eye movements.
Respiratory: Normal respirations.
EMG: Markedly increased chin EMG tone and leg movements during REM sleep. During this REM period, the patient talked, screamed, and made punching and thrashing movements. The behaviors and polysomnographic features are typical of REM sleep behavior disorder.

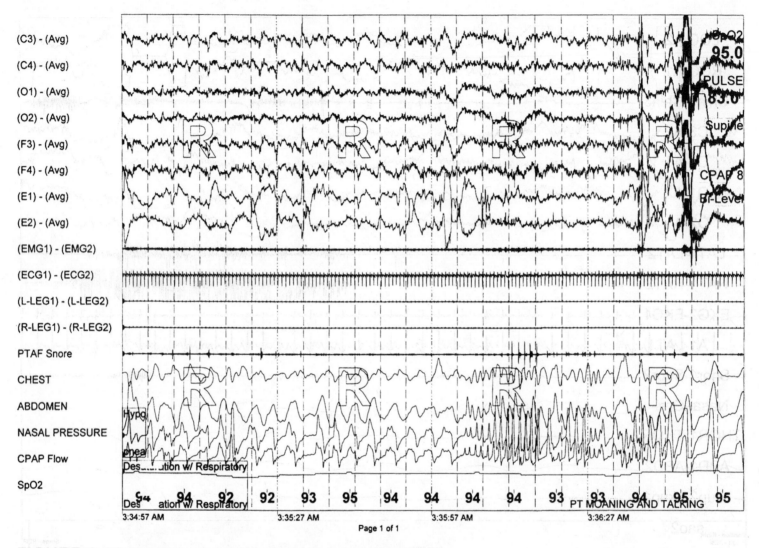

FIGURE 6-15 **Polysomnogram: Standard montage; 120 second page.**
Clinical: 57-year-old man with a history of PTSD and frequent nightmares. The patient awoke with reports of a nightmare about drowning. This was associated with recurrent hypopneas. He stated that this was a common dream. This resolved after effective treatment of the obstructive sleep apnea.
Staging: Stage REM sleep with rapid eye movements with an arousal.
Respiratory: Hypopnea. The obstructive sleep apnea was isolated to REM sleep in this patient.

EEG Abnormalities

James D. Geyer, MD and Paul R. Carney, MD

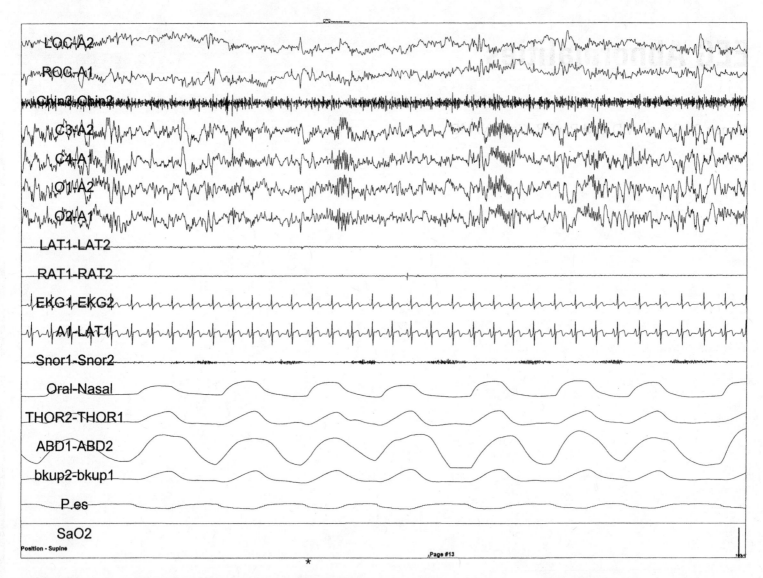

FIGURE 7-1　**Polysomnogram: Standard montage with intrathoracic pressure monitoring (prior display montage); 30 second page.**

Clinical: 29-year-old woman with complex partial seizures, snoring, and excessive daytime sleepiness.

Staging: Stage 2 sleep.

Respiratory: Snoring with normal respirations.

EEG: Subtle right hemispheric sharp waves (*) during stage 2 sleep with sleep spindles, K-complexes, and POSTs.

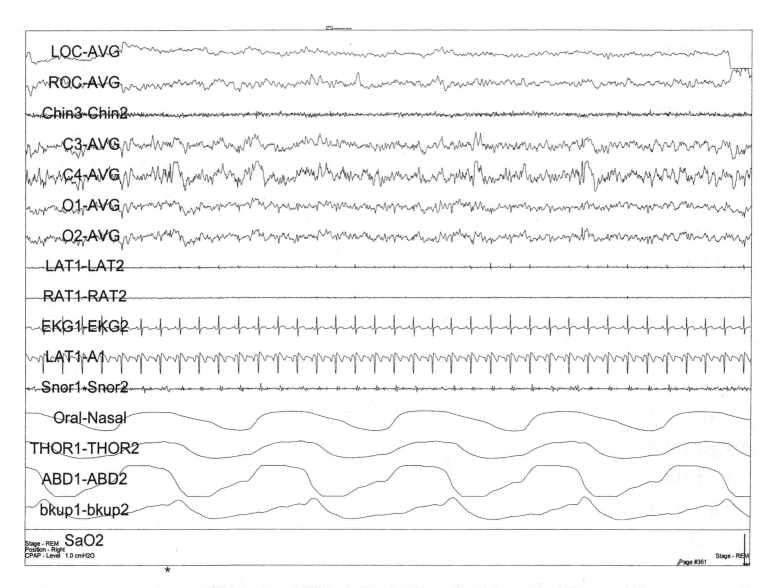

FIGURE 7-2   **Polysomnogram: Standard montage (prior display montage); 30 second page.**
Clinical: 44-year-old man with a right frontal glioma, epilepsy, and excessive daytime sleepiness.
Staging: Stage REM sleep.
Respiratory: Normal respirations.
EEG: Right hemispheric sharp and slow waves most prominent in the C4 electrode (*). The sharp wave can also be seen in the O2-avg derivation.

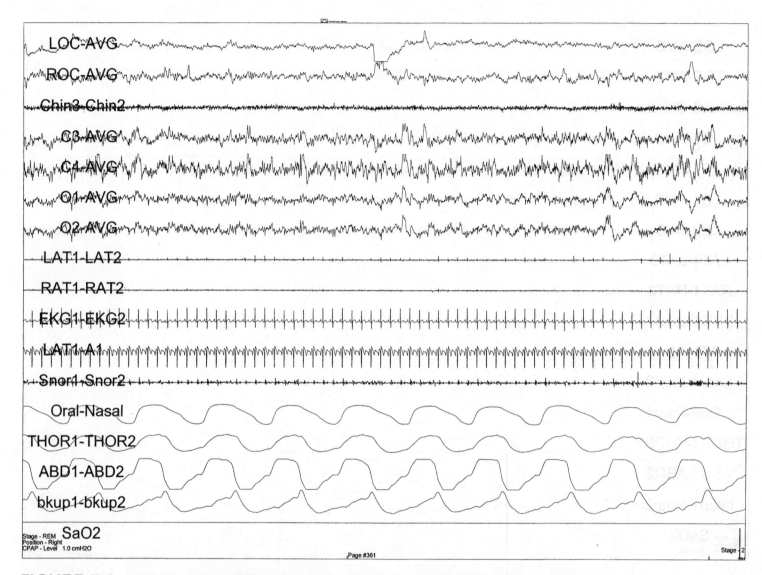

FIGURE 7-3   **Polysomnogram: Standard montage (prior display montage); 60 second page.**
Clinical: 44-year-old man with a right frontal glioma, epilepsy, and excessive daytime sleepiness.
Staging: Stage REM sleep.
Respiratory: Normal respirations.
EEG: Right hemispheric (electrode C4) sharp and slow waves. When compared to the previous figure with a 30-second time base, the abnormality is more difficult to identify because of time compression.

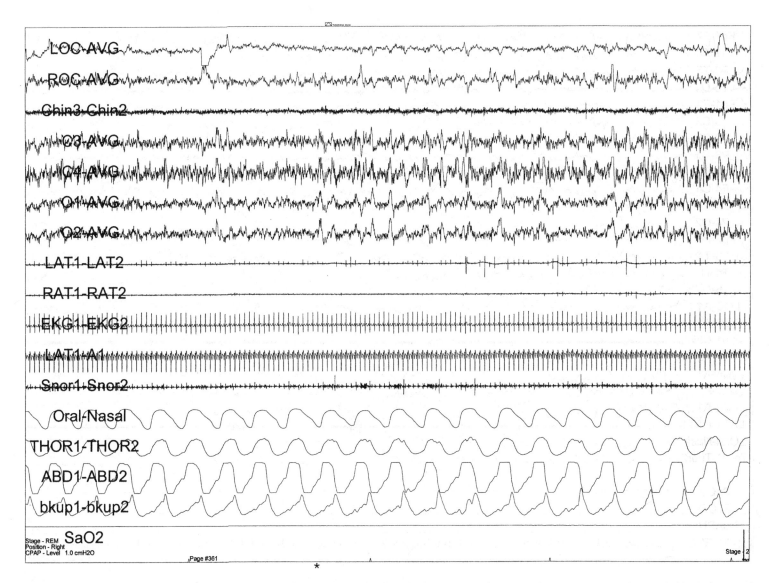

FIGURE 7-4 **Polysomnogram: Standard montage (prior display montage); 120 second page.**
Clinical: 44-year-old man with a right frontal glioma, epilepsy, and excessive daytime sleepiness.
Staging: Stage REM sleep.
Respiratory: Normal respirations.
EEG: Right hemispheric (electrode C4) sharp and slow waves (*). When compared to the previous two figures, the abnormality is almost impossible to identify because of time compression.

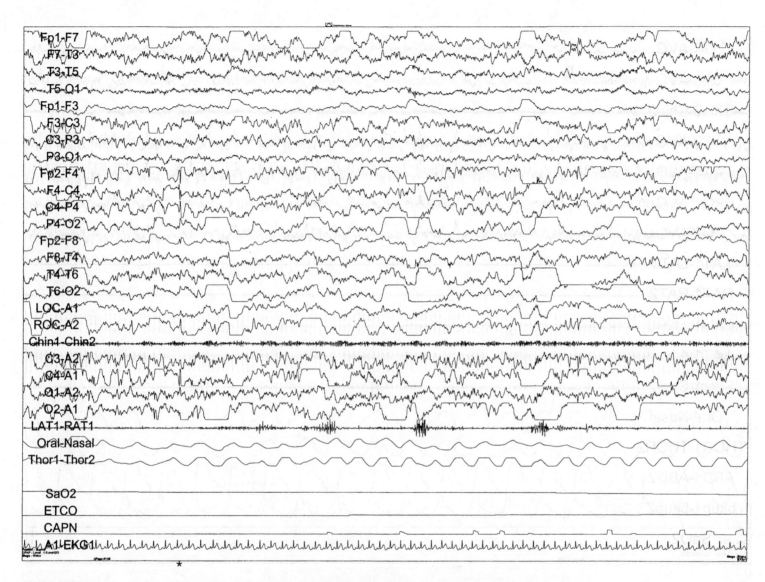

FIGURE 7-5 **Polysomnogram: Expanded montage (prior display montage); 60 second page.**
Clinical: 4-year-old with symptomatic generalized epilepsy and witnessed apneas.
Staging: Stage 2 sleep.
Respiratory: Normal respirations.
EEG: Right frontal sharp and slow waves maximal at electrodes F4 and C4 (*). The expanded EEG montage permits localization of the discharge.

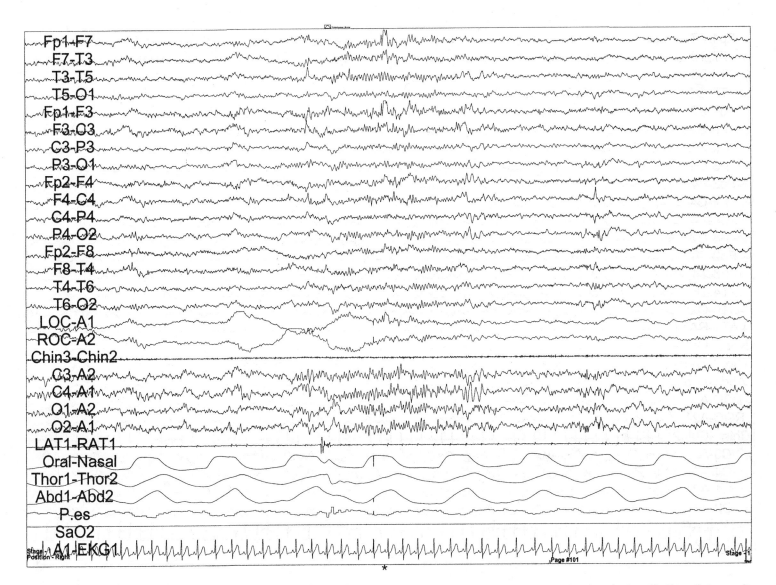

FIGURE 7-6   **Polysomnogram: Expanded EEG montage with intrathoracic pressure monitoring (prior display montage); 30 second page.**

Clinical: 28-year-old with frontal epilepsy and episodes of apnea and snoring.

Staging: Stage 1 sleep.

Respiratory: Normal respirations.

EEG: A left frontal spike and wave is maximal at electrode Fp1 (*). It is not seen in the standard sleep staging channels (C3-A2, C4-A1, O1-A2, O2-A1) but has a subtle representation in the LOC (left eye) channel.

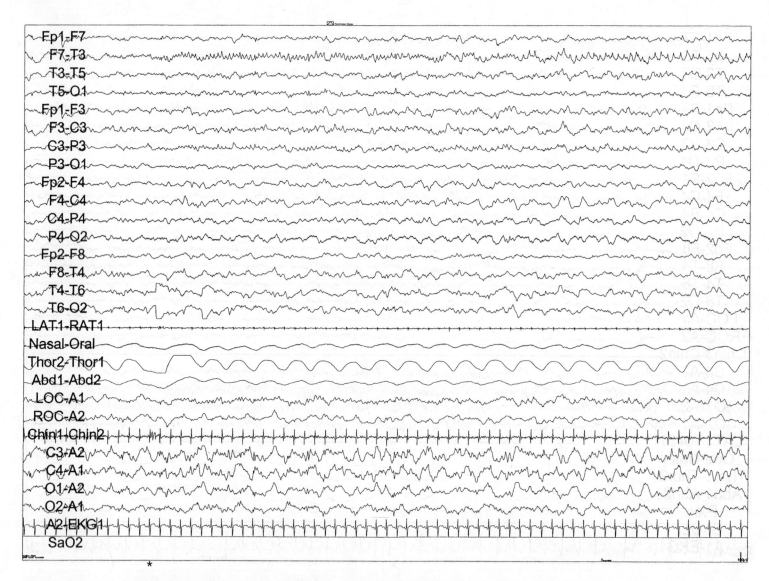

FIGURE 7-7   **Polysomnogram: Expanded EEG montage (prior display montage); 60 second page.**

Clinical: 18-month-old boy with seizures and apnea.

Staging: Stage 2 sleep. This page is difficult to stage because of seizure activity.

Respiratory: Increased respiratory effort at the onset of seizure activity.

EEG: Onset (*) of a focal seizure with medium amplitude rhythmic sharp waves maximal in channels F7-T3 and C3-P3. As commonly occurs with focal seizures, the frequency of the ictal activity gradually decreases and the amplitude gradually increases.

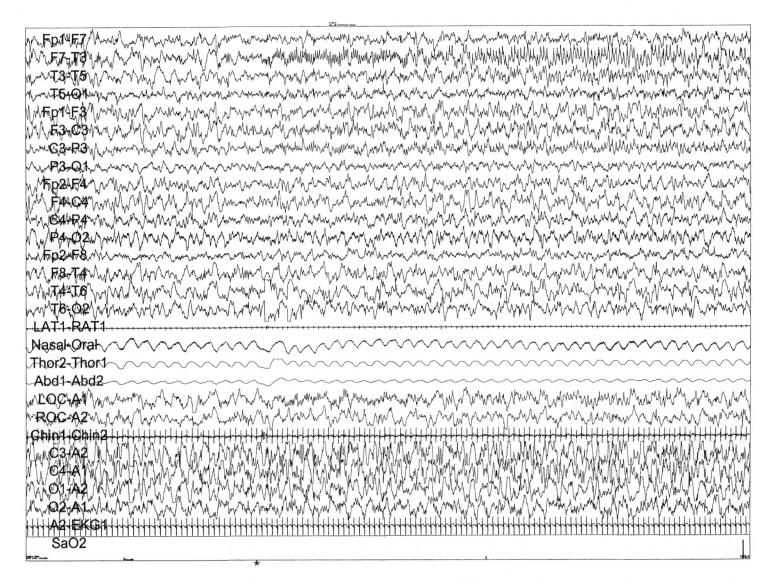

FIGURE 7-8   Polysomnogram: Expanded EEG montage (prior display montage); 120 second page.

Clinical: 18-month-old boy with seizures and apnea.

Staging: Stage 2 sleep. This page is difficult to stage because of seizure activity.

Respiratory: Increased respiratory effort at the onset of seizure activity.

EEG: Onset (*) of a focal seizure with medium amplitude rhythmic sharp waves maximal in channels F7-T3 and C3-P3. The evolution of ictal activity is readily apparent with the compressed time base.

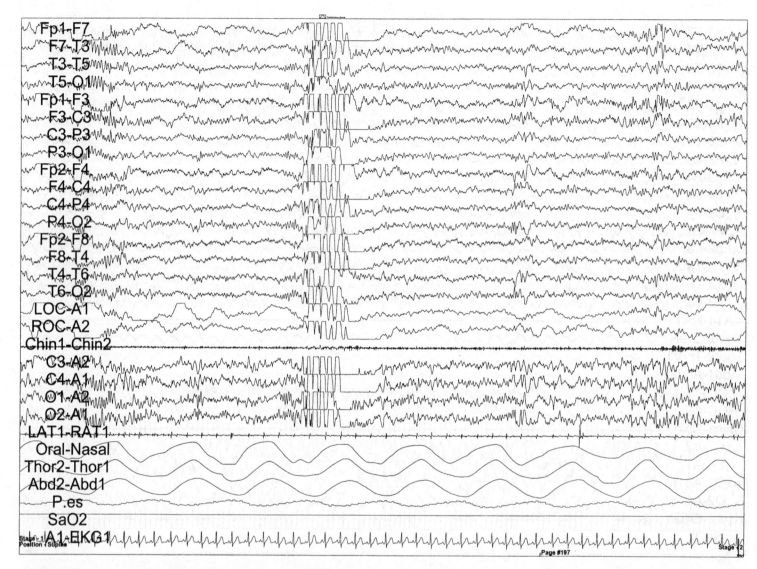

FIGURE 7-9 **Polysomnogram: Expanded EEG montage with intrathoracic pressure monitoring (prior display montage); 30 second page.**

Clinical: 18-year-old patient with primary generalized epilepsy and excessive daytime sleepiness.

Staging: Stage 1 sleep.

Respiratory: Normal respirations.

EEG: Generalized, high-amplitude spike and wave discharges are recorded in all EEG channels and in the EOG channels. The very high amplitudes are cut off in the display.

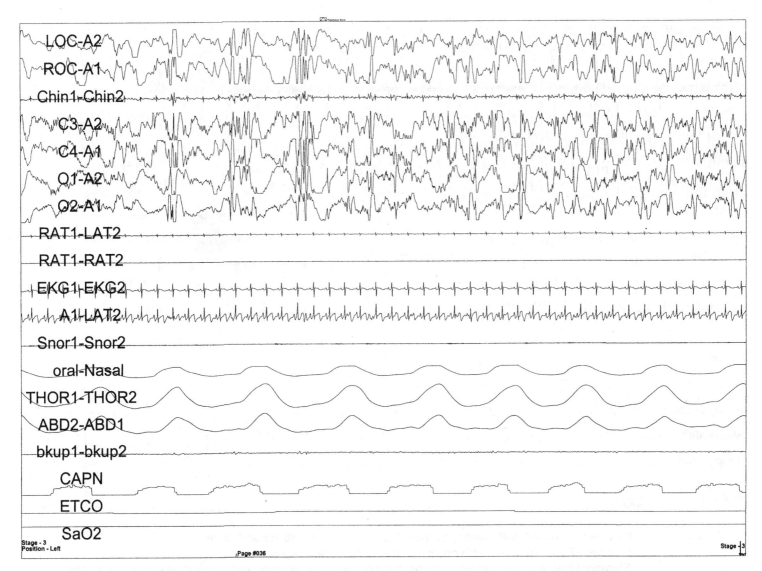

FIGURE 7-10 **Polysomnogram: Standard montage with CO₂ monitoring (prior display montage); 30 second page.**
Clinical: 7-year-old boy with symptomatic generalized epilepsy and episodes of apnea.
Staging: Stage 3 sleep. Staging is difficult with such severe EEG abnormalities.
Respiratory: Normal respirations.
EEG: Multifocal independent spike and wave discharges and generalized spike and wave discharges.

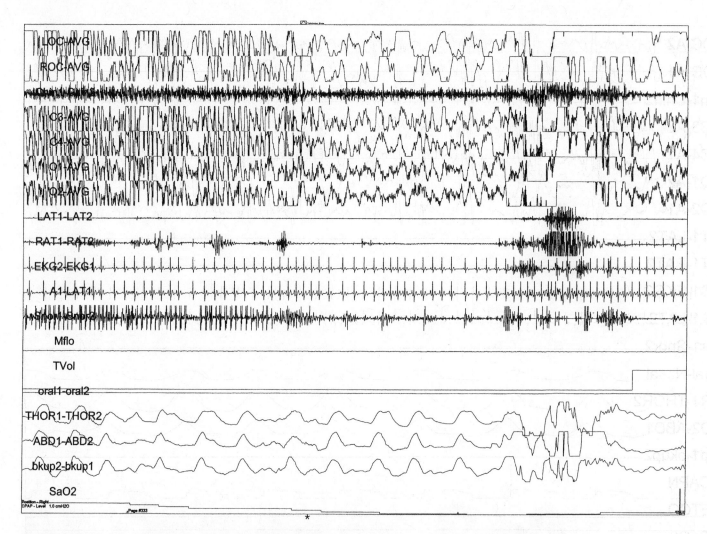

FIGURE 7-11   Polysomnogram: CPAP montage (prior display montage); 30 second page.

Clinical: 17-year-old man with epilepsy and obstructive sleep apnea.

Staging: Unable to accurately stage because of generalized spike and wave discharges during this generalized tonic–clonic seizure and subsequent postictal slowing.

Respiratory: Ictal and postictal obstructive apnea associated with an arousal and an oxygen desaturation.

EEG: Generalized spike and wave discharges. At the end of the seizure (*), there is generalized delta activity during the postictal phase.

Artifact: The tidal volume channel has artifact caused by the mask being pulled from the patient's face during postictal confusion.

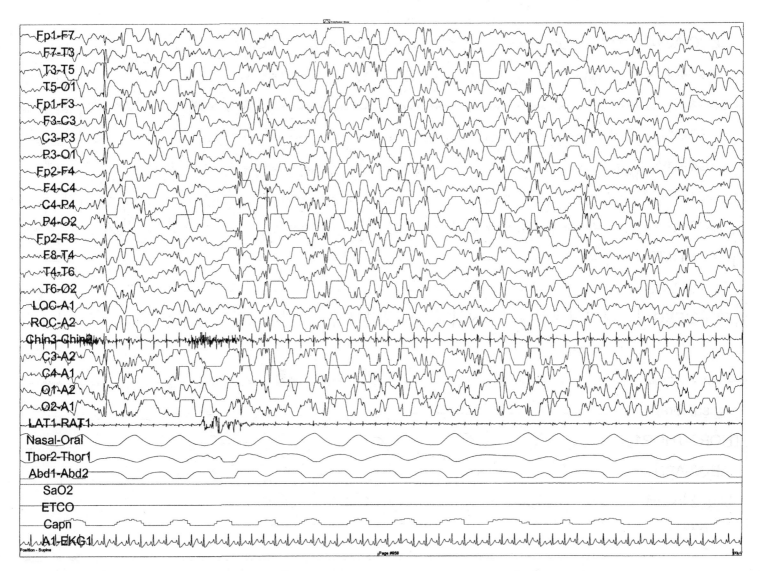

FIGURE 7-12 **Polysomnogram: Expanded EEG montage (prior display montage); 30 second page.**
Clinical: 15-month-old patient with Turner syndrome and infantile spasms.
Staging: Stage 1 sleep. Staging is difficult because of the severely abnormal EEG.
Respiratory: Normal respirations.
EEG: Hypsarrhythmia, generalized spike and wave discharges, slow spike and wave discharges, and a slow and asynchronous background.

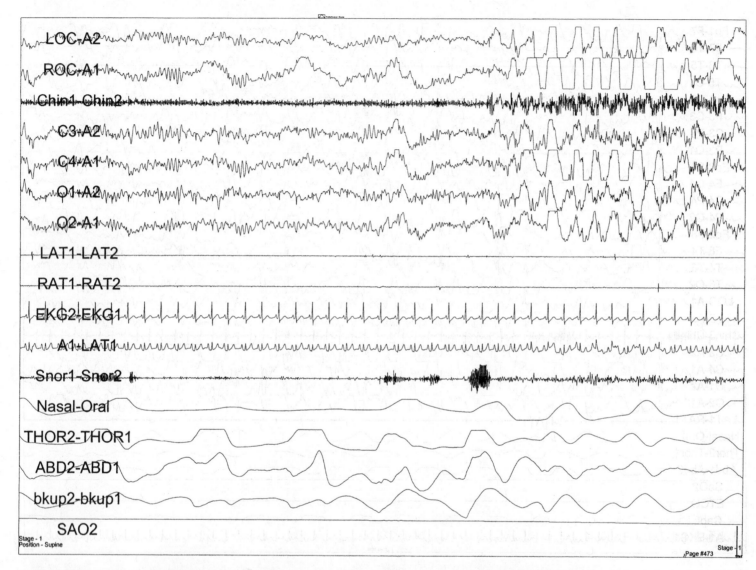

LOC-A2
ROC-A1
Chin1-Chin2
C3-A2
C4-A1
O1-A2
O2-A1
LAT1-LAT2
RAT1-RAT2
EKG2-EKG1
A1-LAT1
Snor1-Snor2
Nasal-Oral
THOR2-THOR1
ABD2-ABD1
bkup2-bkup1
SAO2

Stage - 1
Position - Supine

Page #473   Stage - 1

FIGURE 7-13 **Polysomnogram: Standard montage (prior display montage); 30 second page.**
Clinical: 48-year-old patient with a right frontal glioma and loud snoring.
Staging: Stage 1 sleep with an arousal.
Respiratory: Apnea followed by a snore and an arousal.
EEG: Asymmetric delta activity, greater on the right, during the arousal. Although the tumor is in the right frontal region, the pathologic delta activity is present over the entire right hemisphere and can also be seen in the LOC channel.

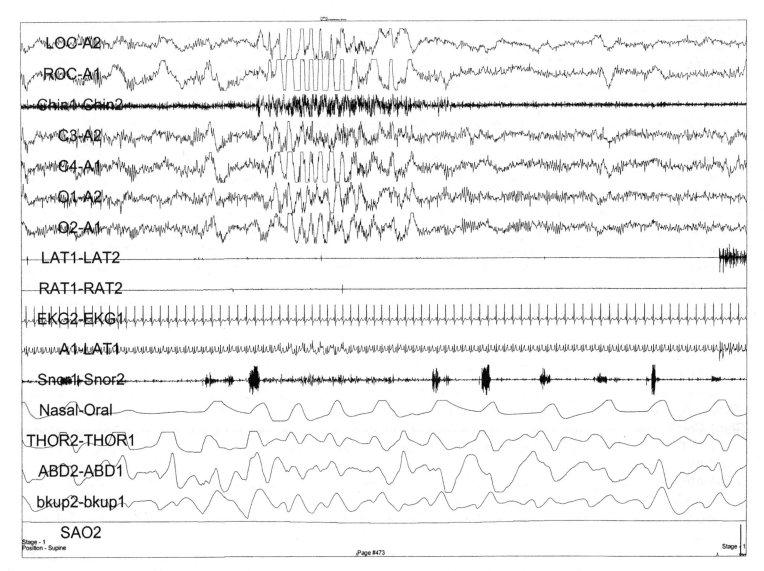

FIGURE 7-14   **Polysomnogram: Standard montage (prior display montage); 60 second page.**

Clinical: 48-year-old patient with a right frontal glioma and loud snoring.

Staging: Stage 1 sleep with an arousal.

Respiratory: Apnea followed by a snore and an arousal.

EEG: Asymmetric delta activity, greater on the right, during the arousal. Although the tumor is in the right frontal region, the pathologic delta activity is present over the entire right hemisphere and can also be seen in the LOC channel.

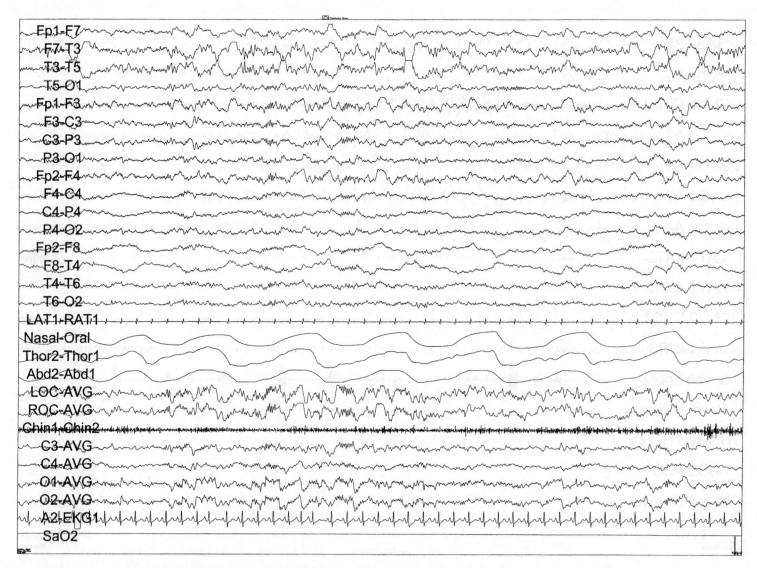

FIGURE 7-15 **Polysomnogram: Expanded EEG montage (prior display montage); 30 second page.**

Clinical: 49-year-old woman status post left frontotemporal arteriovenous malformation resection with excessive daytime sleepiness and disrupted sleep.

Staging: Stage 2 sleep.

Respiratory: Normal respirations.

EEG: Left hemisphere breach rhythm with higher-amplitude and higher-frequency EEG activity especially over the frontotemporal regions.

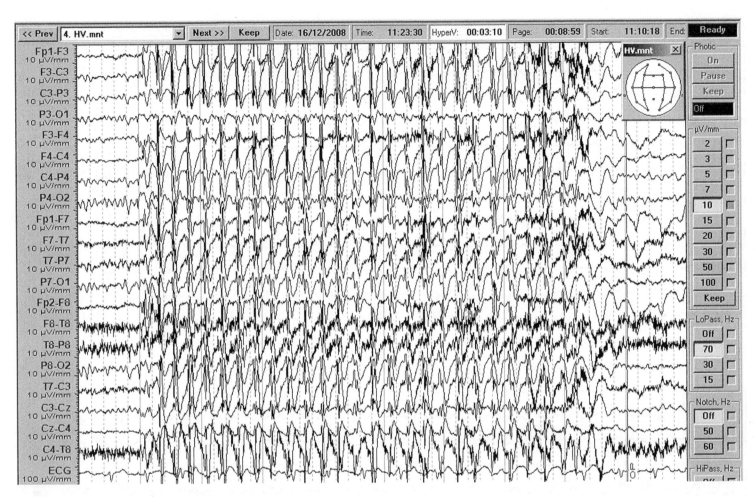

FIGURE 7-16   **EEG; 10 second page.**

Clinical: 8-year-old boy with episodes of staring.

Staging: Stage wake.

EEG: Generalized 3-Hz spike and wave discharges.

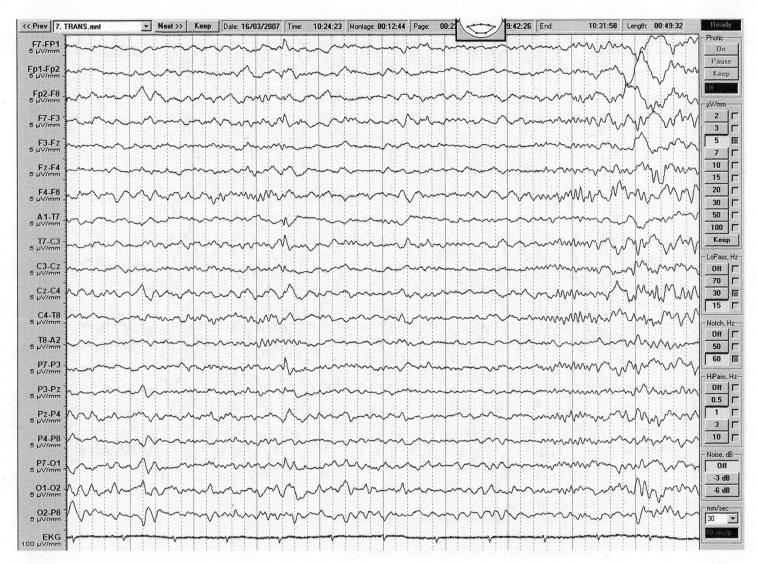

FIGURE 7-17   **EEG; 10 second page.**
Clinical: 7-year-old boy with a nocturnal seizure. Benign Rolandic epilepsy.
EEG: Centrotemporal spikes are present on an otherwise unremarkable background.

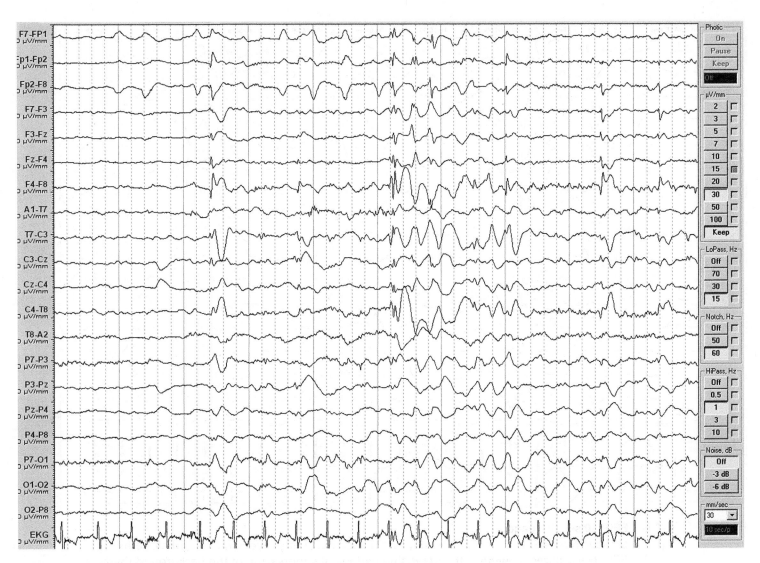

FIGURE 7-18 **EEG; 10 second page.**

Clinical: 3-year-old boy with myoclonic seizures and developmental delay. Dravet syndrome or severe myoclonic epilepsy of infancy.

EEG: Spike and wave and polyspike and wave discharges with background slowing.

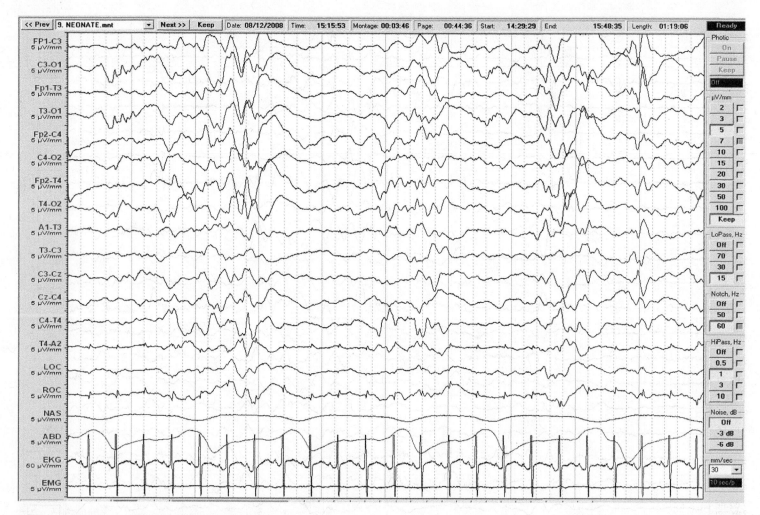

FIGURE 7-19   **EEG; 10 second page.**

Clinical: Neonate with encephalopathy and myoclonus. Early myoclonic encephalopathy.

EEG: Generalized slowing with intervening periods of suppression of the background rhythms.

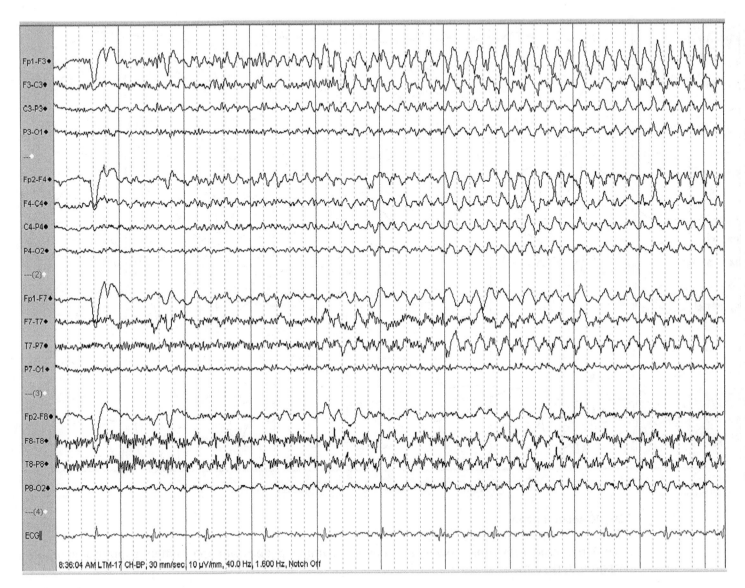

8:36:04 AM LTM-17 CH-BP, 30 mm/sec, 10 μV/mm, 40.0 Hz, 1.600 Hz, Notch Off

FIGURE 7-20   **EEG; 10 second page.**

Clinical: Partial seizure activity occurring in a patient with an intracranial mass. Epilepsia partialis continua (EPC).

EEG: Prolonged seizure activity with an approximately 5-Hz spike and wave and rhythmic theta activity morphology.

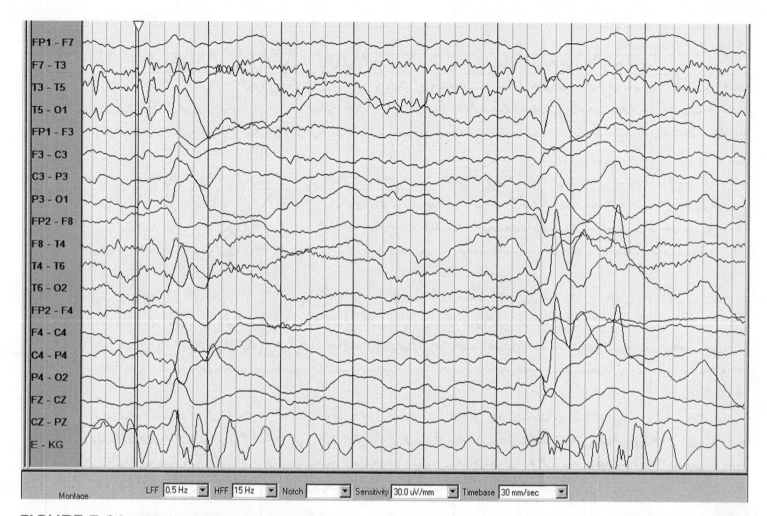

FP1 - F7
F7 - T3
T3 - T5
T5 - O1
FP1 - F3
F3 - C3
C3 - P3
P3 - O1
FP2 - F8
F8 - T4
T4 - T6
T6 - O2
FP2 - F4
F4 - C4
C4 - P4
P4 - O2
FZ - CZ
CZ - PZ
E - KG

Montage   LFF 0.5 Hz HFF 15 Hz Notch Sensitivity 30.0 uV/mm Timebase 30 mm/sec

FIGURE 7-21   EEG; 10 second page.
Clinical: Infant with infantile spasms.
EEG: Generalized arrhythmic slowing and a hypsarrhythmia pattern with intermittent suppression of the background rhythms.

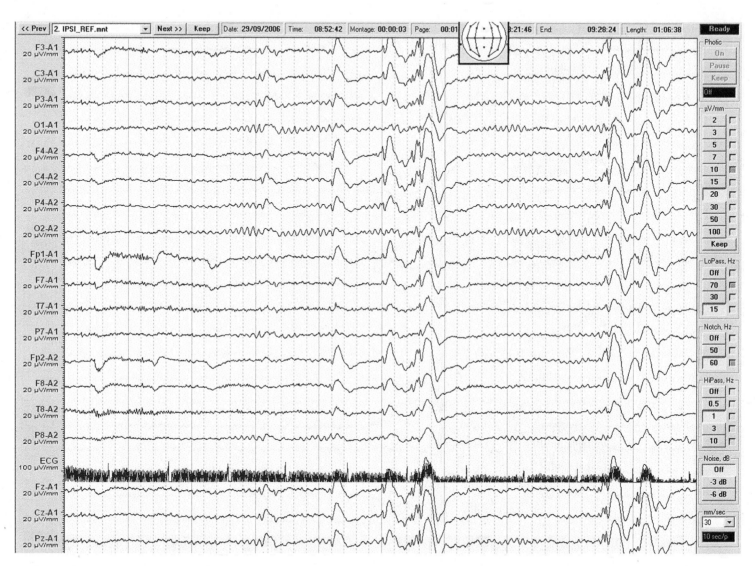

FIGURE 7-22 **EEG; 10 second page.**

Clinical: 14-year-old boy with morning myoclonus and generalized seizures. Juvenile myoclonic epilepsy (JME).

Stage: Stage wake.

EEG: Spike and wave and polyspike and wave discharges superimposed on an otherwise unremarkable background activity.

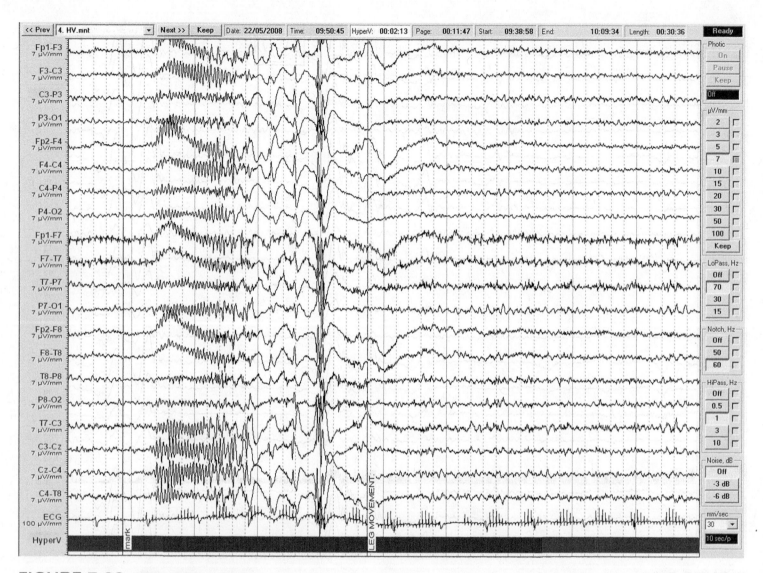

FIGURE 7-23 **EEG; 10 second page.**

Clinical: Lennox-Gastaut syndrome. Lennox-Gastaut syndrome is characterized by a combination of clinical seizures, including myoclonic, atonic, atypical absence, tonic axial, and generalized tonic–clonic seizures.

EEG: The EEG typically shows a generalized spike and wave pattern. The EEG reveals a slow spike wave complex with a frequency of 1 to 2.5 Hz, multifocal spikes, and generalized paroxysmal fast activity (GPFA).

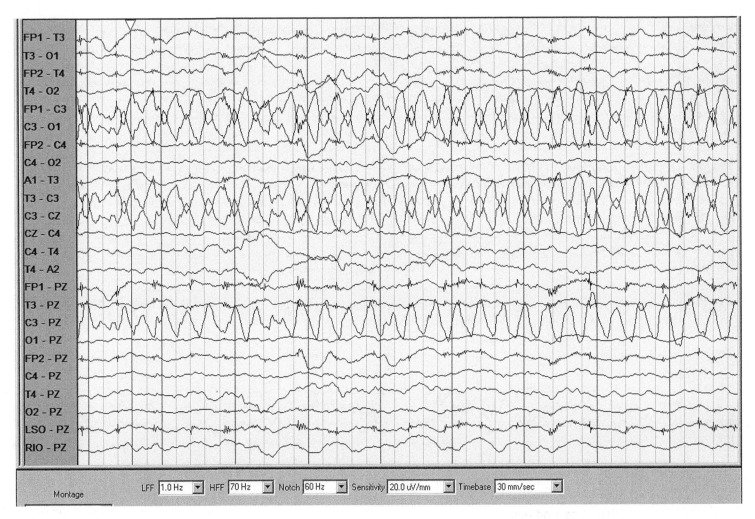

FIGURE 7-24   EEG; 10 second page.
Clinical: Neonate with seizures.
EEG: Seizure activity with centrally predominant rhythmic activity.

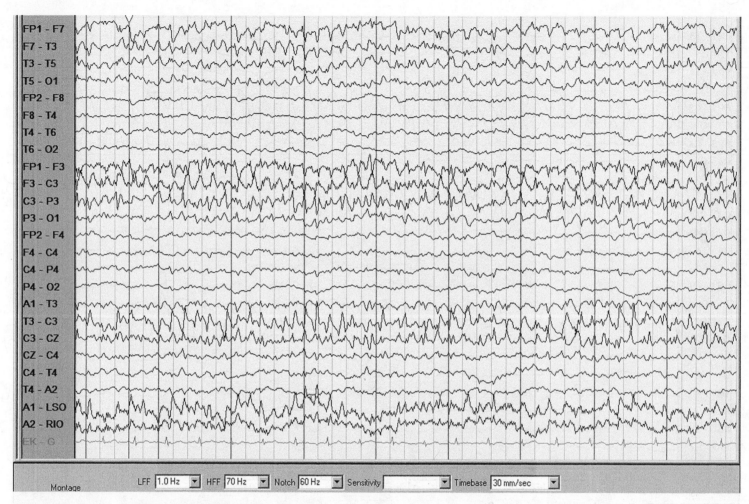

LFF	1.0 Hz	
HFF	70 Hz	
Notch	60 Hz	
Sensitivity		
Timebase	30 mm/sec	

Montage

FIGURE 7-25   **EEG; 10 second page.**

Clinical: 10-year-old girl with partial status epilepticus.

EEG: Epilepsia partialis continua with left frontally predominant spike activity.

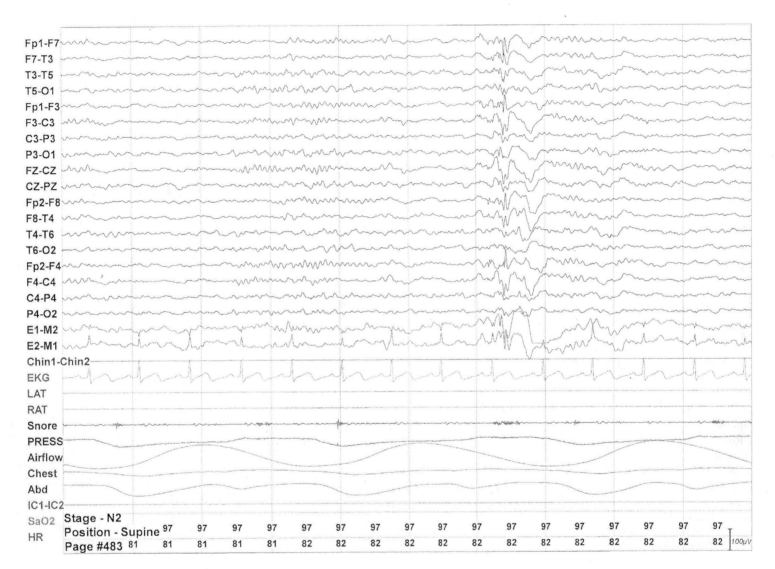

FIGURE 7-26   **Polysomnogram: Expanded EEG montage; 30 second page.**
Clinical: 42-year-old man with poor sleep and a history of epilepsy.
Staging: Stage 2 sleep.
Respiratory: Normal respirations.
EEG: Diffusely distributed spike and wave discharge.

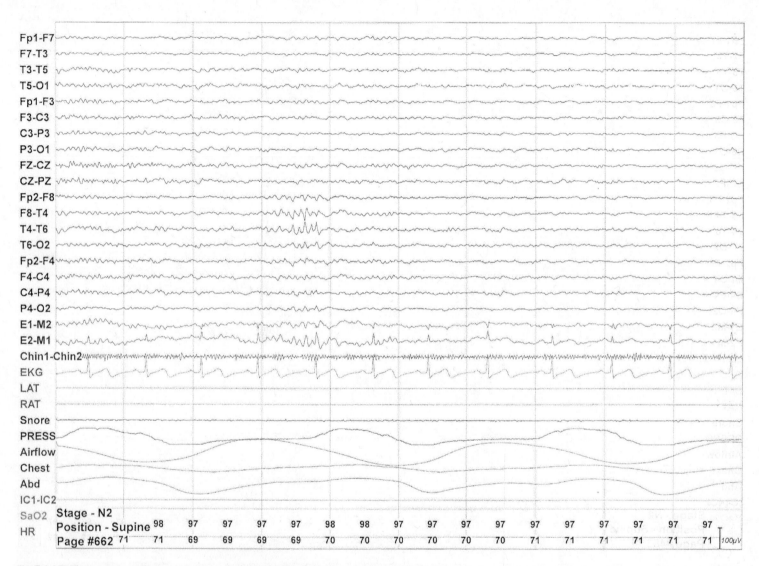

FIGURE 7-27   **Polysomnogram: Expanded EEG montage; 30 second page.**
Clinical: 42-year-old man with poor sleep and a history of epilepsy.
Staging: Stage 2 sleep.
Respiratory: Normal respirations.
EEG: Asymmetric background activity with right hemispheric theta activity.

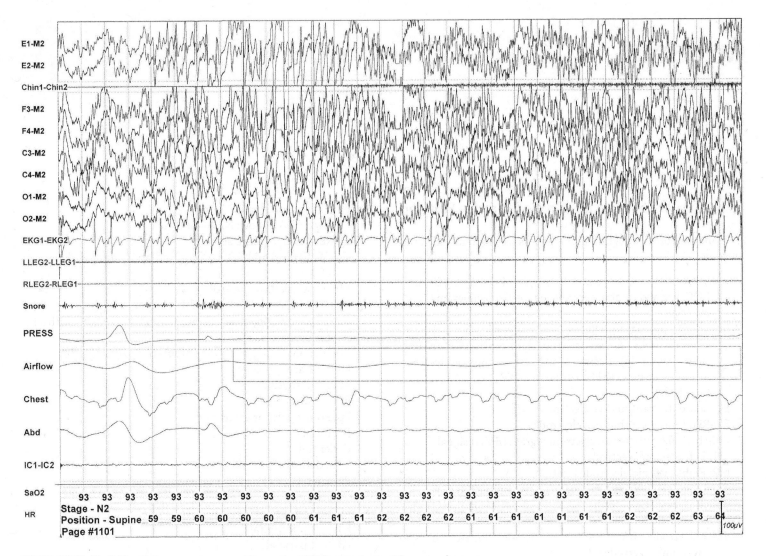

FIGURE 7-28   **Polysomnogram: Expanded EEG montage; 30 second page.**

Clinical: 39-year-old man with witnessed apneas and morning confusion.

Staging: Stage 2 sleep.

Respiratory: Apnea associated with a seizure.

EEG: Seizure activity identified in the EEG and EOG derivations.

Artifacts

James D. Geyer, MD and Paul R. Carney, MD

Key for Channels Used in the Examples Provided

The standard polysomnogram montage was used and included the following:

- Electro-oculogram (left, LOC-A2; right, ROC-A1): LOC and ROC, left and right outer canthus electro-oculogram (EOG) electrodes
- Electroencephalogram (EEG), C3-A2, C4-A1, F3-A2, F4-A1, O1-A2, and O2-A1, left central, right central, left frontal, right frontal, left occipital, and right occipital; electrode location, ground (FPZ), reference (CZ), and A1 and A2 (mastoids)
- E1: Left outer canthus eye electrode
- E2: Right outer canthus eye electrode
- Chin1-Chin2: Submental electromyogram (EMG) signal
- M1: Left mastoid electrode location
- M2: Right mastoid electrode location
- C3, F3, and O1: Left central, frontal, and occipital EEG electrodes
- C4, F4, and O2: Right central, frontal, and occipital EEG electrodes
- EMG electrodes: LAT1-LAT2 and RAT1-RAT2, left and right lower limb electrodes
- Two standard electrocardiogram (ECG) leads are included: ECG1-ECG2, ECG2-ECG3
- SNORE: Snore sensor sound

N/O: Nasal/oral thermistor
ORAL/N/O AIR-flow: Nasal–oral airflow
NPRE: Nasal pressure signal
THOR/CHEST and ABD: Chest and abdominal walls motion effort
MFLO: Mask flow of CPAP
P_{CO_2}: Pressure in mm Hg of carbon dioxide
SpO_2: Percent oxygen desaturation by pulse oximetry with a finger probe
Pt Position: Patient position (supine, left, right, prone)
NPRE: Nasal pressure
Pleth: Plethysmography
EEG electrodes:
Fp: Frontopolar or prefrontal
F: Frontal
C: Central
T: Temporal
P: Parietal
O: Occipital
A: Ear or mastoid
F3: Left midfrontal
P3: Left parietal
T4: Right temporal
A1: Right ear
Cz: Vertex

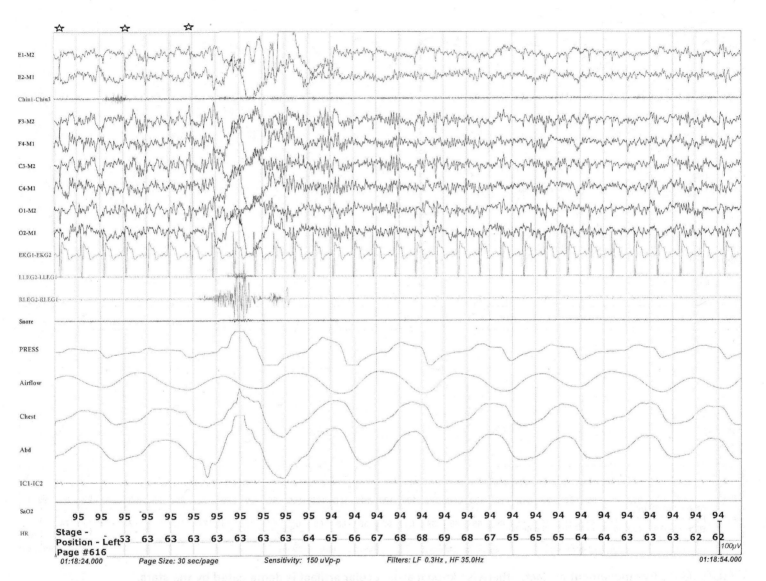

FIGURE 8-1 **ECG artifact in the EEG, EOG, and chin EMG.**
These sharply contoured waveforms can be confirmed as an ECG artifact by their correlation with the ECG channel. (Copyright James Geyer and JNP Media, 2016. Used with permission.)

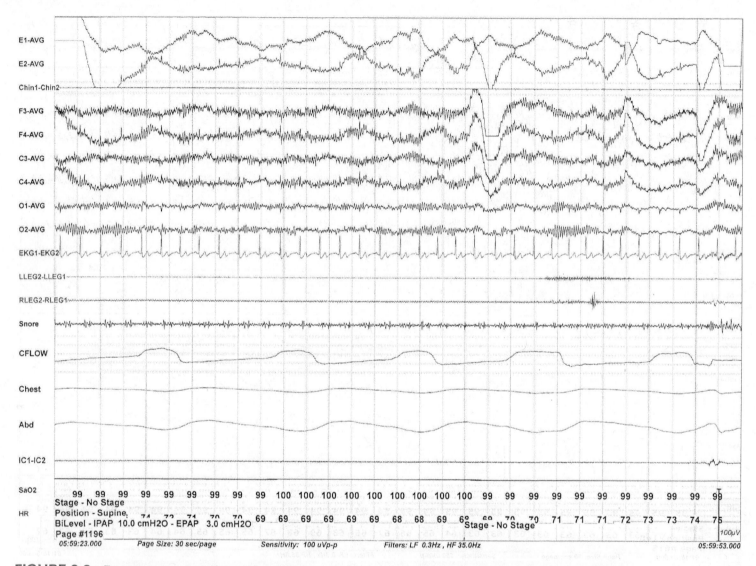

FIGURE 8-2 **Eye movement artifact, otherwise known as an ocular artifact is demarcated by the stars.**
The eye is a charged dipole (much like a battery). The positive pole is at the cornea and the negative pole is at the retina. The EOG consists of a bipolar linkage from the ROC electrode, 1 cm lateral and 1 cm superior to one outer canthus, to the LOC electrode, 1 cm lateral and 1 cm inferior to the other outer canthus. The electrode toward which the eyes move becomes relatively positive and the other relatively negative. (Copyright James Geyer and Neurotexion, 2016. Used with permission.)

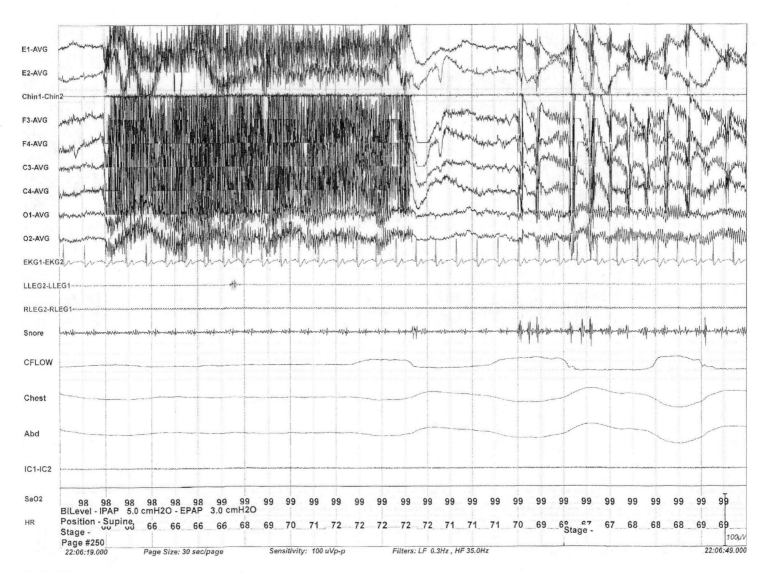

FIGURE 8-3 **Bruxism.**
Bruxism or tooth grinding is a prevalent type of *parafunctional oromotor activity* and is categorized as a sleep-related movement disorder. Sleep bruxism is a stereotyped movement disorder characterized by grinding or clenching of the teeth during sleep. (Copyright James Geyer and JNP Media, 2016. Used with permission.)

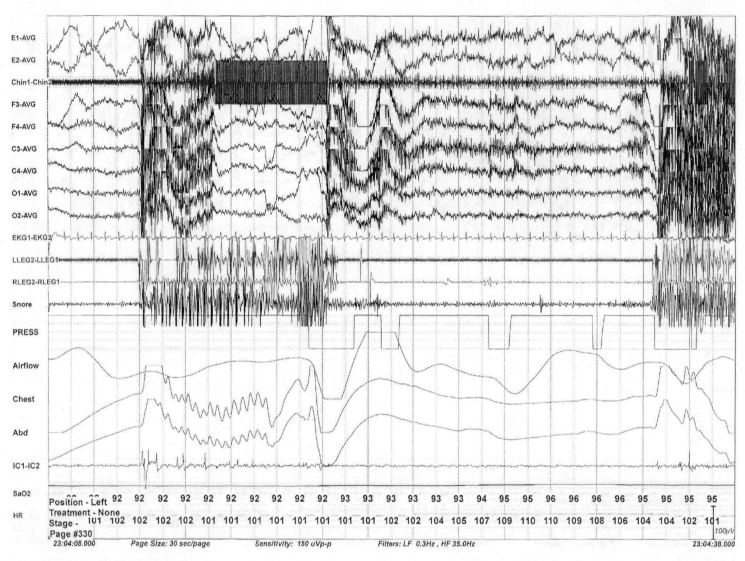

FIGURE 8-4   **Cough artifact.**

The patient has a history of lung cancer which predisposes the patient to coughing. The findings associated with a cough relate in part to the forcefulness of the cough. A hiccup has some similarities but occurs with a sudden contraction of the muscles of inspiration and closure of the glottis, which produces the characteristic sound. (Copyright James Geyer and JNP Media, 2016. Used with permission.)

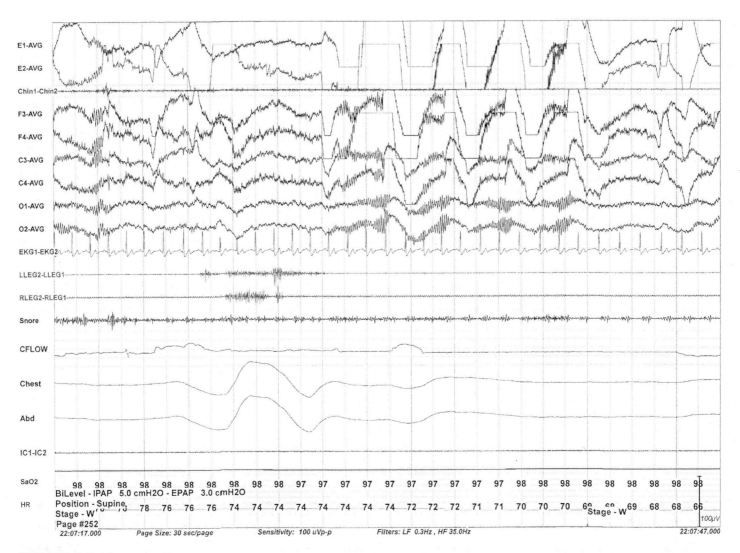

FIGURE 8-5 Sweat artifact.
Sweat artifact is identified by a high amplitude and slow-frequency waveforms typically with superimposed EEG activity. This may sometimes be erroneously labeled as slow-wave sleep (stage N3) by an inexperienced technologist or polysomnographer. The electro-oculogram (EOG) and EEG electrodes are the regions most frequently affected by sweat artifact. The slow frequencies seen with sweat artifact are typically much slower than stage N3 and usually have superimposed faster frequencies. The most appropriate way to correct the artifact is by cooling the patient, removing the electrode or electrodes affected by sweating and drying the area, or even applying an antiperspirant. (Copyright James Geyer and JNP Media, 2016. Used with permission.)

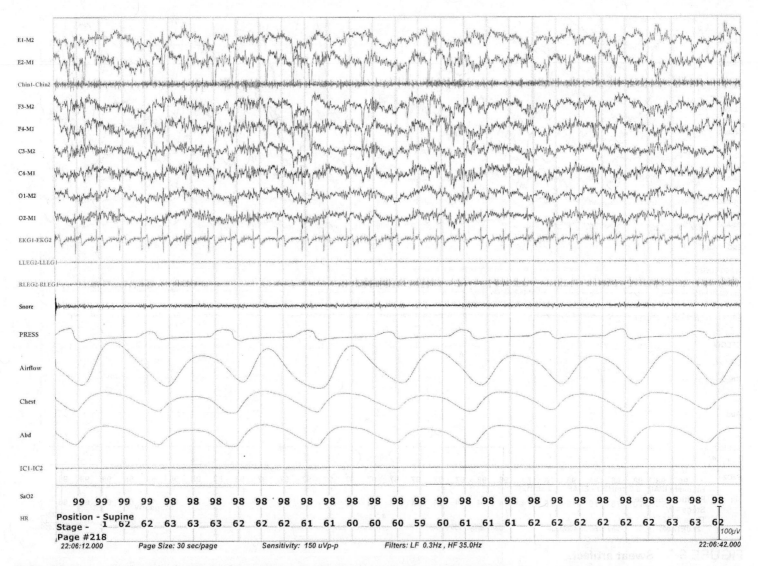

FIGURE 8-6   **Left artificial eye with metallic components and eyelid dysfunction.**
An ocular prosthesis results in a loss of the dipole and therefore the loss of the left EOG signal. Some patients with prosthetic eyes have prosthetic hardware containing metallic components that may act as a dipole generating a typically smaller electrical potential that may appear as a low-amplitude eye movement when compared with the normal eye. (Copyright James Geyer and JNP Media, 2016. Used with permission.)

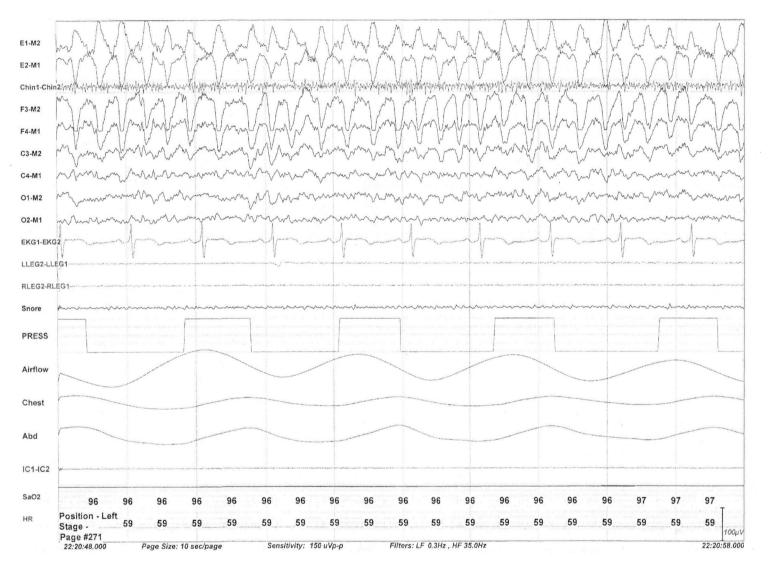

FIGURE 8-7 Eye flutter.
This may be seen with certain ocular disorders and in psychiatric conditions including anxiety and panic.
(Copyright James Geyer and JNP Media, 2016. Used with permission.)

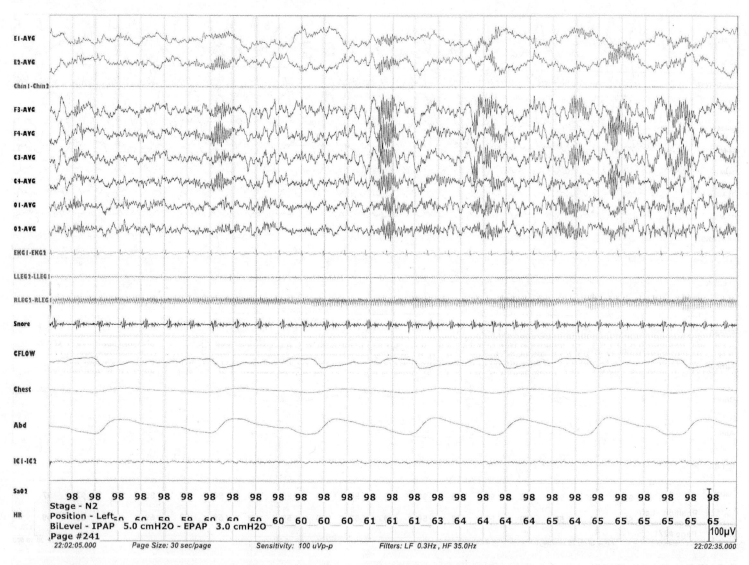

FIGURE 8-8 **Abnormal eye movements related to selective serotonin reuptake inhibitor use, revealed in the EOG channels.** Prominent eye movements are seen during non-REM (NREM) stage N2 sleep. These abnormal eye movements during NREM sleep have been described in patients taking SSRIs such as fluoxetine, paroxetine, citalopram, and escitalopram. (Copyright James Geyer and JNP Media, 2016. Used with permission.)

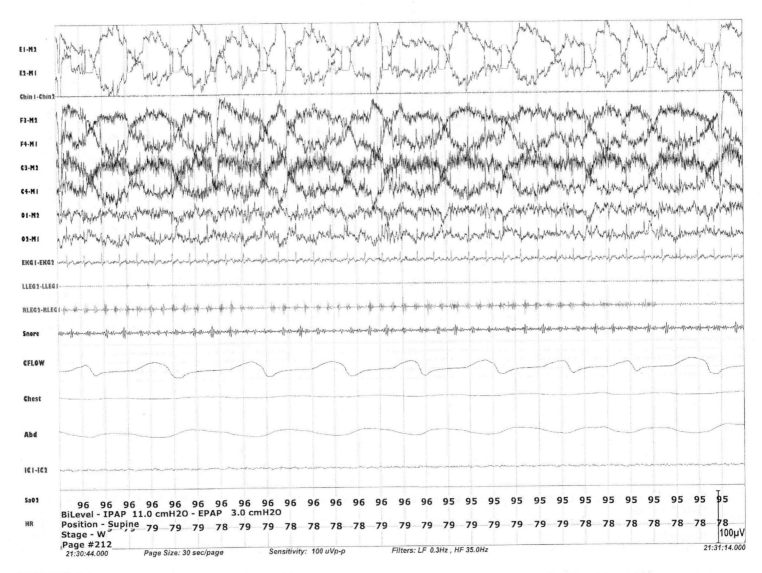

FIGURE 8-9   Reading artifact in the ocular leads.
The unique feature of this artifact is demonstrated by the repetitive rhythmic pattern compatible with reading. (Copyright James Geyer and JNP Media, 2016. Used with permission.)

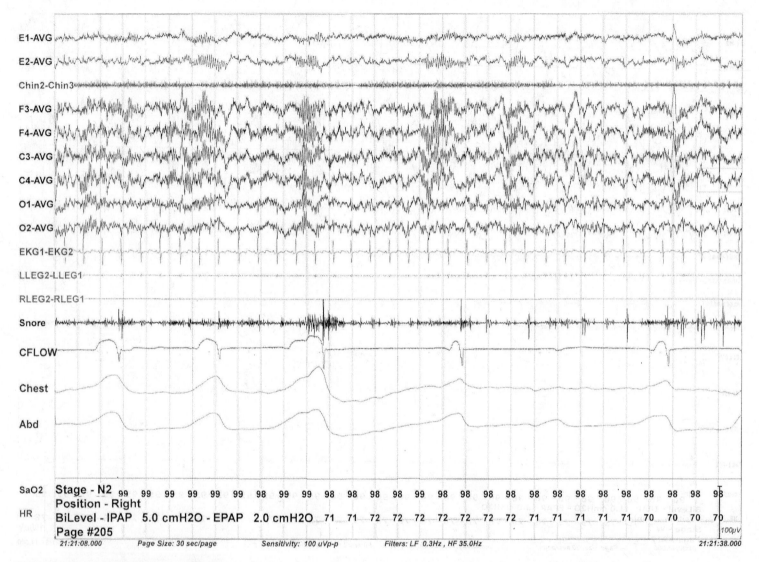

FIGURE 8-10 Mask flow artifact.
The morphology of the mask flow channel displays the characteristic sharp dip at the end of each breath below the baseline level. (Copyright James Geyer and JNP Media, 2016. Used with permission.)

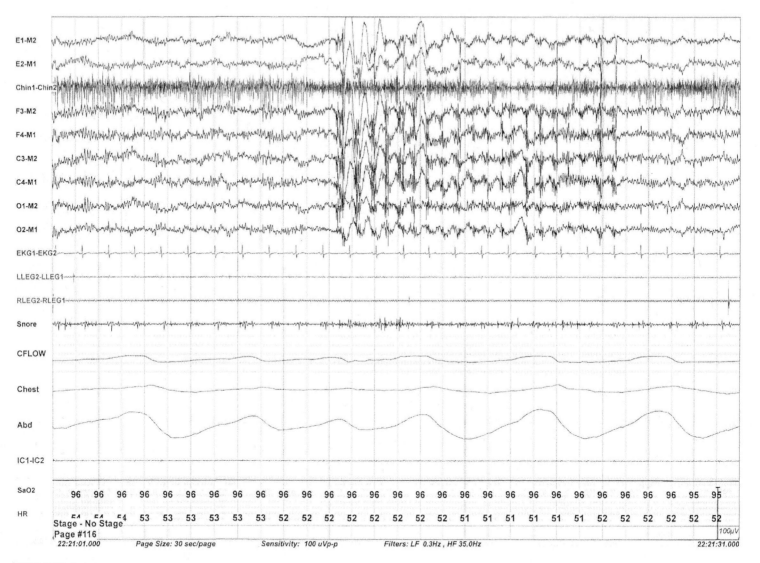

FIGURE 8-11 **Chewing artifact from the patient eating.**
The chewing motion, occurring during wakefulness, originates in the chin with spread to the other EEG electrodes, which is similar to the pattern seen with bruxism. (Copyright James Geyer and JNP Media, 2016. Used with permission.)

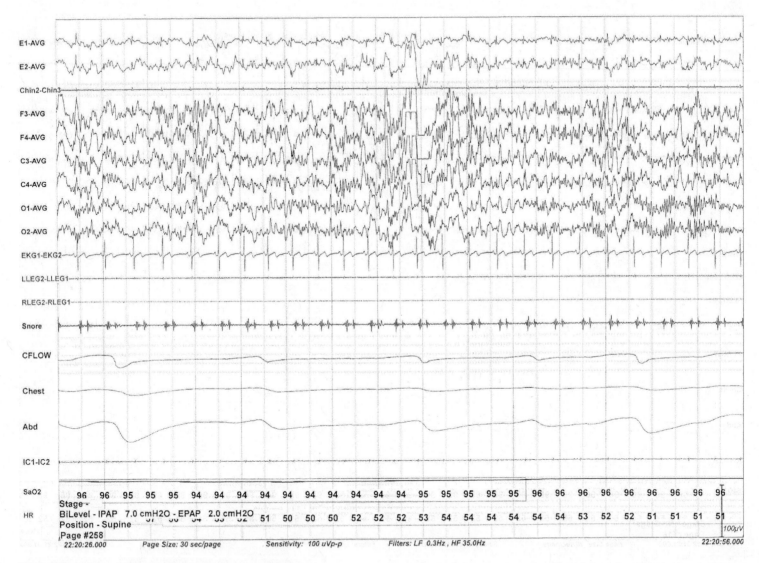

FIGURE 8-12   **Pulse artifact in the snore lead.**

It comes after each QRS complex. It is not at the exact time of the QRS. (Copyright James Geyer and JNP Media, 2016. Used with permission.)

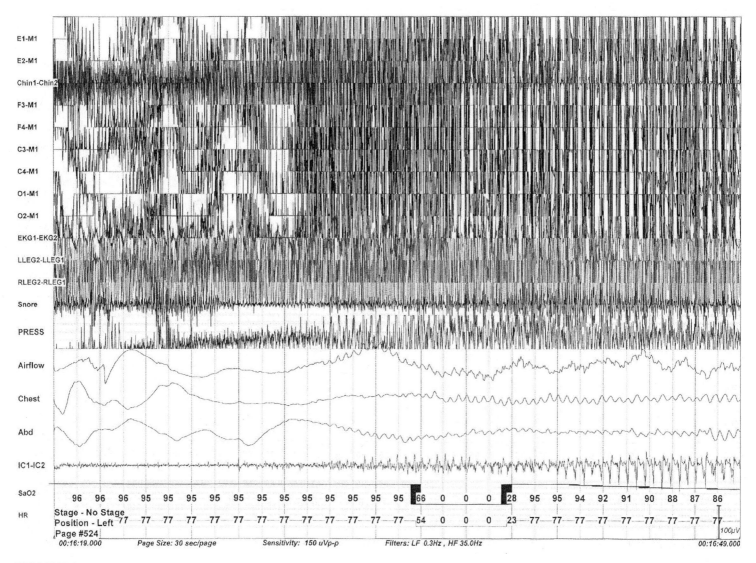

FIGURE 8-13 **Muscle artifact caused by seizure activity.** (Copyright James Geyer and Neurotexion, 2016. Used with permission.)

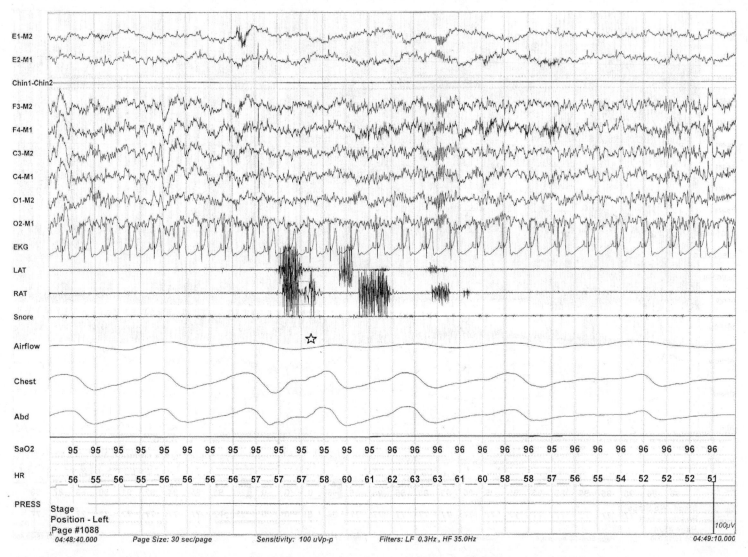

FIGURE 8-14 **The thermocouple is not picking up the necessary temperature differential (denoted by the star in the airflow channel).**
The nasal/oral (N/O) signal is derived from a thermocouple and is qualitative as opposed to quantitative; it allows recording of the fluctuations in temperature that occur during inspiration of relatively cooler air and expiration of relatively warmer air. (Copyright James Geyer and Neurotexion, 2016. Used with permission.)

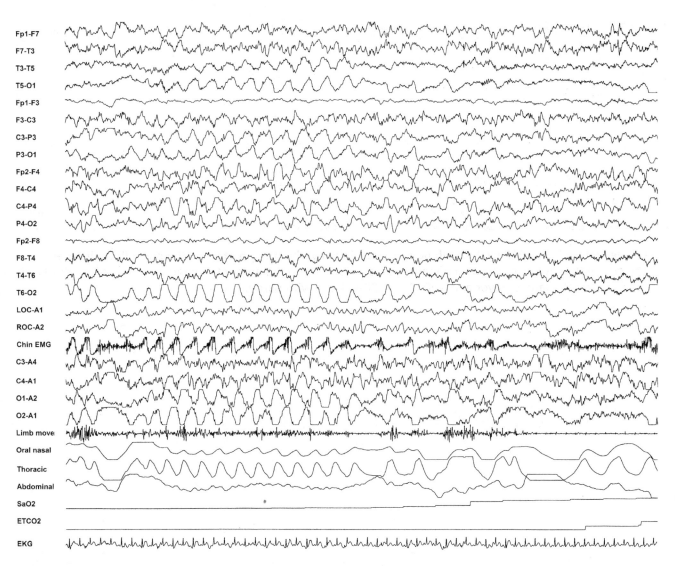

FIGURE 8-15 Patting artifact.
A 16-month-old girl has episodes of possible pauses in breathing during sleep reported by her parents.
She had difficulty falling asleep with the monitors in place. (Copyright James Geyer and JNP Media, 2016.
Used with permission.)

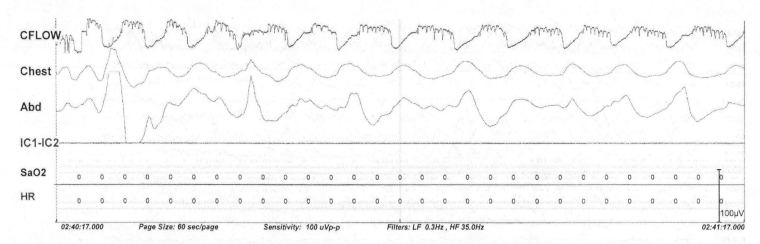

FIGURE 8-16 **Condensation in the PAP system tubing can result in a reverberating pattern in the mask flow channel.**
The size of the reverberation on inspiration depends in part on the amount of condensation and on the mask flow. (Copyright James Geyer and JNP Media, 2016. Used with permission.)

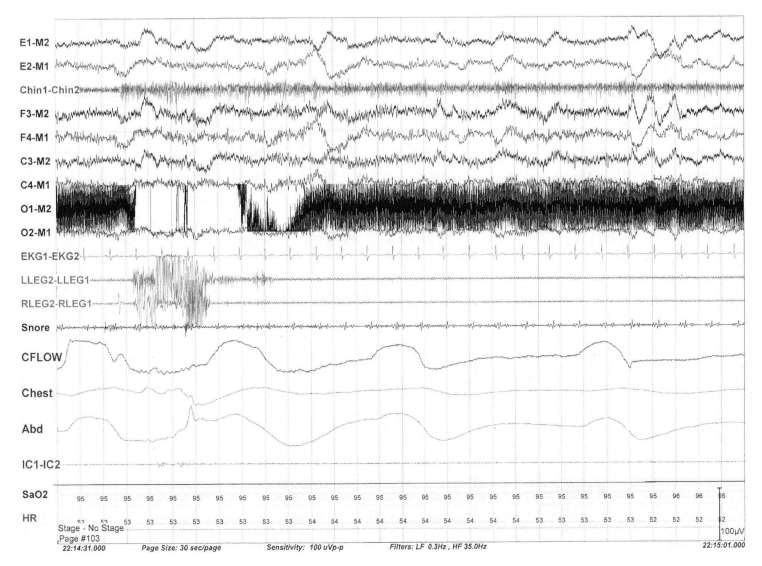

FIGURE 8-17 **Loose connection at the O1 electrode.** (Copyright James Geyer and JNP Media, 2016. Used with permission.)

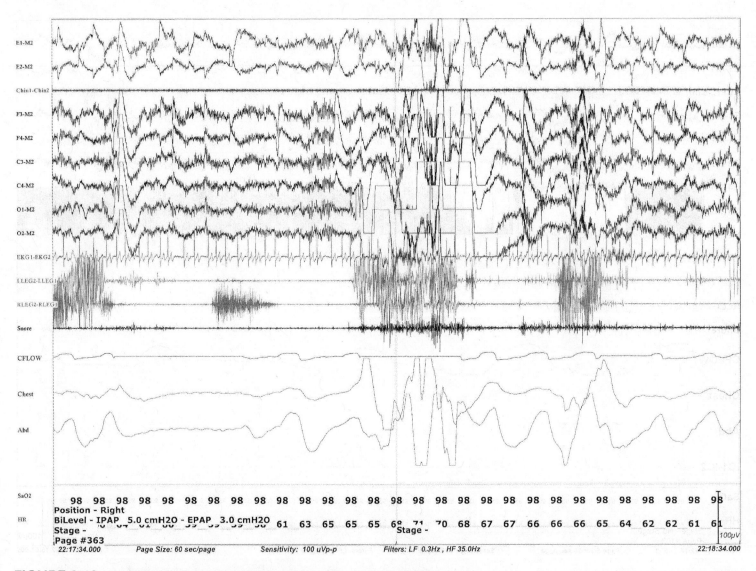

FIGURE 8-18 **Cardioballistic artifact during an episode of central sleep apnea.**
Cardioballistic artifact corresponds to cardiac pulsations, which are transmitted through the rib cage and are typically most apparent in the thoracic channel. It may also be picked up by the EEG electrodes. (Copyright James Geyer and JNP Media, 2016. Used with permission.)

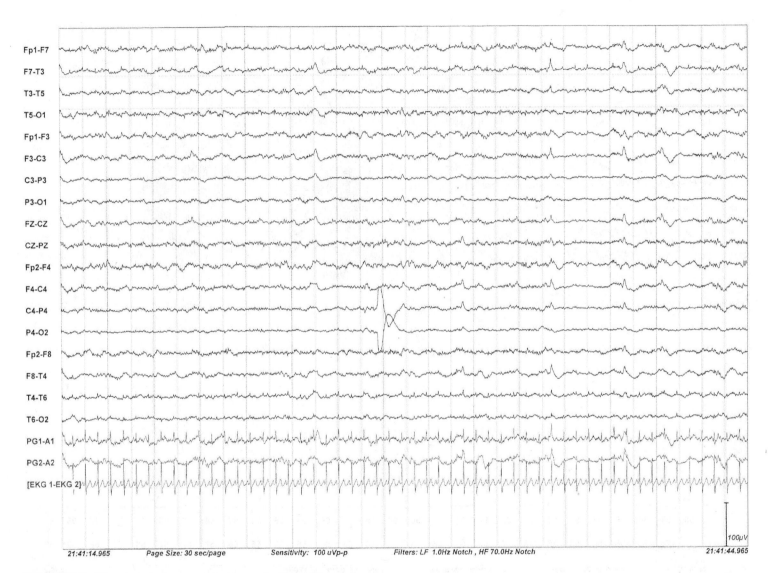

FIGURE 8-19   Electrode pop at electrode P4, which is loose.
Electrode pop artifact is caused by an electrode that may be unstable because of insufficient conductive paste, poor or intermittent contact of the electrode with the skin, or a faulty electrode cup or wire. This creates a capacitance effect. (Copyright James Geyer and Neurotexion, 2016. Used with permission.)

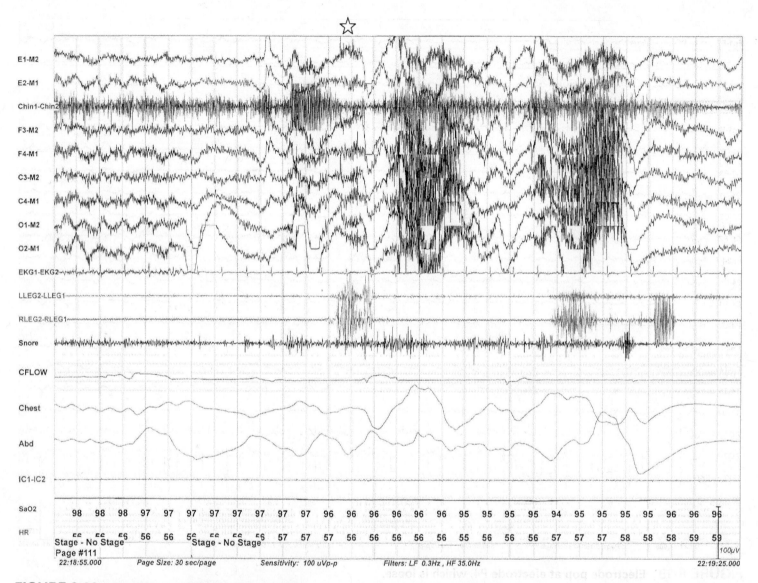

FIGURE 8-20 **Swallow or glossokinetic artifact.**
Like the eyeball, the tongue also functions as a dipole, with the tip being negative (–) with respect to the base (+). The tip of the tongue is relatively more mobile with respect to the tongue base. (Copyright James Geyer and JNP Media, 2016. Used with permission.)

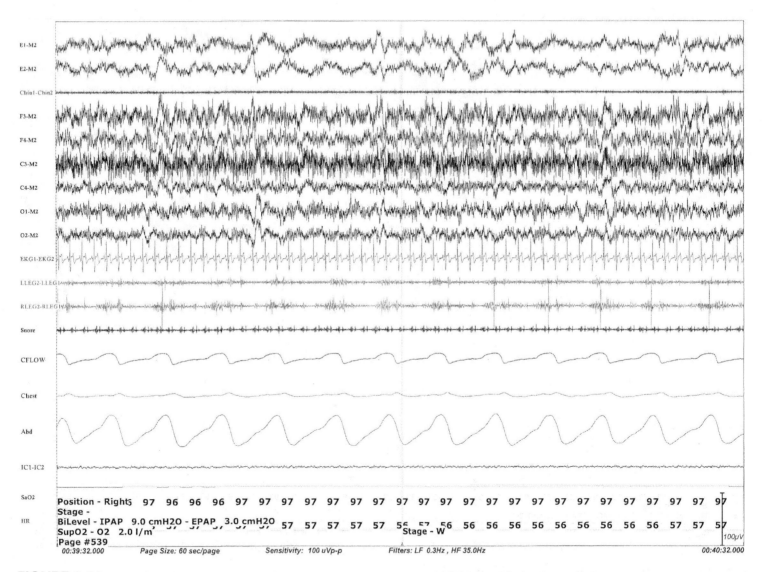

FIGURE 8-21   **60-Hz artifact.** (Copyright James Geyer and JNP Media, 2016. Used with permission.)

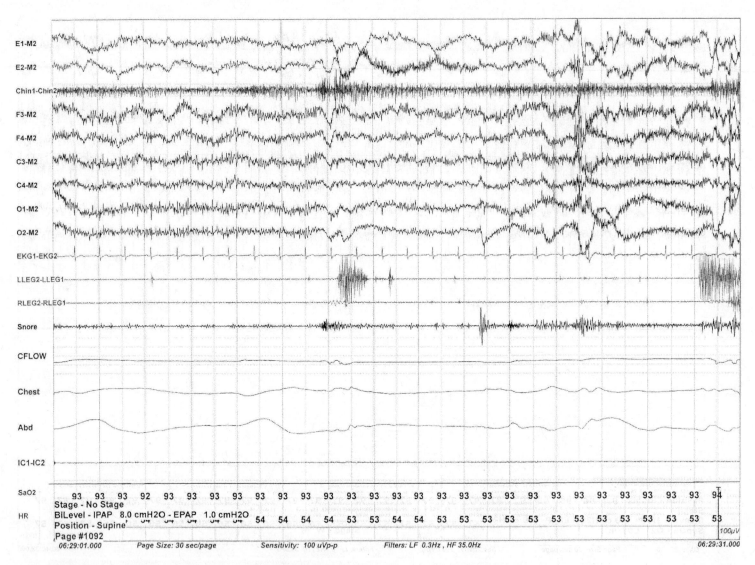

FIGURE 8-22   **Reading with poor focus on the paper.**
Notice that the eye movements have two different slope morphologies: one that is faster returning to the next line, and the slower as the line is read. Reading artifact can be confirmed by viewing the corresponding video image. (Copyright James Geyer and JNP Media, 2016. Used with permission.)

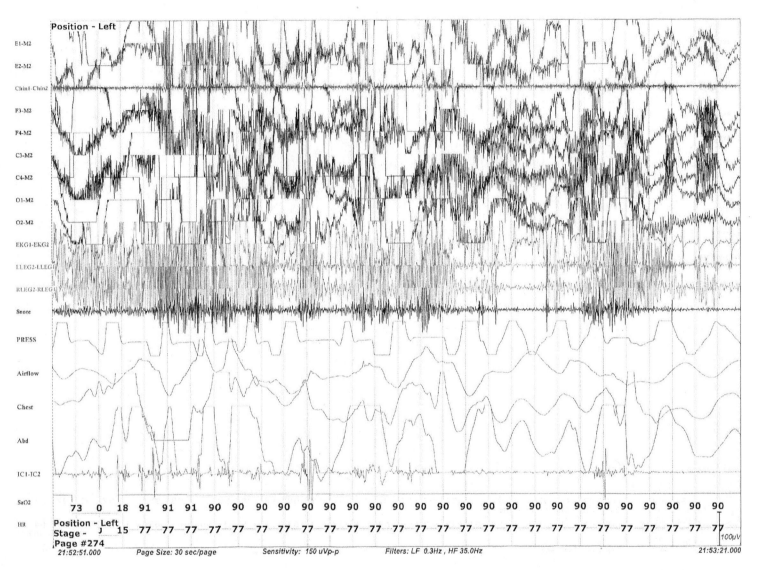

FIGURE 8-23 Movement artifact from the patient getting settled.
This consists of motor activity that does not represent any specific rhythm but that of the patient's normal movement at the time of recording. (Copyright James Geyer and JNP Media, 2016. Used with permission.)

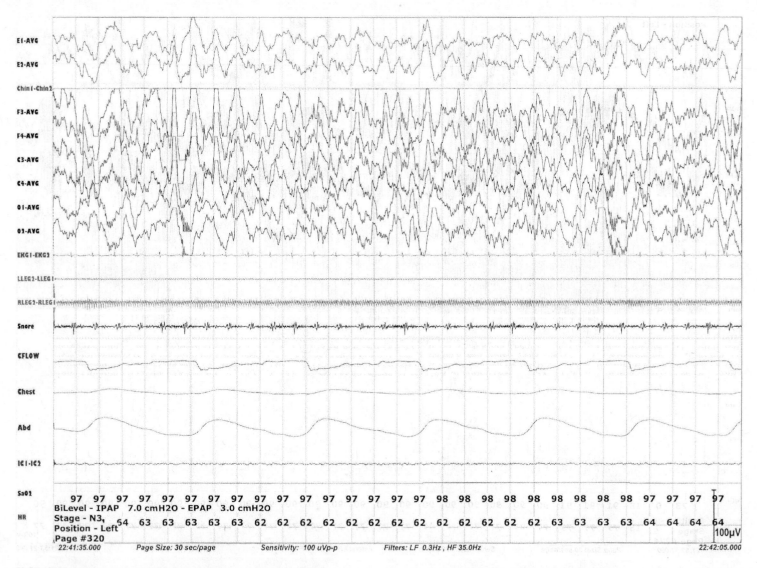

FIGURE 8-24 **Stage 3 delta activity in the eye leads.** (Copyright James Geyer and JNP Media, 2016. Used with permission.)

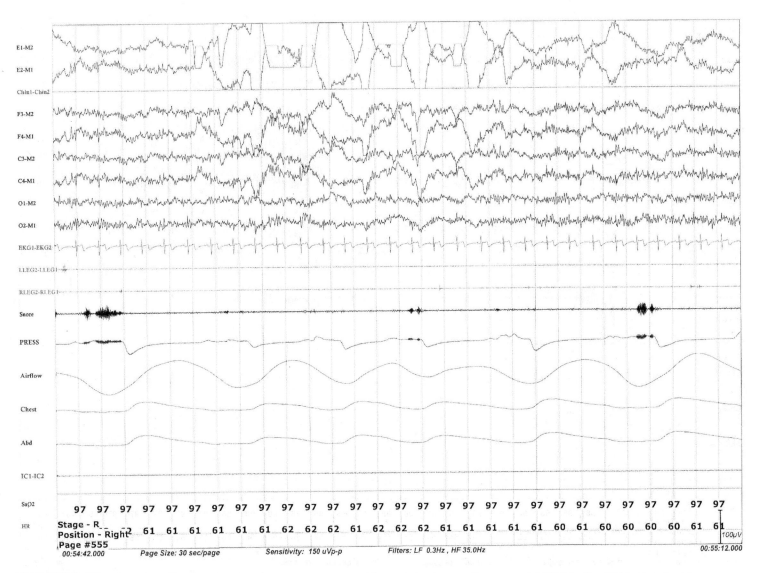

FIGURE 8-25 **Snore artifact in the nasal pressure sensor.** (Copyright James Geyer and JNP Media, 2016. Used with permission.)

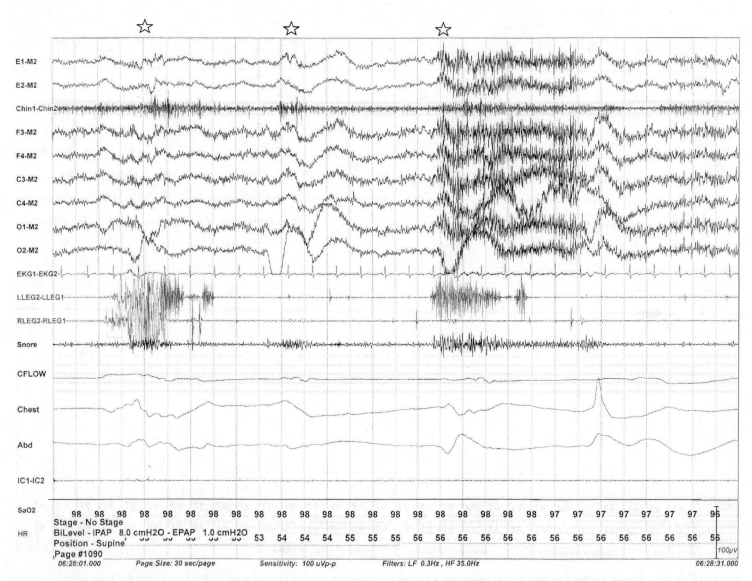

FIGURE 8-26   **Scratching.** (Copyright James Geyer and JNP Media, 2016. Used with permission.)

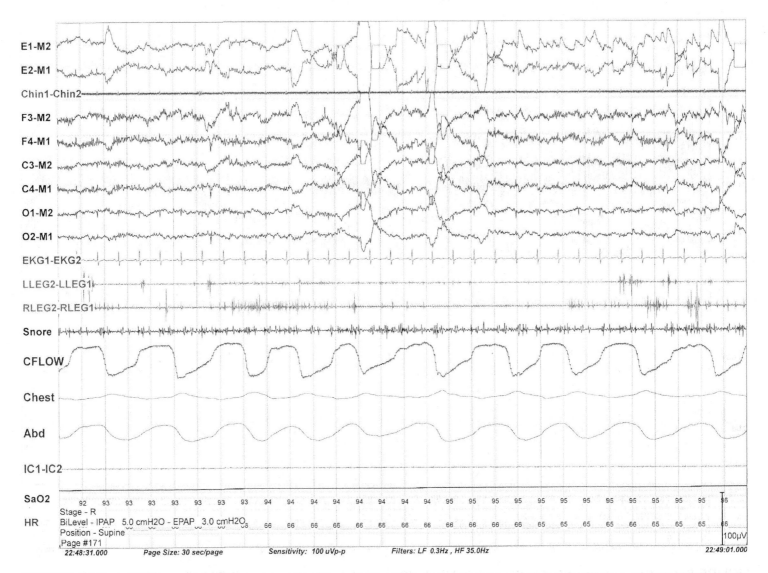

FIGURE 8-27 **REM sleep with eye movement artifacts in the EEG channels.** (Copyright James Geyer and JNP Media, 2016. Used with permission.)

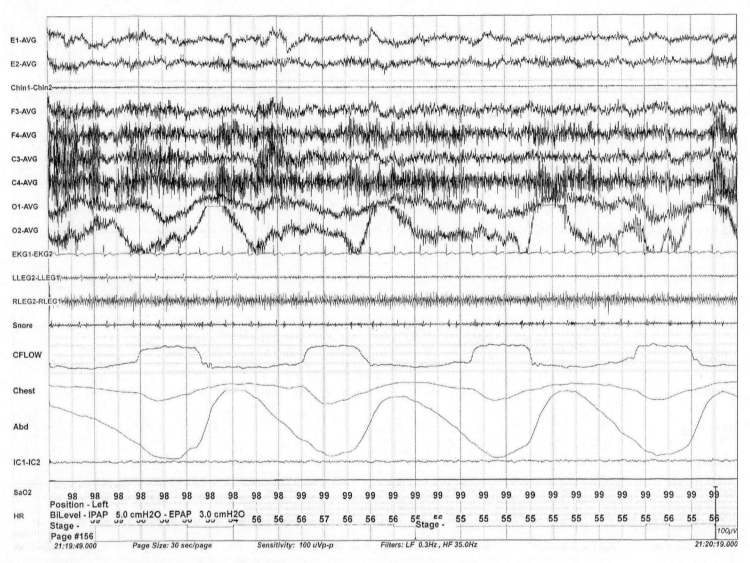

FIGURE 8-28 **Respiratory artifact in the occipital leads.** (Copyright James Geyer and JNP Media, 2016. Used with permission.)

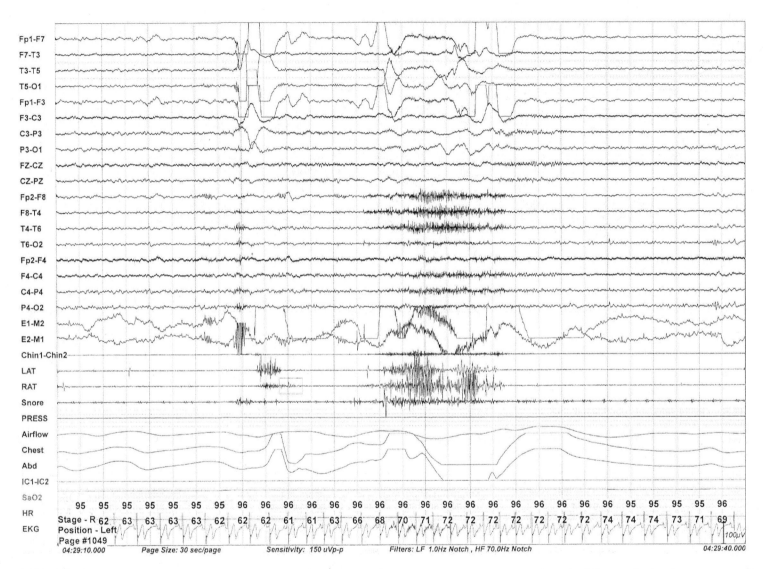

FIGURE 8-29 **RBD with motion artifact.** (Copyright James Geyer and JNP Media, 2016. Used with permission.)

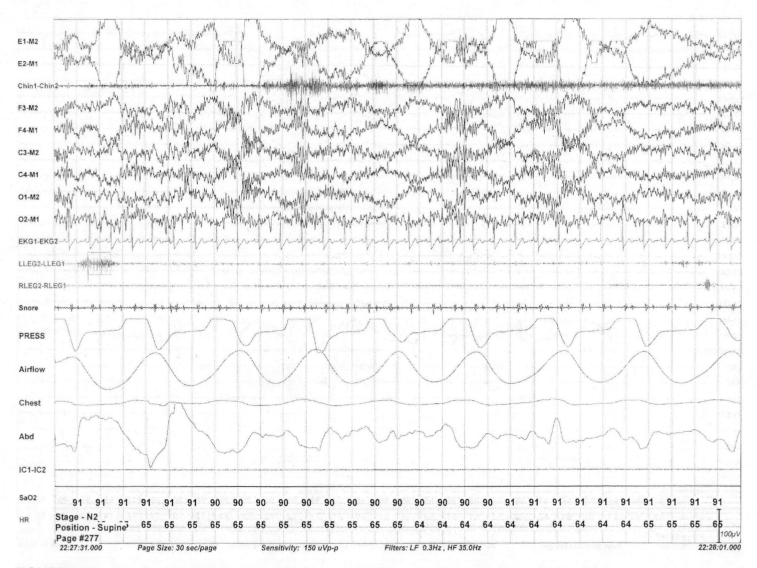

FIGURE 8-30 **Pressure sensor clipping artifact.** (Copyright James Geyer and JNP Media, 2016. Used with permission.)

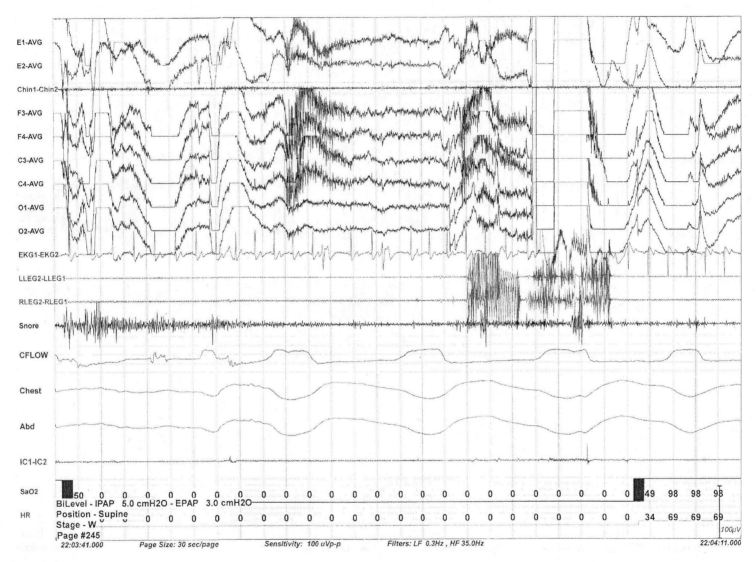

FIGURE 8-31 **Oxygen saturation probe malfunction.** (Copyright James Geyer and JNP Media, 2016. Used with permission.)

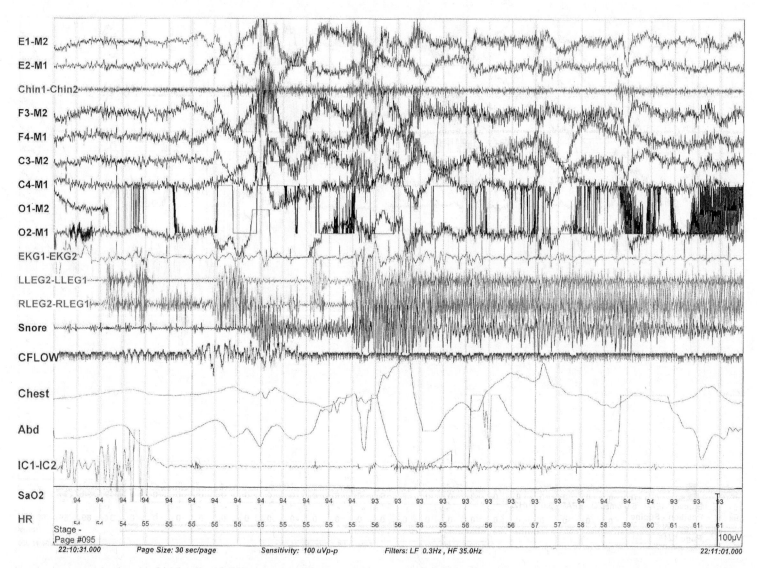

FIGURE 8-32   Movement artifact from getting settled. (Copyright James Geyer and JNP Media, 2016. Used with permission.)

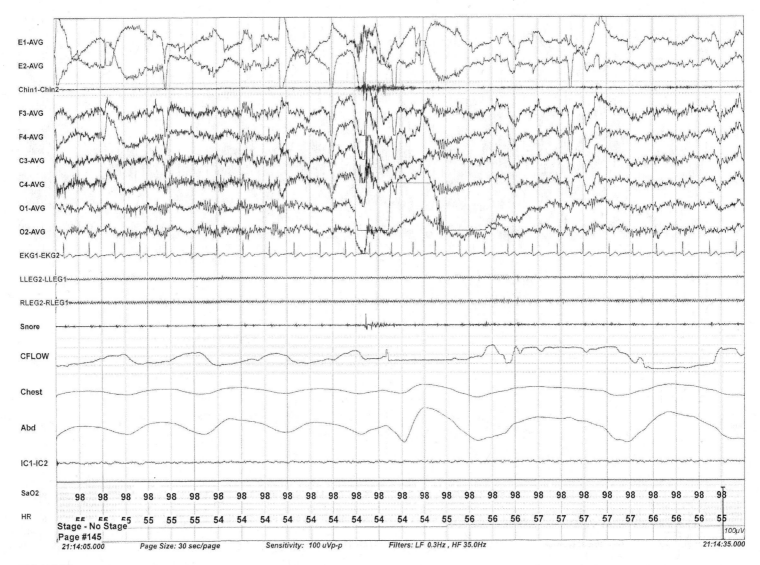

FIGURE 8-33 **Loss of mask flow with motion artifact.** (Copyright James Geyer and JNP Media, 2016. Used with permission.)

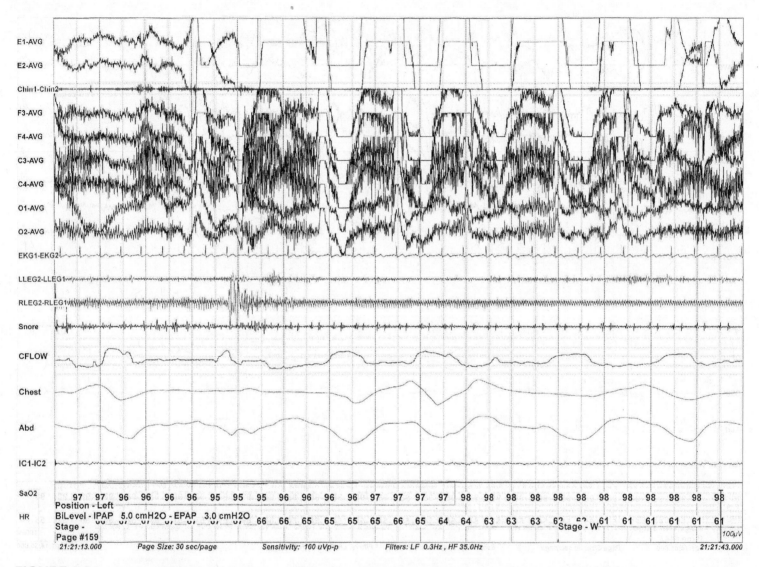

FIGURE 8-34 **Head rolling.** (Copyright James Geyer and JNP Media, 2016. Used with permission.)

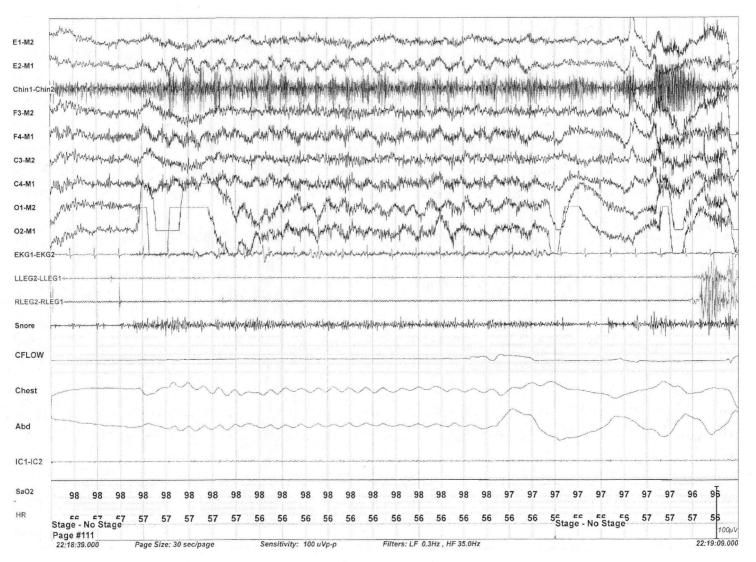

FIGURE 8-35   **Face rubbing.** (Copyright James Geyer and JNP Media, 2016. Used with permission.)

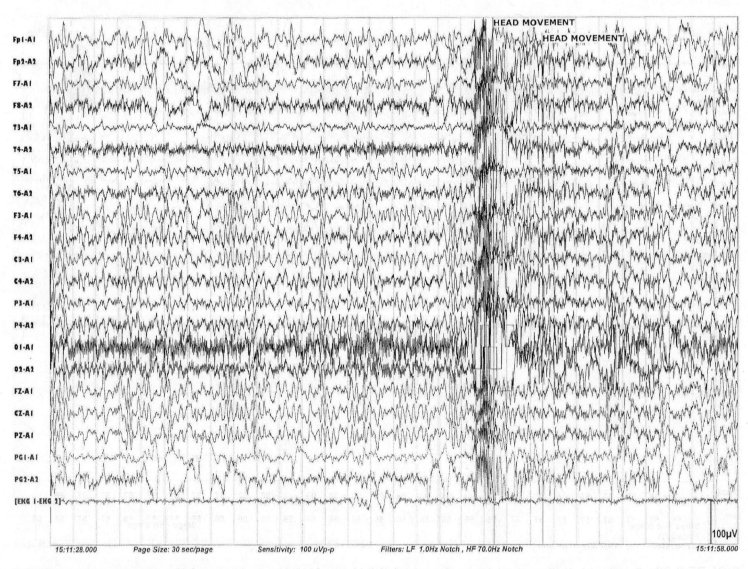

FIGURE 8-36 **Awake slowing in a patient with dementia.** (Copyright James Geyer and Neurotexion, 2016. Used with permission.)

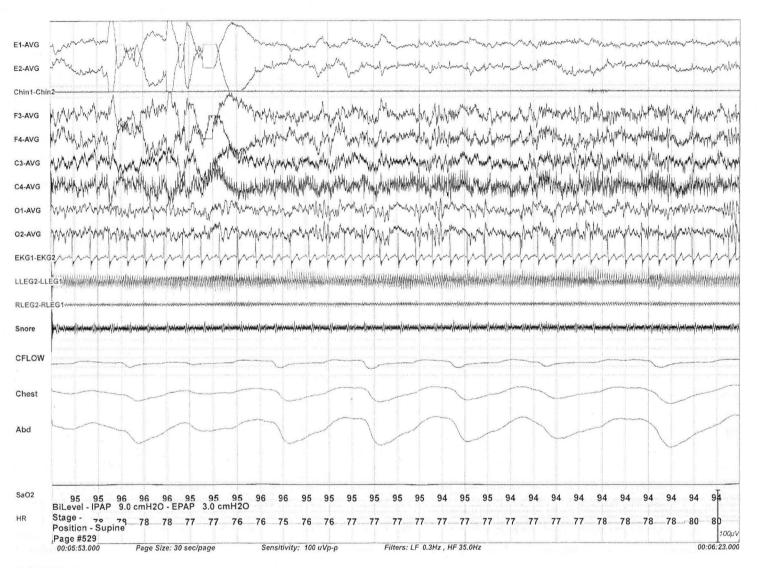

FIGURE 8-37 **Heated tubing.** (Copyright James Geyer and JNP Media, 2016. Used with permission.)

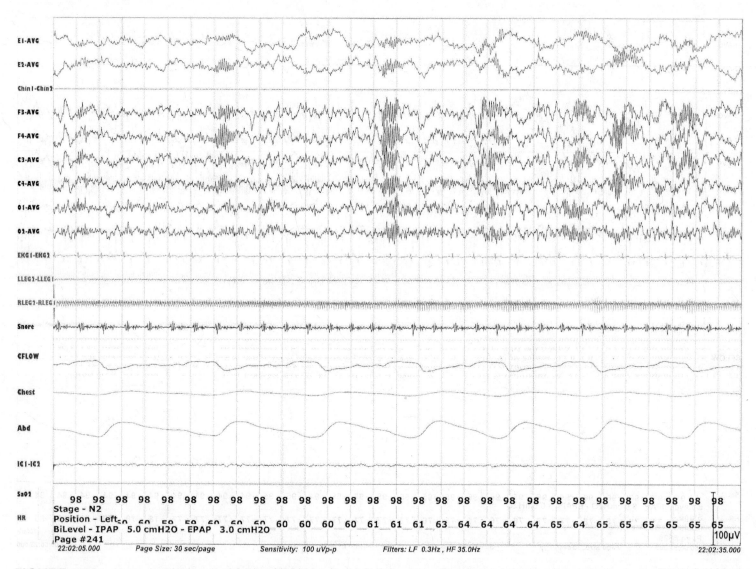

FIGURE 8-38   Sleep spindles in the EOG. (Copyright James Geyer and JNP Media, 2016. Used with permission.)

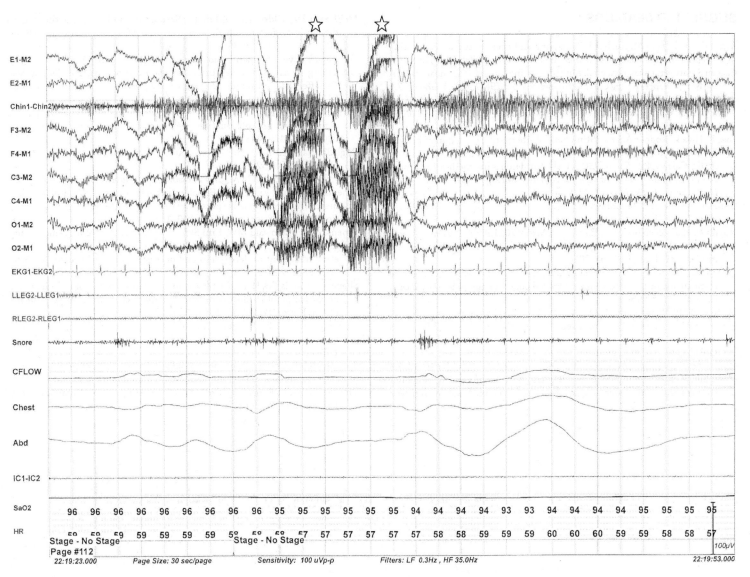

FIGURE 8-39 **Tight eye closure.** (Copyright James Geyer and JNP Media, 2016. Used with permission.)

SUGGESTED READINGS

Armitage R, Trivedi M, Rush AJ. Fluoxetine and oculomotor activity during sleep in depressed patients. *Neuropsychopharmacology* 1995;12(2):159–165.

Cazeau S, Ritter P, Lazarus A, et al. Multisite pacing for end-stage heart failure: Early experience. *Pacing Clin Electrophysiol* 1996;19(11 Pt 2):1748–1757.

de la Hoz-Aizpurua JL, Díaz-Alonso E, LaTouche-Arbizu R, et al. Sleep bruxism. Conceptual review and update. *Med Oral Patol Oral Cir Bucal* 2011;16(2):e231–e238.

Fass R, Higa L, Kodner A, et al. Stimulus and site specific induction of hiccups in the oesophagus of normal subjects. *Gut* 1997;41(5):590–593.

Geyer JD, Carney PR, Dillard SC, et al. Antidepressant medications, neuroleptics, and prominent eye movements during NREM sleep. *J Clin Neurophysiol* 2009;26(1):39–44.

Gordon N. Review: Juvenile myoclonic epilepsy. *Child Care Health Dev* 1994;20(2):71–76.

Huynh N, et al. Sleep bruxism. *Handb Clin Neurol* 2011;99:901–911.

International Classification of Sleep Disorders. 3rd Ed. Westchester, IL: American Academy of Sleep Medicine, 2014.

Lavigne GJ, Rompre PH, Montplaisir JY. Sleep bruxism: Validity of clinical research diagnostic criteria in a controlled polysomnographic study. *J Dent Res* 1996;75(1):546–552.

Mahowald MW. Parasomnias. *Med Clin North Am* 2004;88(3):669–678, ix.

Mahowald M, Schenck C. REM sleep parasomnias. In: Kryger MH, Roth T, Dement WC, eds. *Principles and Practice of Sleep Medicine.* 3rd Ed. Philadelphia, PA: WB Saunders, 2000:724–737.

Marai I, Levi Y. The diverse etiology of hiccups. *Harefuah* 2003;142(1):10–13, 79.

Marshall JB, Landreneau RJ, Beyer KL. Hiccups: Esophageal manometric features and relationship to gastroesophageal reflux. *Am J Gastroenterol* 1990;85(9):1172–1175.

McElreath DP, Olden KW, Aduli F. Hiccups: A subtle sign in the clinical diagnosis of gastric volvulus and a review of the literature. *Dig Dis Sci* 2008;53(11):3033–3036.

O'Regan JK. Eye movements and reading. *Rev Oculomot Res* 1990;4:395–453.

Oksenberg A, Arons E. Sleep bruxism related to obstructive sleep apnea: The effect of continuous positive airway pressure. *Sleep Med* 2002;3(6):513–515.

Ranieri AL, Tufik S, de Siqueira JT. Refractory cluster headache in a patient with bruxism and obstructive sleep apnea: A case report. *Sleep Breath* 2009;13(4):429–433.

Rugh JD, Harlan J. Nocturnal bruxism and temporomandibular disorders. *Adv Neurol* 1988;49:329–341.

Schenck CH, Mahowald MW. REM parasomnias. *Neurol Clin* 1996;14:697–720.

Schenck CH, Mahowald MW. REM sleep behavior disorder: Clinical, developmental, and neuroscience perspectives 16 years after its formal identification in SLEEP. *Sleep* 2002;25(2):120–138.

Schenck CH, Mahowald MW, Kim SW, et al. Prominent eye movements during NREM sleep and REM sleep behavior disorder associated with fluoxetine treatment of depression and obsessive-compulsive disorder. *Sleep* 1992;15(3):226–235.

Shepard J, Harris CD, Hauri PJ. Miscellaneous polysomnographic findings and nocturnal penile tumescence. In: Shepard J, ed. *Atlas of Sleep Medicine.* Mount Kisco, NY: Futura, 1991:215–240.

Siddiqui F, Osuna E, Walters AS, et al. Sweat artifact and respiratory artifact occurring simultaneously in polysomnogram. *Sleep Med* 2006;7(2):197–199.

Spriggs WH. *Essentials of Polysomnography: A Training Guide and Reference for Sleep Technicians.* Carrollton, TX: Sleep Ed., 2008.

The Atlas Task Force. Recording and scoring leg movements. *Sleep* 1993;16(8):748–759.

CHAPTER 9

EKG

James D. Geyer, MD and Paul R. Carney, MD

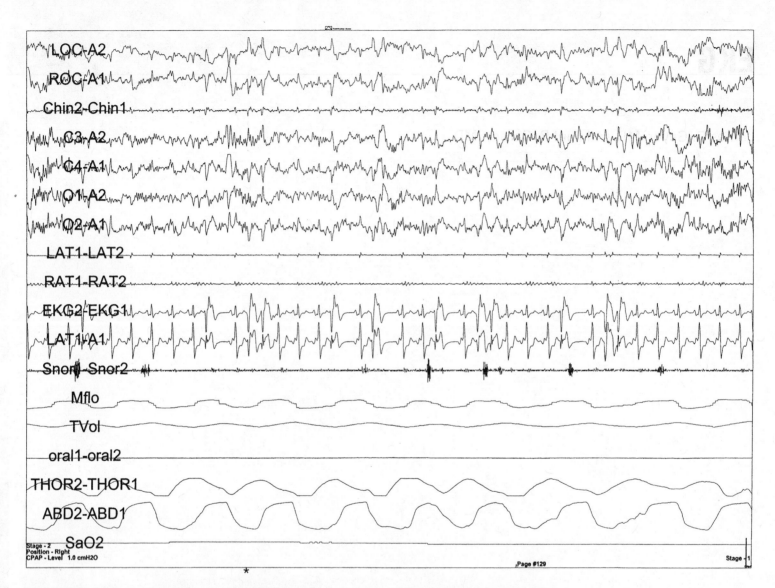

FIGURE 9-1   **Polysomnogram: CPAP montage (prior display montage); 30 second page.**
Clinical: 56-year-old man with snoring and excessive daytime sleepiness.
Staging: Stage 2 sleep.
Respiratory: Intermittent snoring.
EKG: Frequent premature ventricular complexes (PVCs) with couplets (*).

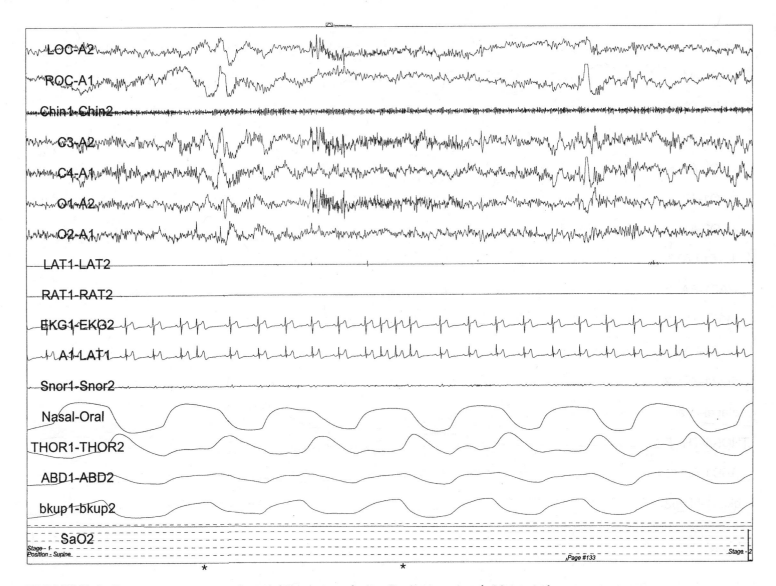

FIGURE 9-2 **Polysomnogram: Standard montage (prior display montage); 30 second page.**

Clinical: 48-year-old woman with intermittent snoring and witnessed apneas.

Staging: Stage 1 sleep.

Respiratory: Normal respirations.

EKG: Narrow premature complexes (*) without definite P waves.

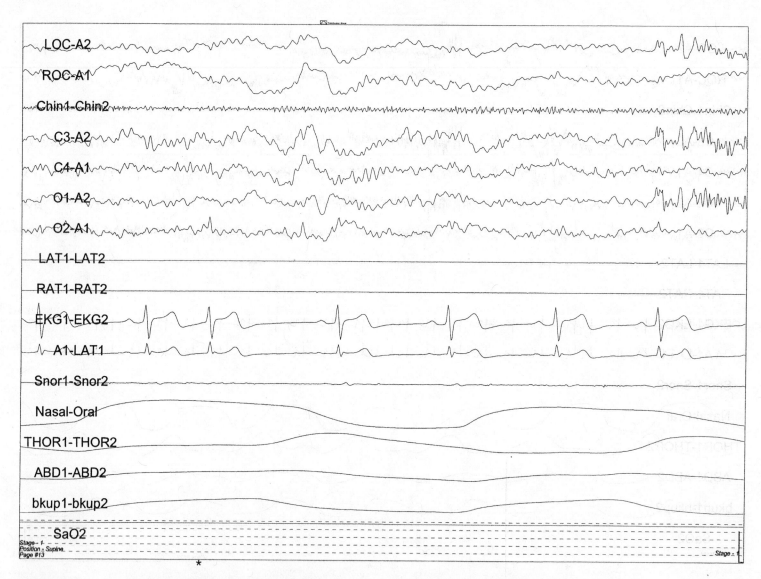

FIGURE 9-3   Polysomnogram: Standard montage (prior display montage); 10 second page.
Clinical: 48-year-old woman with intermittent snoring and witnessed apneas.
Staging: Stage 1 sleep.
Respiratory: Normal respirations.
EKG: Narrow premature complexes (*) without definite P waves.

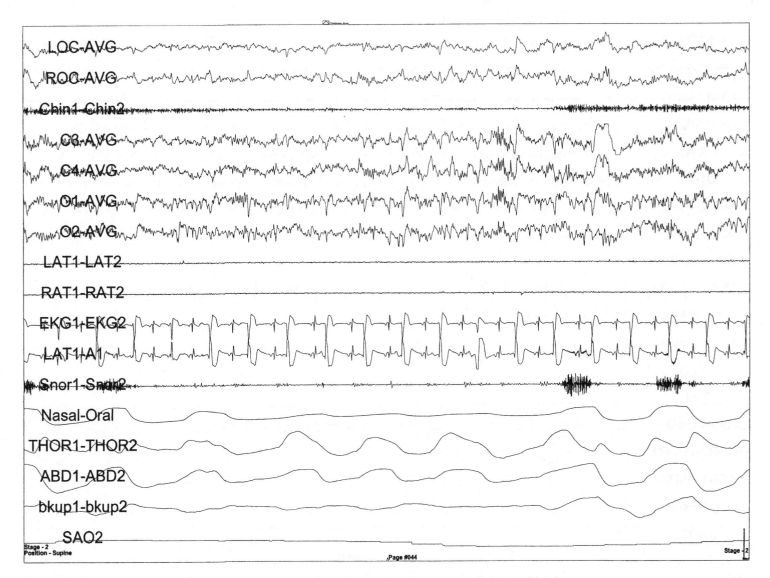

FIGURE 9-4   **Polysomnogram: Standard montage (prior display montage); 30 second page.**
Clinical: 27-year-old man with obstructive sleep apnea.
Staging: Stage 2 sleep.
Respiratory: Apnea followed by an arousal, snoring, and an oxygen desaturation.
EKG: Ventricular bigeminy.

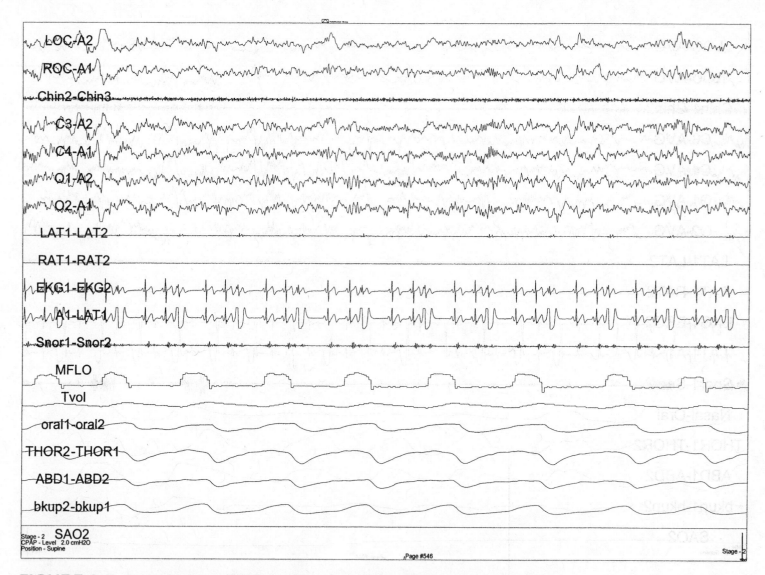

FIGURE 9-5   **Polysomnogram: CPAP montage (prior display montage); 30 second page.**

Clinical: 31-year-old man with obstructive sleep apnea.

Staging: Stage 2 sleep.

Respiratory: Normal respirations.

EKG: Ventricular trigeminy.

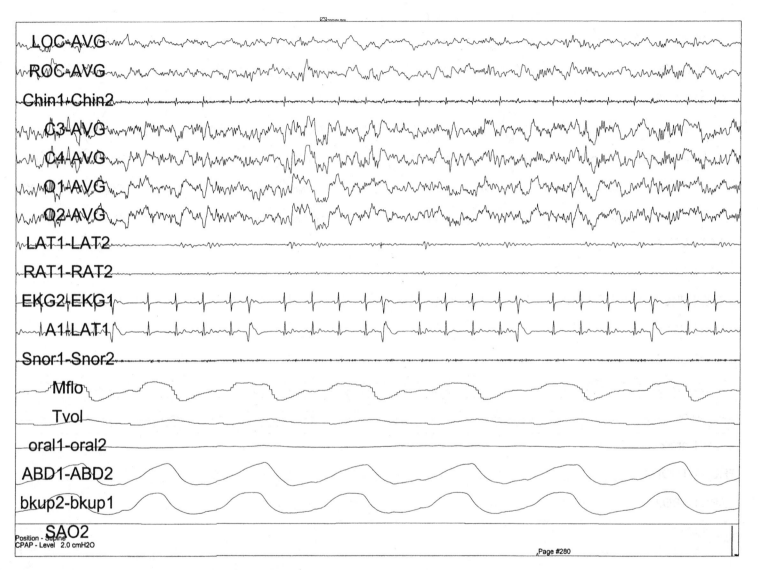

FIGURE 9-6   **Polysomnogram: CPAP montage (prior display montage); 30 second page.**

Clinical: 71-year-old man with obstructive sleep apnea.
Staging: Stage 2 sleep.
Respiratory: Normal respirations.
EKG: Ventricular quintigeminy.

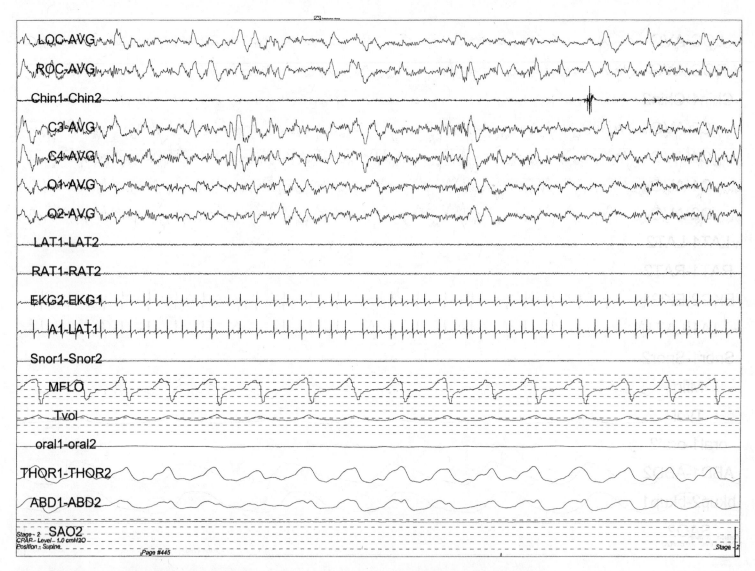

FIGURE 9-7 **Polysomnogram: CPAP montage (prior display montage); 60 second page.**
Clinical: 69-year-old man with obstructive sleep apnea and atrial fibrillation.
Staging: Stage 2 sleep.
Respiratory: Mild variations in respiratory effort.
EKG: Atrial fibrillation.

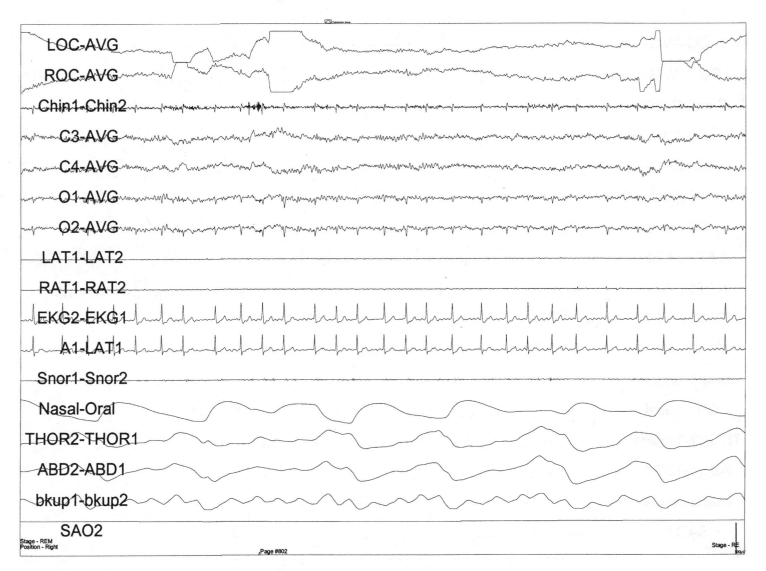

FIGURE 9-8 **Polysomnogram: Standard montage (prior display montage); 30 second page.**
Clinical: 52-year-old man with excessive daytime sleepiness and intermittent atrial fibrillation.
Staging: Stage REM sleep.
EKG: Atrial fibrillation.

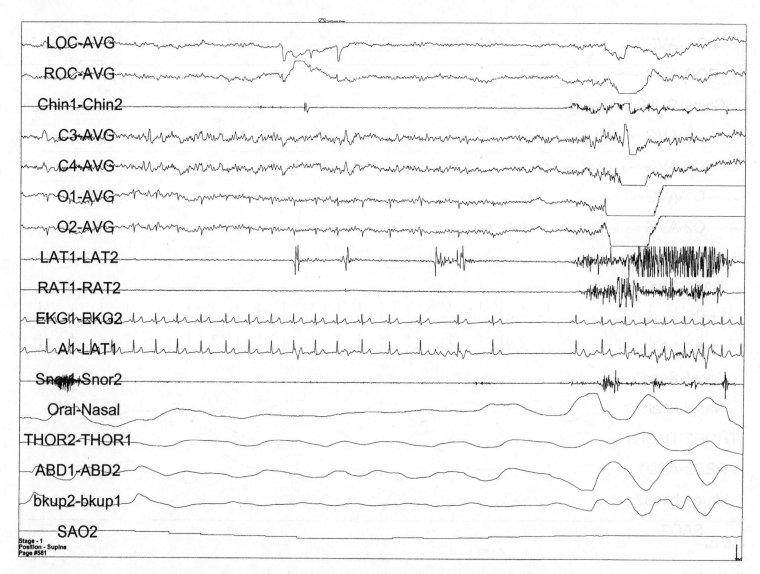

FIGURE 9-9   **Polysomnogram: Standard montage (prior display montage); 30 second page.**
Clinical: 40-year-old woman with obstructive sleep apnea.
Staging: Stage REM sleep with an arousal.
Respiratory: Apnea followed by an arousal and an oxygen desaturation. The oxygen desaturation on this page was caused by an apnea from the preceding page of the record.
EKG: Bradycardia with the apnea. There is a 3-second asystole at the end of the apnea.

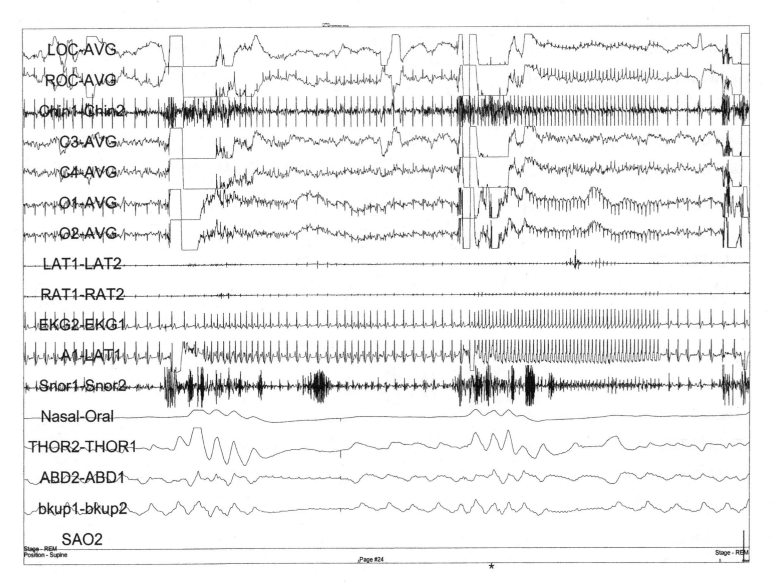

FIGURE 9-10   **Polysomnogram: Standard montage (prior display montage); 60 second page.**

Clinical: 50-year-old man with obstructive sleep apnea and hypertension.

Staging: Stage REM sleep with arousals.

Respiratory: Mixed apneas followed by arousals.

EKG: Wide-complex tachycardia with a rate of greater than 160 beats per minute accompanies the second arousal (*).

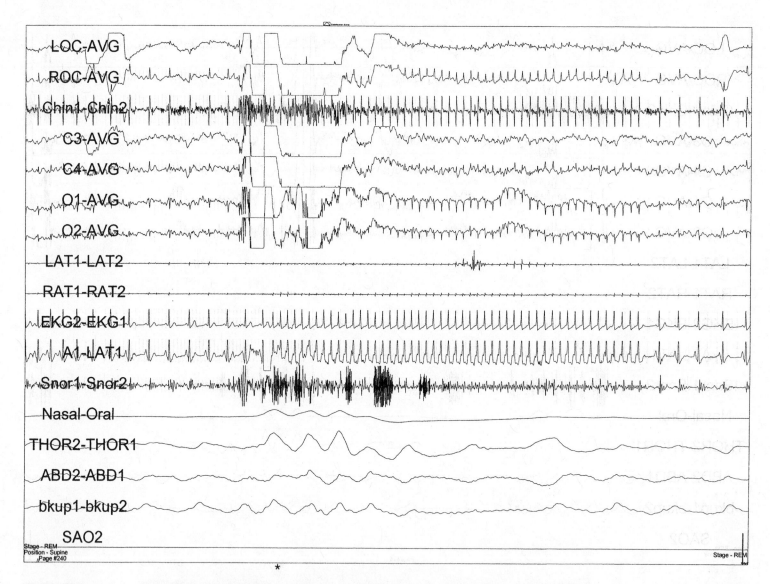

FIGURE 9-11   **Polysomnogram: Standard montage (prior display montage); 30 second page.**

Clinical: 50-year-old man with obstructive sleep apnea and hypertension.

Staging: Stage REM sleep with an arousal.

Respiratory: Mixed apnea followed by an arousal.

EKG: Wide-complex tachycardia with a rate of greater than 160 beats per minute accompanies the arousal (*).

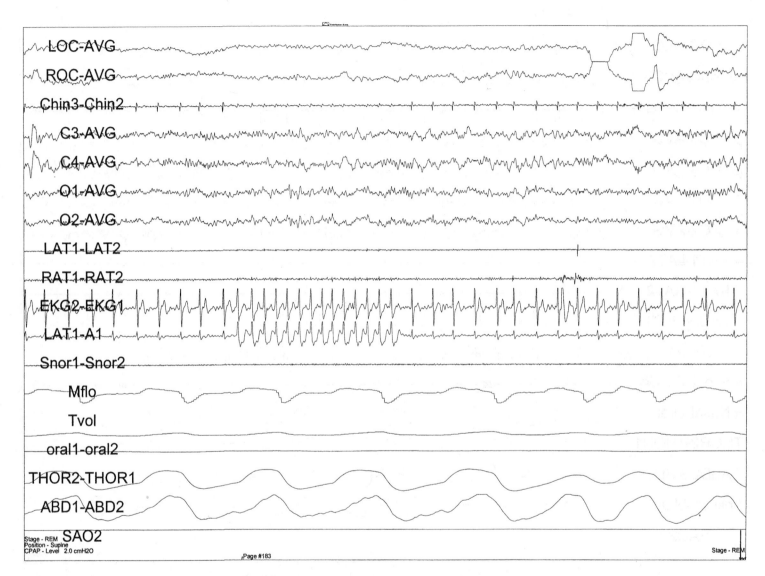

FIGURE 9-12   Polysomnogram: Standard montage (prior display montage); 30 second page.

Clinical: 58-year-old man with obstructive sleep apnea.

Staging: Stage REM sleep with an arousal.

Respiratory: Mixed apnea followed by an arousal.

EKG: Ventricular tachycardia.

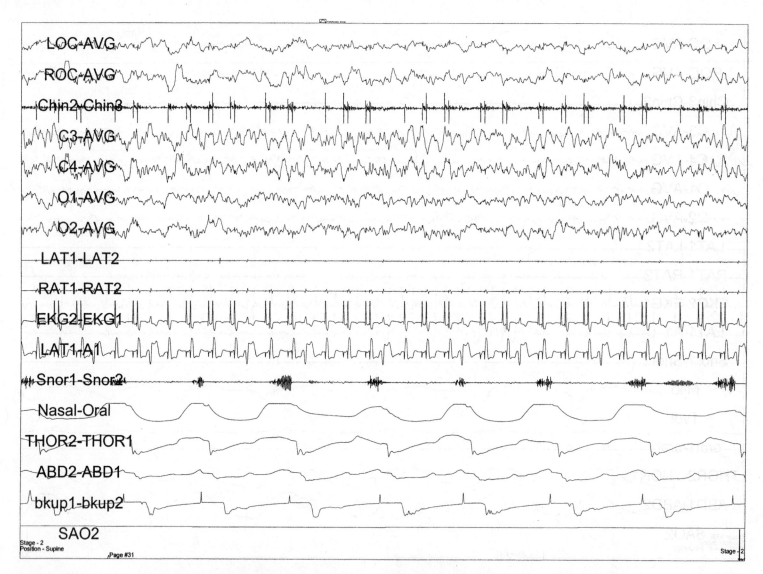

FIGURE 9-13   **Polysomnogram: Standard montage (prior display montage); 30 second page.**
Clinical: 69-year-old man with excessive daytime sleepiness and third-degree A-V block.
Staging: Stage 2 sleep.
Respiratory: Normal respirations.
EKG: Third-degree A-V block. Pacemaker spikes precede several of the QRS complexes and can also be seen in the backup respiratory channel.

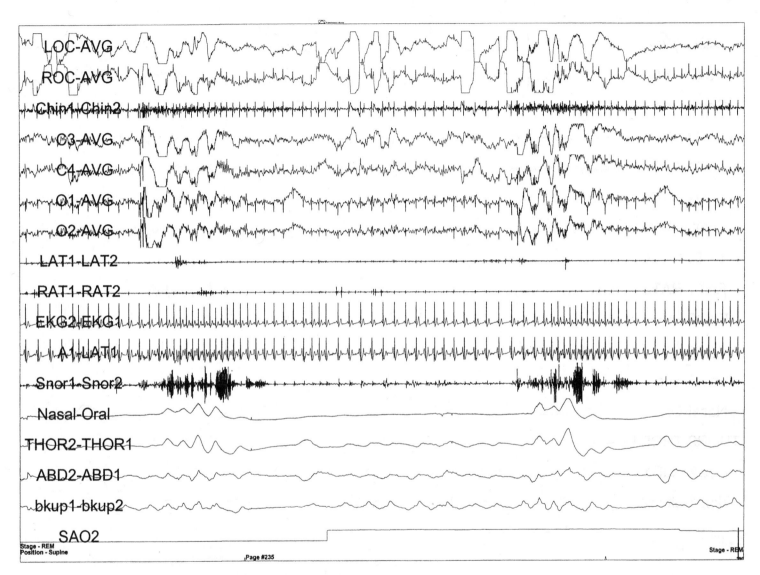

FIGURE 9-14 **Polysomnogram: Standard montage (prior display montage); 60 second page.**

Clinical: 40-year-old man with obstructive sleep apnea.

Staging: Stage REM sleep with arousals.

Respiratory: Repeated apneas followed by arousals. The pulse oximetry channel is contaminated by artifact.

EKG: Bradycardia accompanies the apnea. Tachycardia occurs with the arousal.

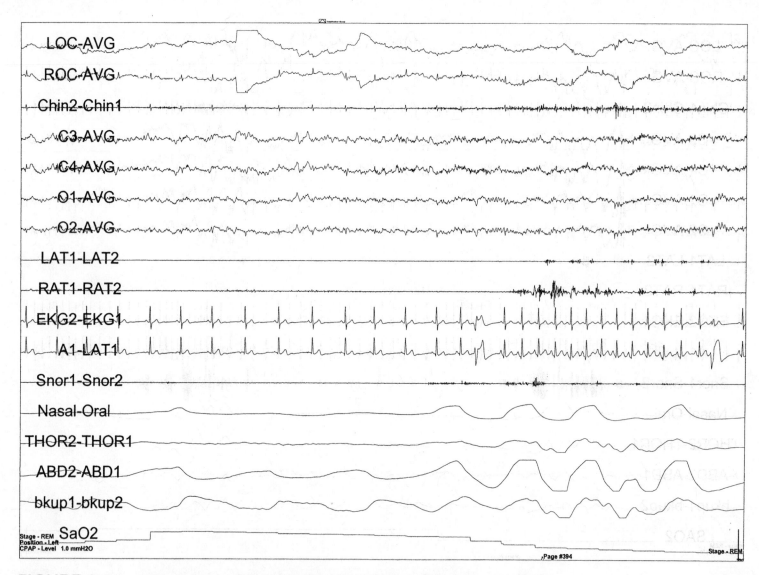

LOC-AVG

ROC-AVG

Chin2-Chin1

C3-AVG

C4-AVG

O1-AVG

O2-AVG

LAT1-LAT2

RAT1-RAT2

EKG2-EKG1

A1-LAT1

Snor1-Snor2

Nasal-Oral

THOR2-THOR1

ABD2-ABD1

bkup1-bkup2

SaO2

Stage - REM
Position - Left
CPAP - Level 1.0 mmH2O

Page #394

Stage - REM

FIGURE 9-15   **Polysomnogram: CPAP montage (prior display montage); 30 second page.**
Clinical: 59-year-old man with obstructive sleep apnea.
Staging: Stage REM sleep with an arousal.
Respiratory: Apnea with paradoxical respirations followed by an arousal and an oxygen desaturation.
EKG: Bradycardia accompanies the apnea, while tachycardia occurs with the arousal. Occasional PVCs are evident.

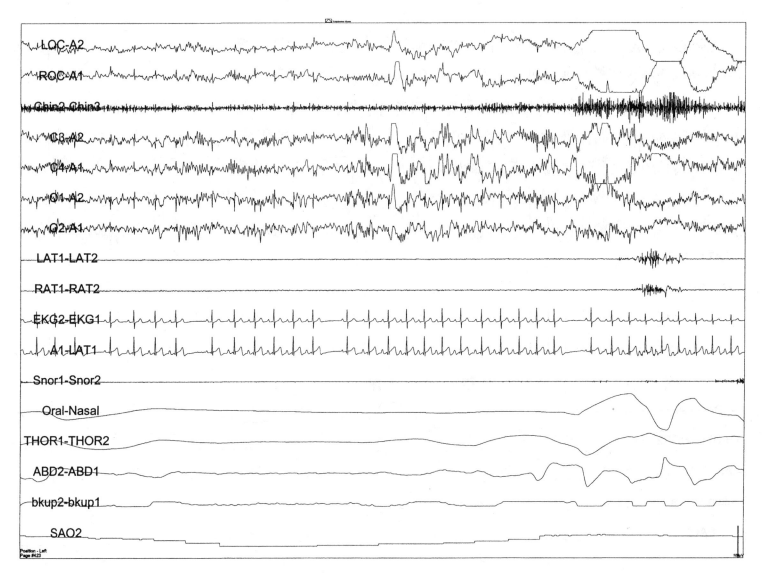

FIGURE 9-16 **Polysomnogram: Standard montage (prior display montage); 30 second page.**
Clinical: 71-year-old man with obstructive sleep apnea and hypertension.
Staging: Stage 2 sleep with an arousal.
Respiratory: Mixed apnea associated with an arousal and an oxygen desaturation from 93% to 87%.
EKG: Sinus arrhythmia.

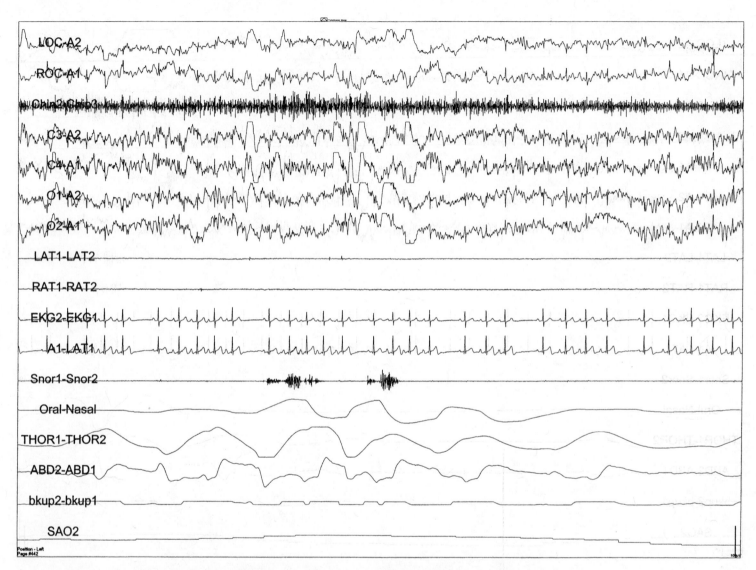

FIGURE 9-17   **Polysomnogram: Standard montage (prior display montage); 30 second page.**
Clinical: 38-year-old obese woman with obstructive sleep apnea.
Staging: Stage 2 sleep with an arousal.
Respiratory: Repeated apneas with associated arousals, snorts, and oxygen desaturations.
EKG: Sinus arrhythmia and first-degree A-V block.

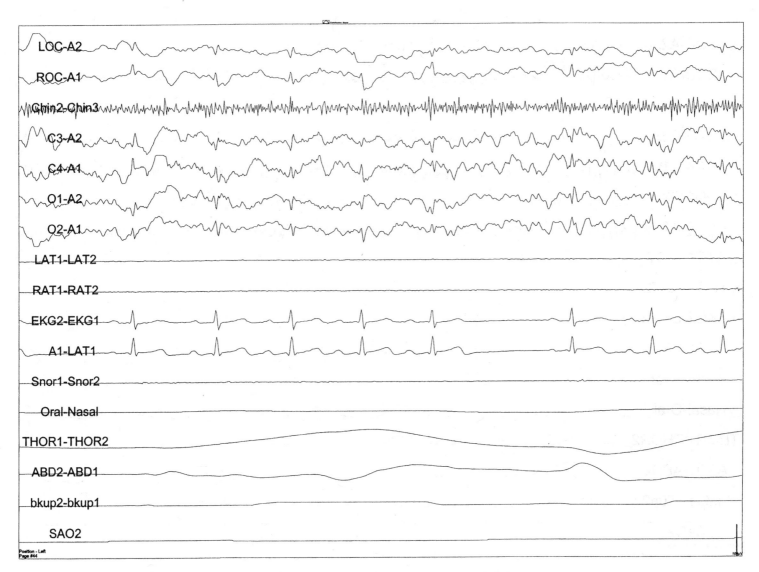

FIGURE 9-18 **Polysomnogram: Standard montage (prior display montage); 10 second page.**

Clinical: 38-year-old obese woman with obstructive sleep apnea.

Staging: Stage 2 sleep with an arousal.

Respiratory: Repeated apneas with associated arousals, snorts, and oxygen desaturations.

EKG: Sinus arrhythmia and first-degree A-V block.

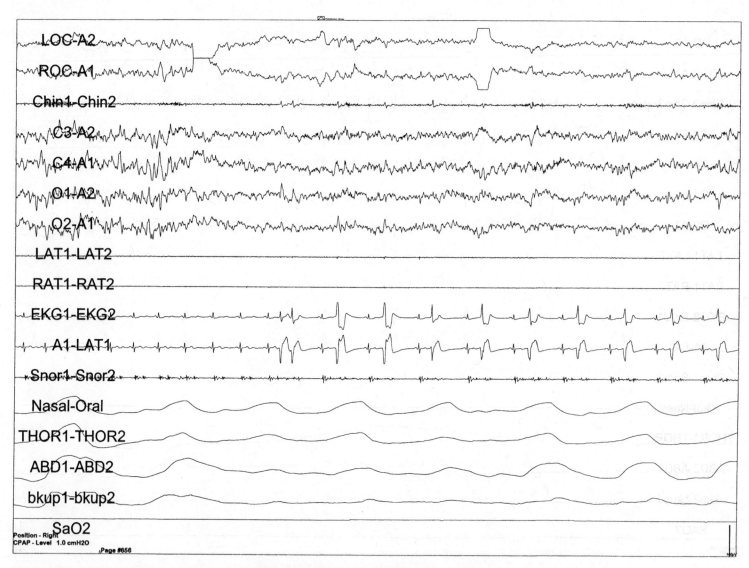

FIGURE 9-19   **Polysomnogram: Standard montage (prior display montage); 30 second page.**
Clinical: 46-year-old man with excessive daytime sleepiness.
Staging: Stage REM sleep.
Respiratory: Variable respiratory effort characteristic of phasic REM sleep.
EKG: Bigeminy occurring in conjunction with phasic REM sleep.

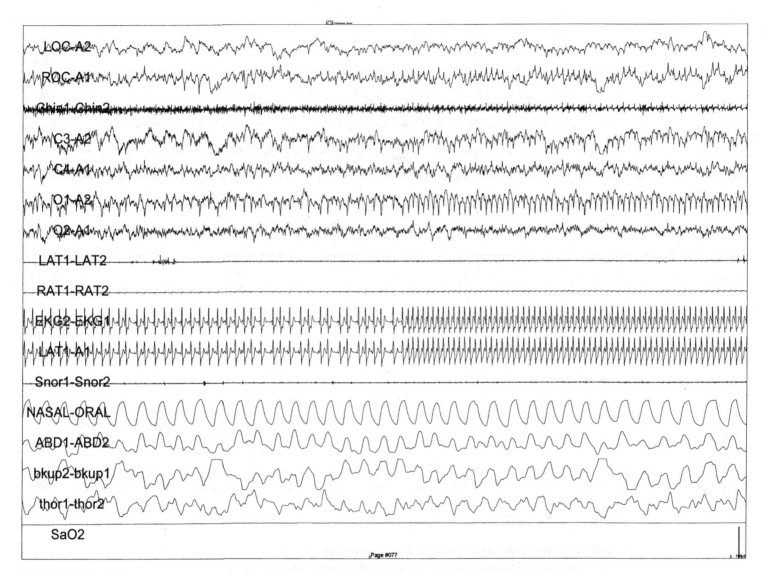

FIGURE 9-20   **Polysomnogram: Standard montage (prior display montage); 60 second page.**
Clinical: 49-year-old woman with snoring and excessive daytime sleepiness.
Staging: Stage 2 sleep.
Respiratory: Normal respirations.
EKG: Supraventricular tachycardia.

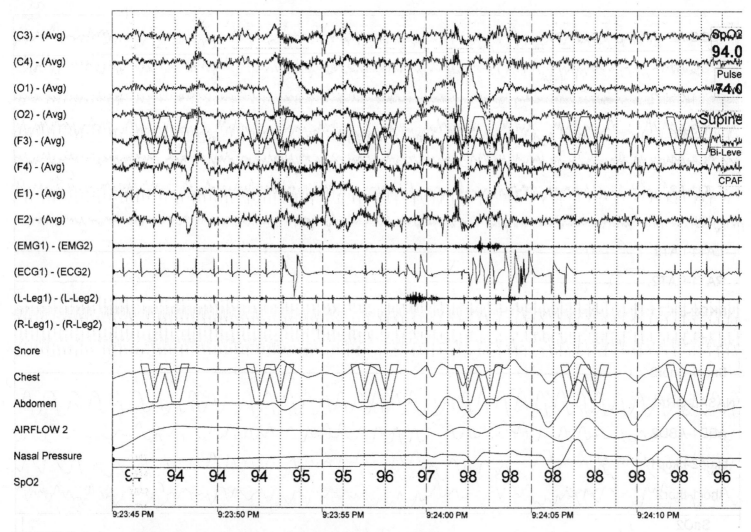

FIGURE 9-21 **Polysomnogram: Standard montage; 30 second page.**
Clinical: 55-year-old woman with snoring and excessive daytime sleepiness.
Staging: Stage wake.
Respiratory: Normal respirations.
EKG: EKG artifact not ventricular tachycardia.

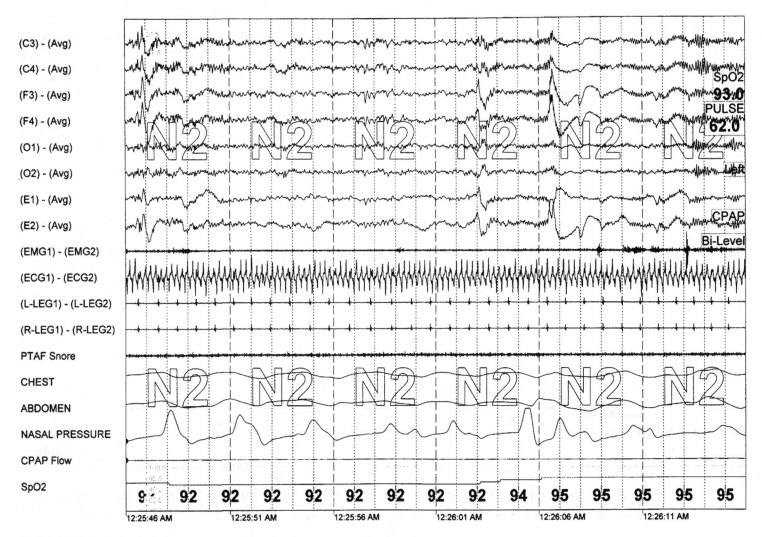

FIGURE 9-22   **Polysomnogram: Standard montage; 30 second page.**

Clinical: 35-year-old man with excessive daytime sleepiness.

Staging: Stage 2 sleep.

Respiratory: The changes in the nasal pressure waveform suggest a respiratory event related arousal.

EKG: The EKG is bad resulting in a waveform suggestive of ventricular tachycardia.

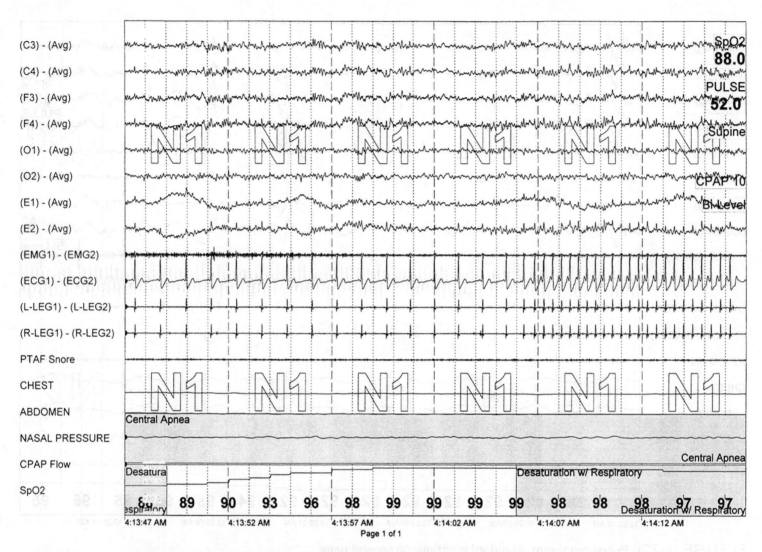

FIGURE 9-23 **Polysomnogram: Standard montage; 30 second page.**
Clinical: 58-year-old woman with heart failure and apneas.
Staging: Stage 1 sleep.
Respiratory: Central apnea.
EKG: Supraventricular tachycardia.

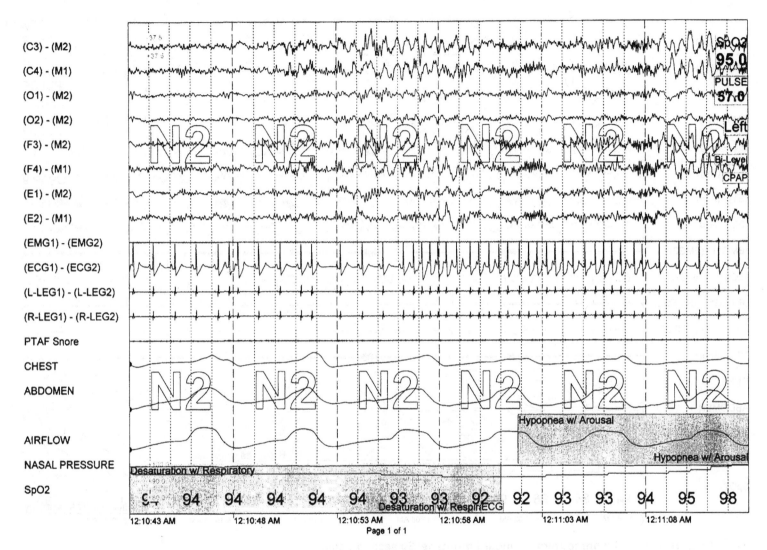

FIGURE 9-24   **Polysomnogram: Standard montage; 30 second page.**
Clinical: 47-year-old man with COPD, snoring, and excessive daytime sleepiness.
Staging: Stage 2 sleep.
Respiratory: Hypopnea. The oxygen desaturation is secondary to the hypopnea from the preceding page.
EKG: Narrow-complex tachycardia.

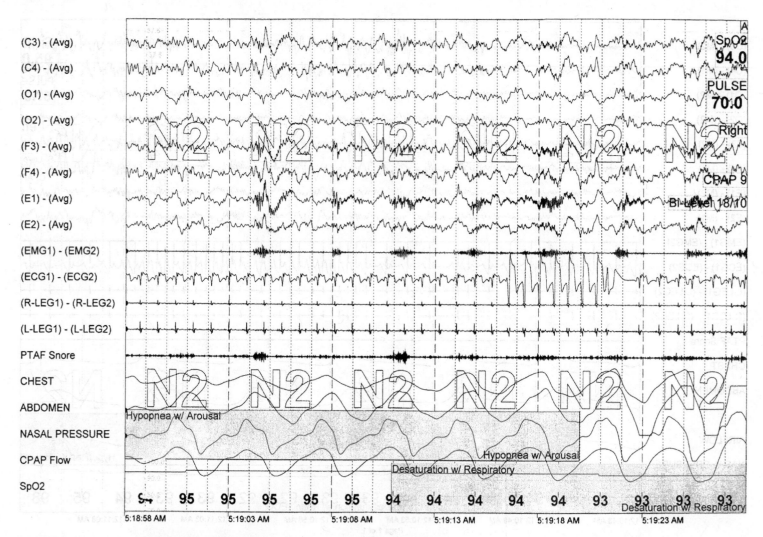

FIGURE 9-25 **Polysomnogram: Standard montage; 30 second page.**
Clinical: 62-year-old man with snoring and fatigue.
Staging: Stage 2 sleep.
Respiratory: Hypopnea.
Snoring: There is artifact from the snoring in the chin EMG and in the EEG channels.
EKG: Ventricular tachycardia.

Calibrations

James D. Geyer, MD and Paul R. Carney, MD

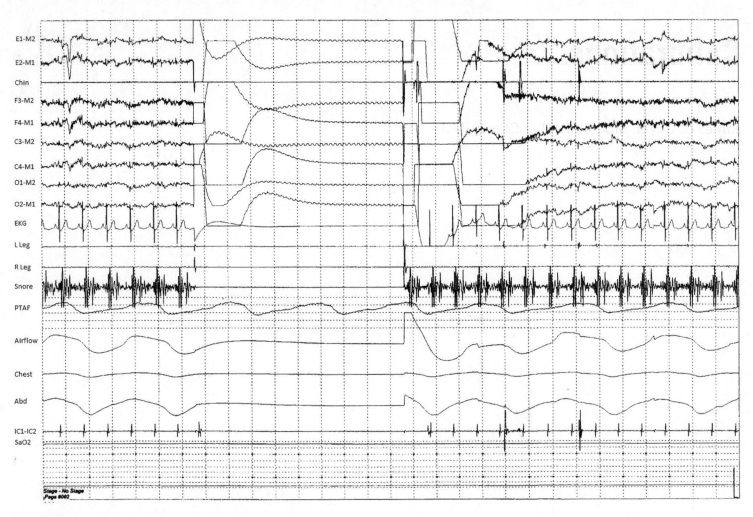

FIGURE 10-1   Machine calibrations.

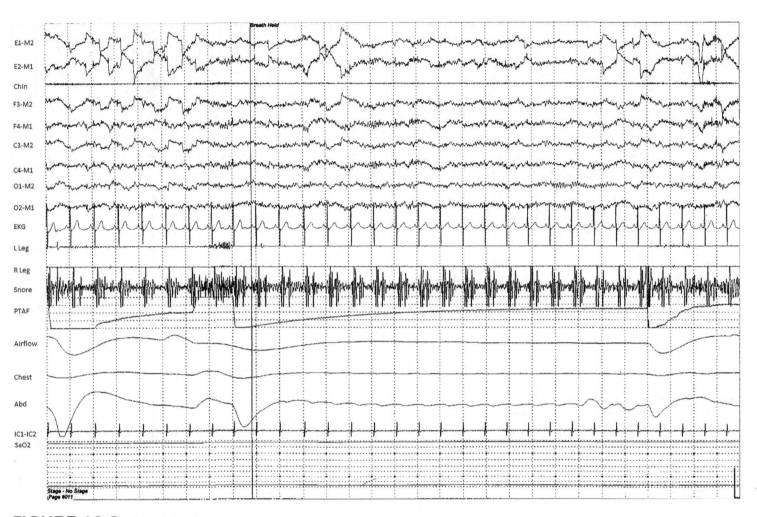

FIGURE 10-2   Breath hold.

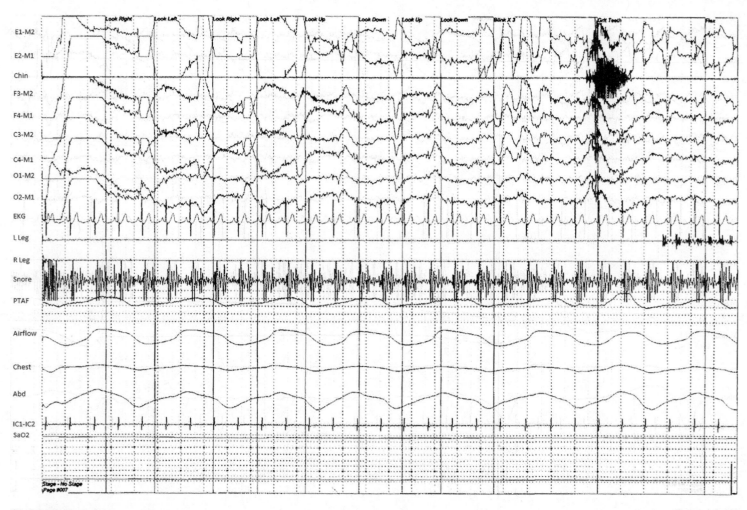

FIGURE 10-3 Grit teeth.

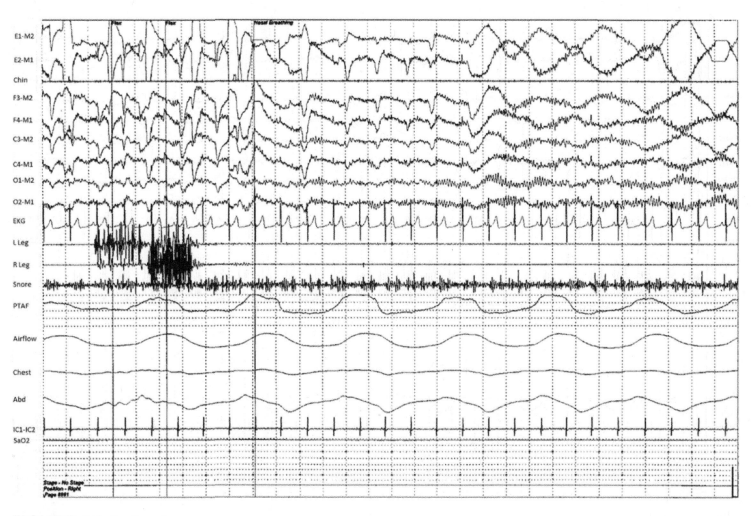

FIGURE 10-4   Foot flex.

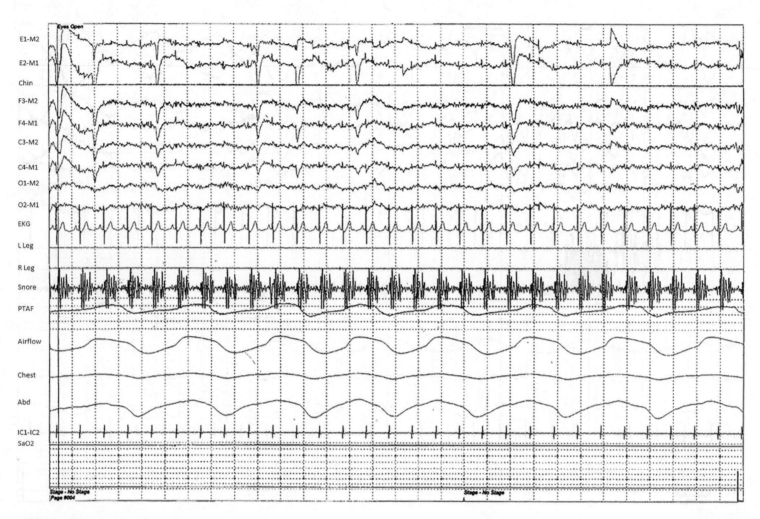

FIGURE 10-5   Eyes open.

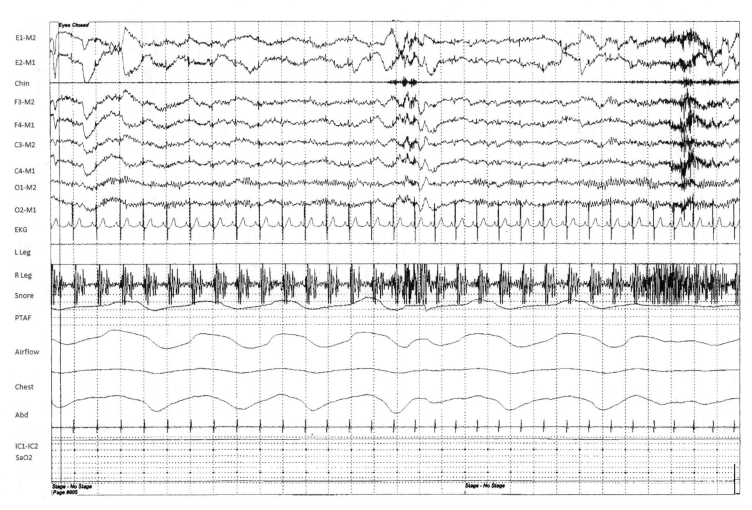

FIGURE 10-6 Eyes closed.

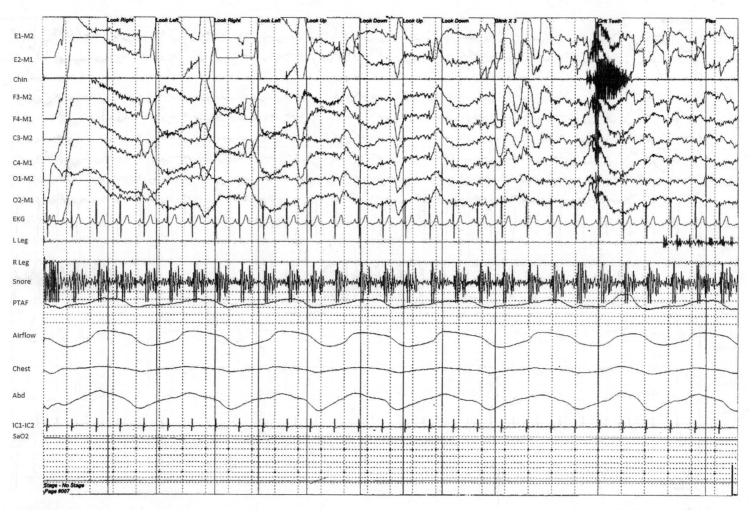

FIGURE 10-7 Eye movements.

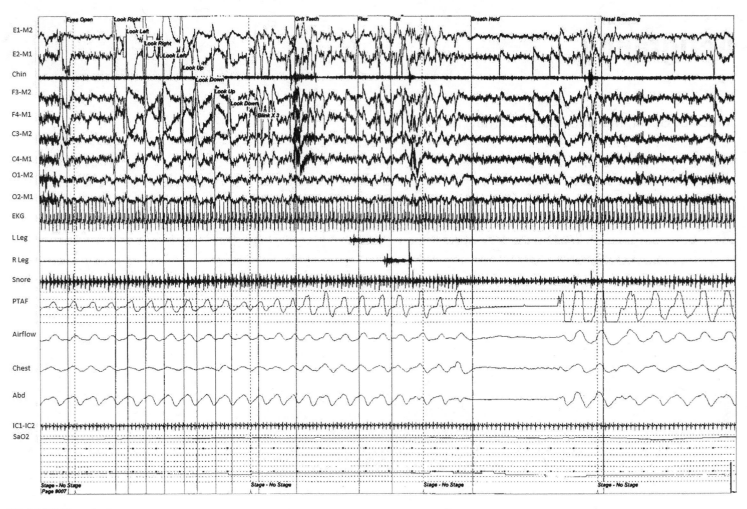

FIGURE 10-8   Calibration sequence at 120 second page.

Actigraphy

James D. Geyer, MD and Paul R. Carney, MD

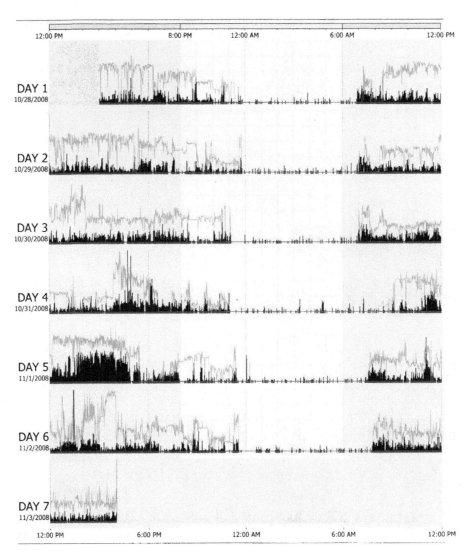

FIGURE 11-1   Actigraphy in a normal subject.

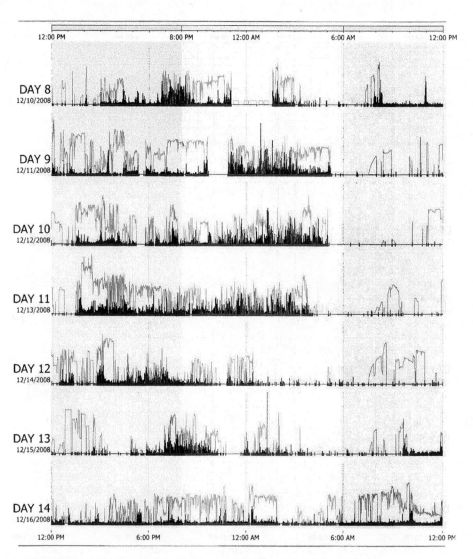

FIGURE 11-2 Actigraphy in a patient with insomnia.

Home Sleep Apnea Monitoring

James D. Geyer, MD and Paul R. Carney, MD

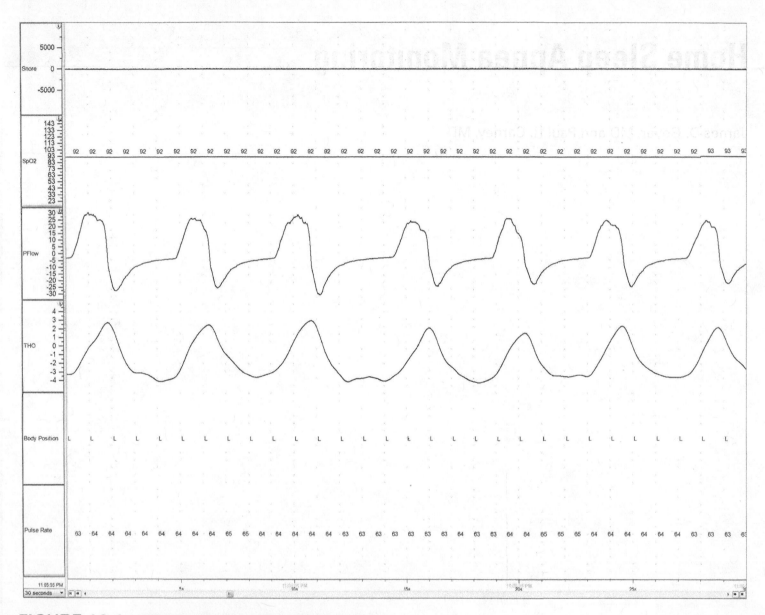

FIGURE 12-1   **HSAT: Standard montage; 30 second page.**
Clinical: 36-year-old overweight man with daytime sleepiness.
Respiratory: Normal respirations with no snoring.

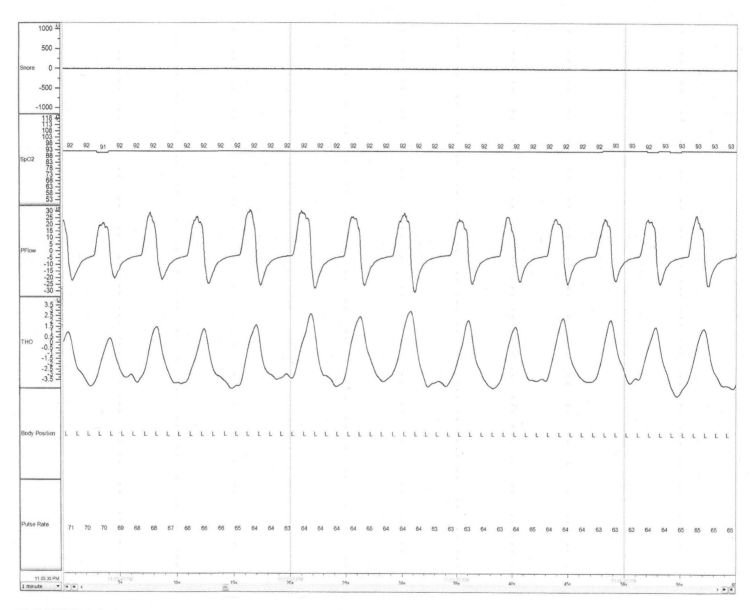

FIGURE 12-2   **HSAT: Standard montage; 60 second page.**
Clinical: 36-year-old overweight man with daytime sleepiness.
Respiratory: Normal respirations with no snoring.

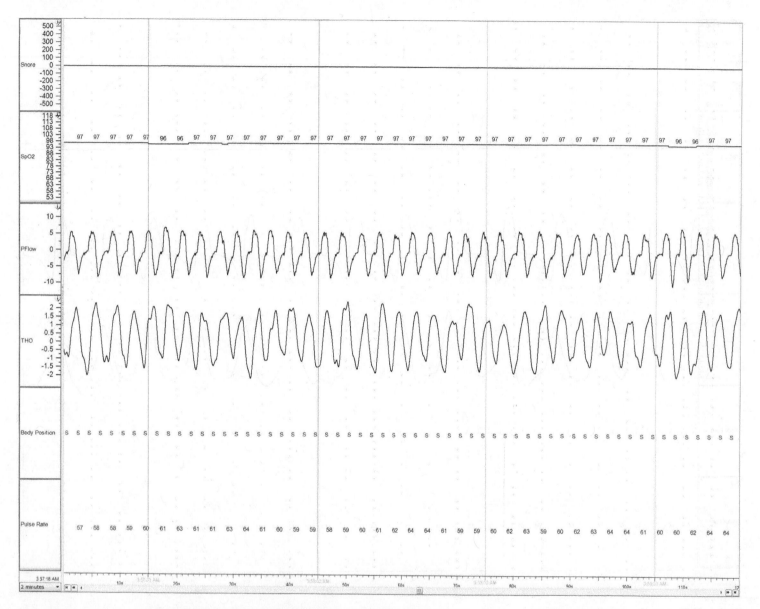

FIGURE 12-3   **HSAT: Standard montage; 120 second page.**
Clinical: 36-year-old overweight man with daytime sleepiness.
Respiratory: Normal respirations with no snoring.

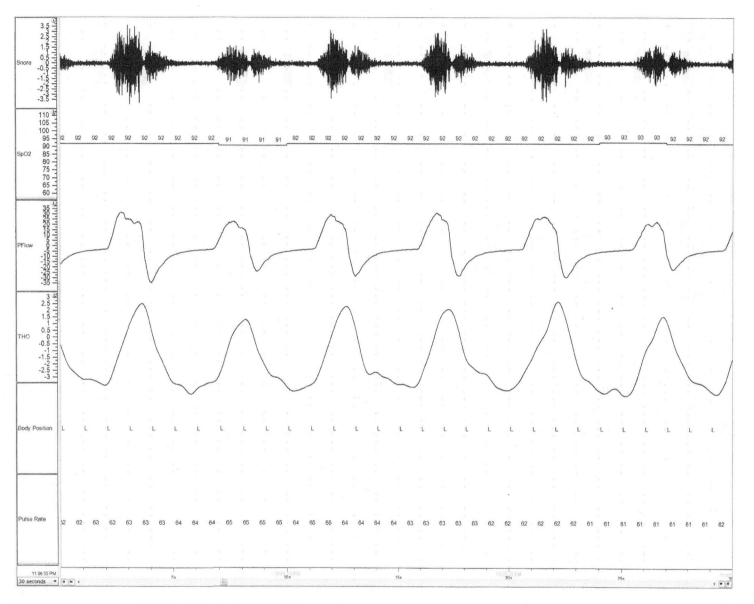

FIGURE 12-4 **HSAT: Standard montage; 30 second page.**
Clinical: 47-year-old woman with fatigue and snoring.
Respiratory: Normal respirations with snoring.

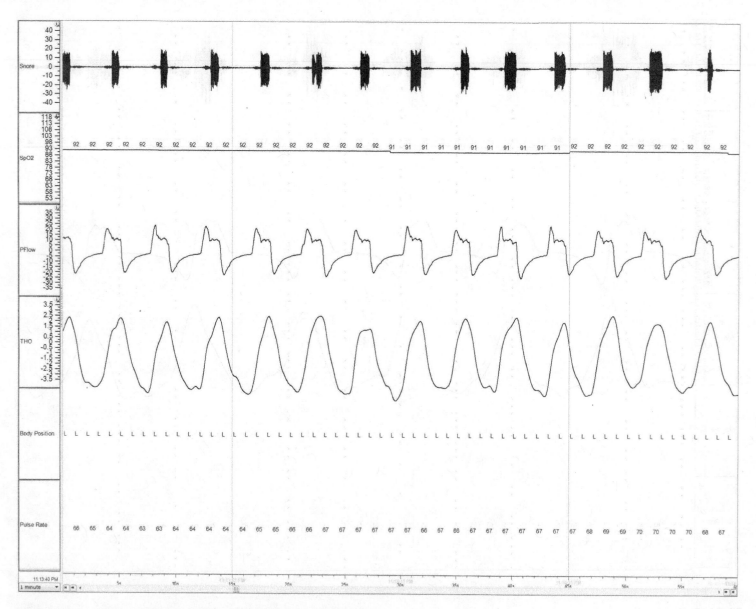

FIGURE 12-5 **HSAT: Standard montage; 60 second page.**
Clinical: 47-year-old woman with fatigue and snoring.
Respiratory: Normal respirations with snoring.

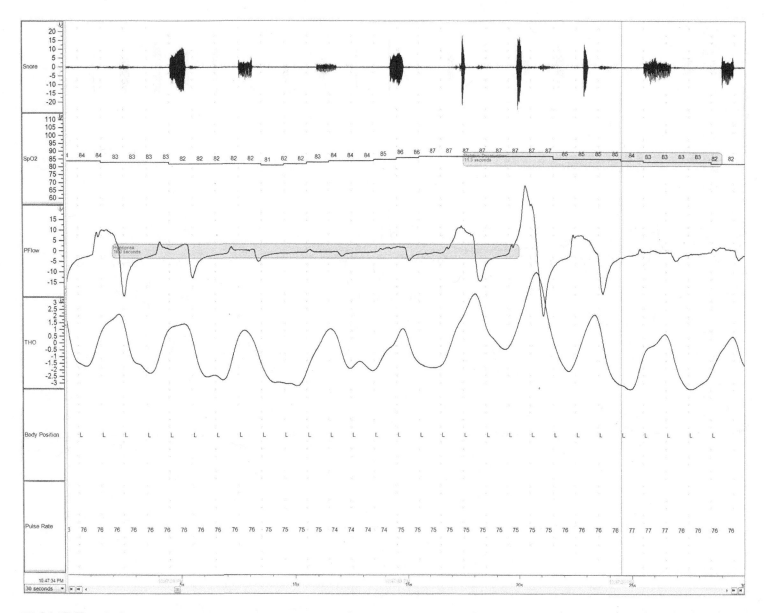

FIGURE 12-6   **HSAT: Standard montage; 30 second page.**
Clinical: 46-year-old obese man with suspected obstructive sleep apnea.
Respiratory: Hypopnea.

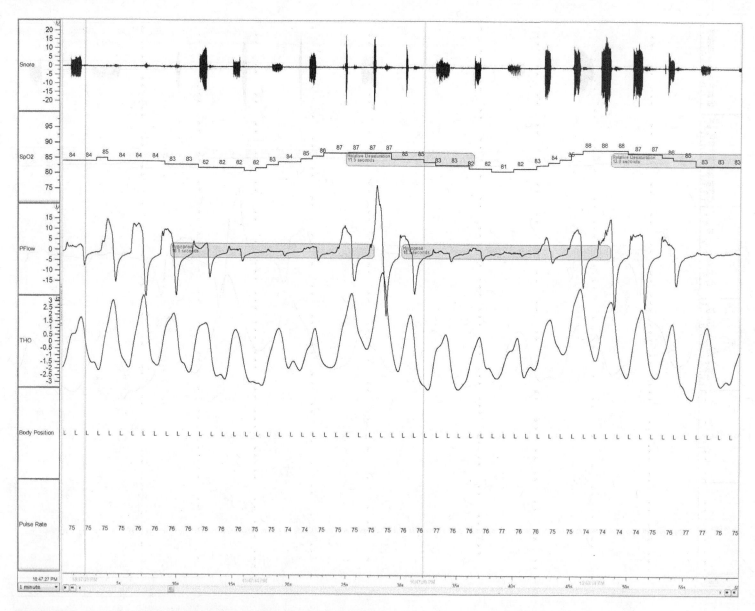

FIGURE 12-7   HSAT: Standard montage; 60 second page.
Clinical: 46-year-old obese man with suspected obstructive sleep apnea.
Respiratory: Hypopnea.

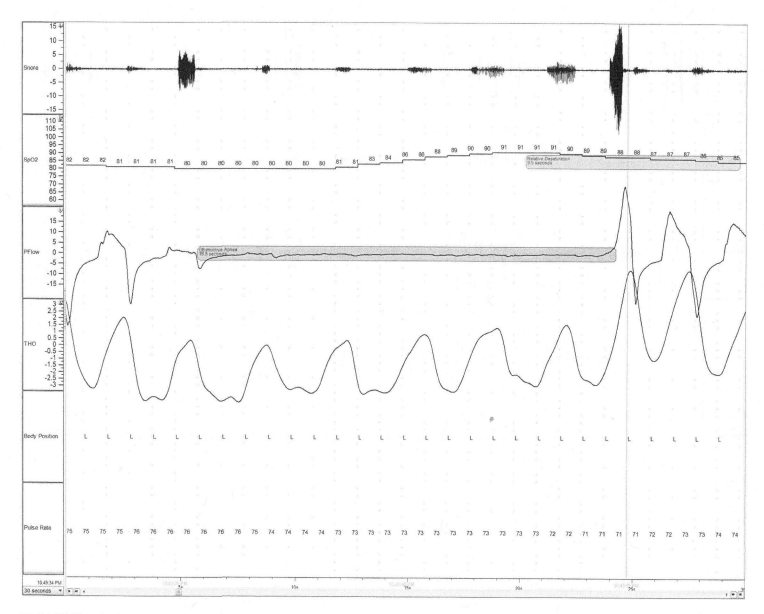

FIGURE 12-8   **HSAT: Standard montage; 30 second page.**
Clinical: 52-year-old man with snoring, sleepiness, and a history of facial trauma.
Respiratory: Obstructive apnea.

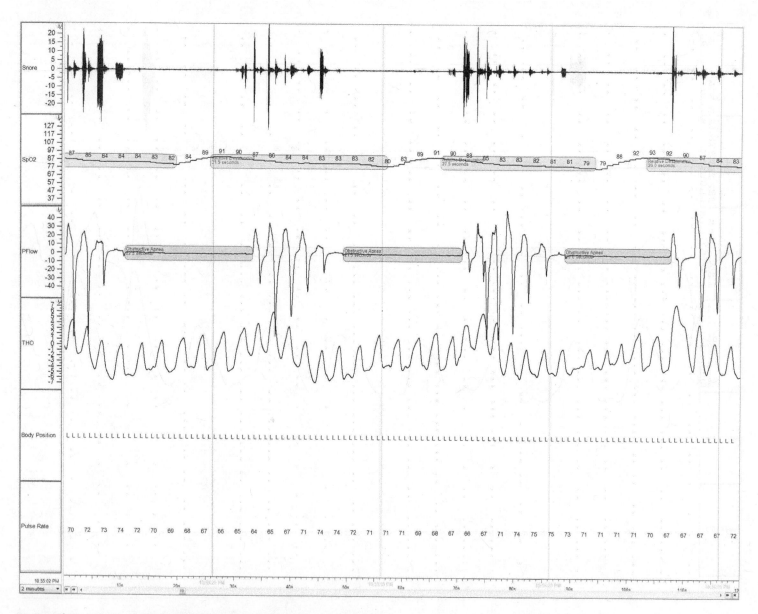

FIGURE 12-9   HSAT: Standard montage; 120 second page.
Clinical: 41-year-old obese man with suspected obstructive sleep apnea.
Respiratory: Obstructive apnea.

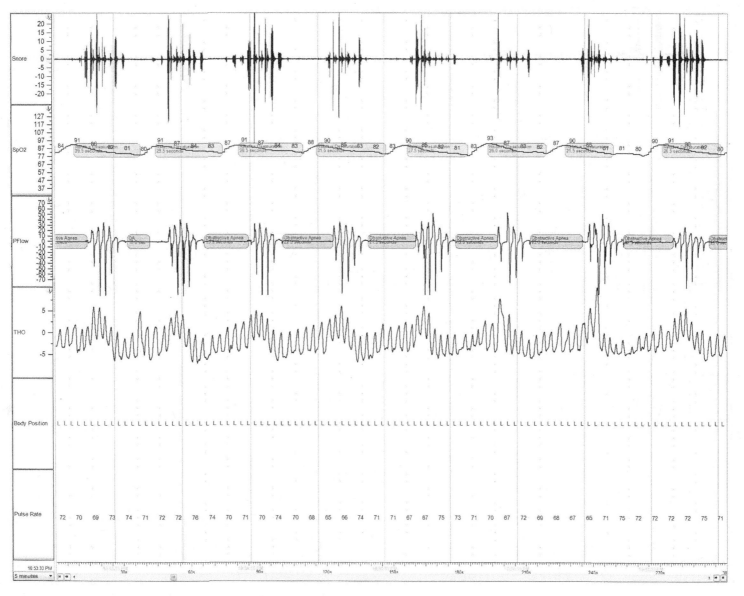

FIGURE 12-10 **HSAT: Standard montage; 5 minute page.**
Clinical: 41-year-old obese man with suspected obstructive sleep apnea.
Respiratory: Obstructive apnea.

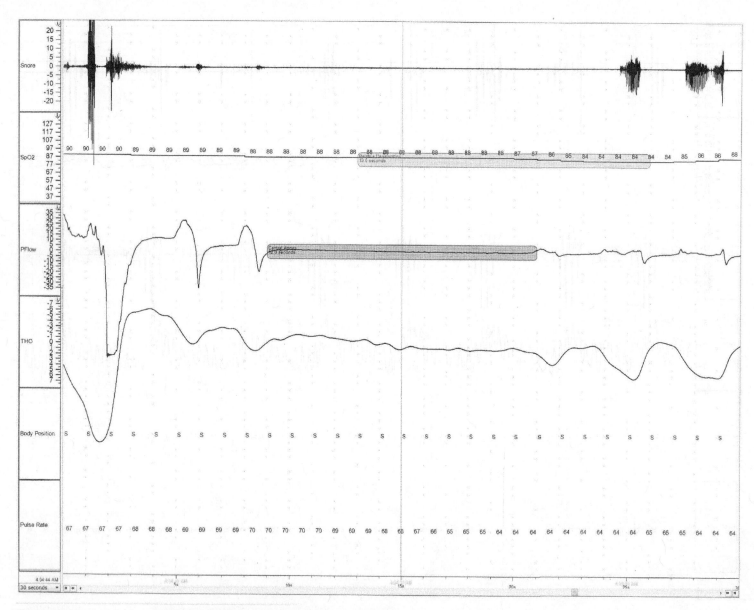

FIGURE 12-11   HSAT: Standard montage; 60 second page.
Clinical: 53-year-old obese man with reported sleep apnea.
Respiratory: Central apnea.

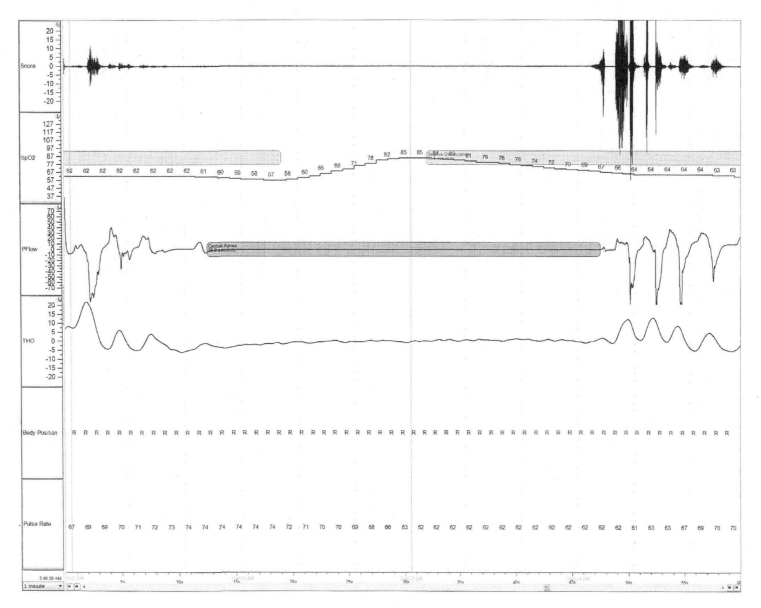

FIGURE 12-12   **HSAT: Standard montage; 60 second page.**
Clinical: 53-year-old obese man with reported sleep apnea.
Respiratory: Central apnea.

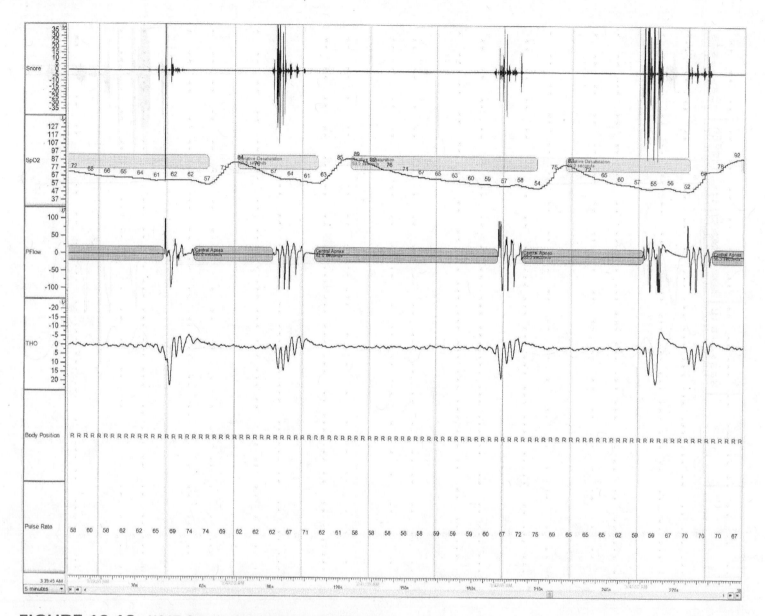

FIGURE 12-13   HSAT: Standard montage; 5 minute page.
Clinical: 53-year-old obese man with reported sleep apnea.
Respiratory: Central apnea.

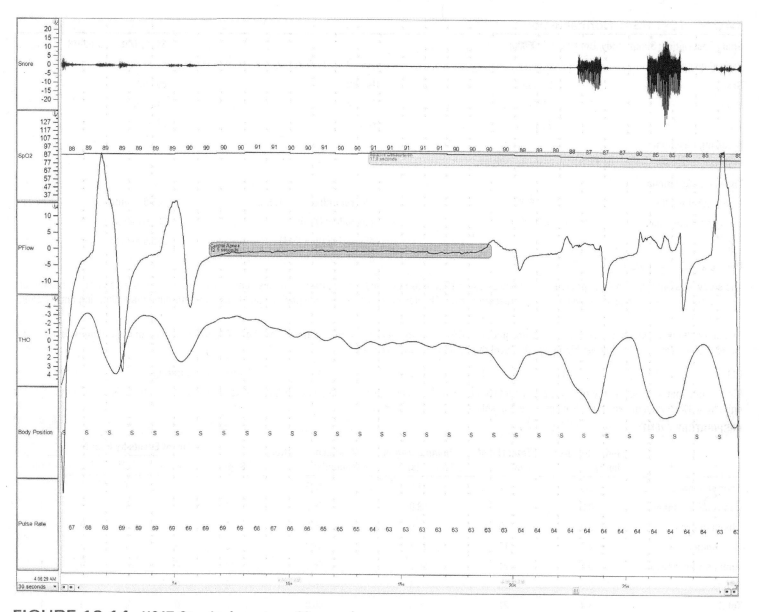

FIGURE 12-14 **HSAT: Standard montage; 30 second page.**
Clinical: 61-year-old man with heart failure and witnessed apnea.
Respiratory: Central apnea/Cheyne-Stokes respirations.

TABLE 12-1 HSAT Normal Report

Study Description: Sleep Study, Unattended (95806)		Study Date: 12/3/2016	
Patient name:		Recording device:	No. 1002
Sex:	Female	Height:	69 inch
D.O.B.:	11/24/1992	Weight:	210 pounds
Age:	24 years	BMI:	31.01

Referring Physician:

Indications: Apnea, unspecified (G47.30). Snoring (R06.83).

Times and Durations

Lights off clock time:	12:36:03 AM	Total recording time (TRT):	381.6 minutes
Lights on clock time:	6:57:39 AM	Time in bed (TIB):	381.6 minutes
		Monitoring time (MT):	375.6 minutes

Device and Sensor Details

The study was recorded on an approved type III device using 1 RIP effort belt and a pressure-based flow sensor. The heart rate is derived from the oximeter sensor, and the snore signal is derived from the pressure sensor. The device also records body position and uses it to determine the monitoring time (sleep/wake periods).

Summary: REI is the number of respiratory events per hour. OAI is the number of obstructive apneas per hour. CAI is the number of central apneas per hour. Lowest desaturation is the lowest blood oxygen level that lasted at least 2 seconds.

REI	3.4	OAI	0.3	CAI	0.3	Lowest desaturation	92

Please note that the "REI" in the report is consistent with the alternative hypopnea definition according to AASM criteria where there is a greater than or equal to a 3% oxygen desaturation from pre-event baseline.

RESPIRATORY EVENTS

	Index (no. per hour)	Total No. of Events	Mean Duration (seconds)	Maximum Duration (seconds)	No. of Events by Position				
					Supine	Prone	Left	Right	Up
Central apneas	0.3	2	11.5	12.5	1	0	1	0	0
Obstructive apneas	0.3	2	38.0	66.0	1	0	0	0	1
Mixed apneas	0.0	0	0.0	0.0	0	0	0	0	0
Hypopneas	2.7	17	27.4	52.0	15	0	1	1	0
Apneas + hypopneas	3.4	21	26.9	66.0	17	0	2	1	1
RERAs	0.0	0	0.0	0.0	0	0	0	0	0
Total	3.4	21	26.9	66.0	17	0	2	1	1
Time in position					264.3	0.1	96.2	12.3	4.8
REI in position					3.9	0.0	1.2	4.9	27.3

Oximetry Summary

	Duration (minutes)	% TIB
<90%	0.0	0.0
<85%	0.0	0.0
<80%	0.0	0.0
<70%	0.0	0.0
Total duration (minutes) < 0		minutes
Average (%)		**97**
Total no. of desaturations		9
Desaturation index (no. per hour)		1.4
Desaturation maximum (%)		6
Desaturation maximum duration (seconds)		45.5
Lowest SpO$_2$ % during sleep		**92**
Duration of minutes SpO$_2$ (seconds)		5
Highest SpO$_2$ % during sleep		**99**
Duration of maximum SpO$_2$ (seconds)		26

Heart Rate Stats

Mean HR during sleep	62.7 (bpm)
Highest HR during sleep	108 (bpm)
Highest HR during TIB	108 (bpm)
Lowest HR during sleep	51 (bpm)
Lowest HR during TIB	51 (bpm)

Snoring Summary

Mild

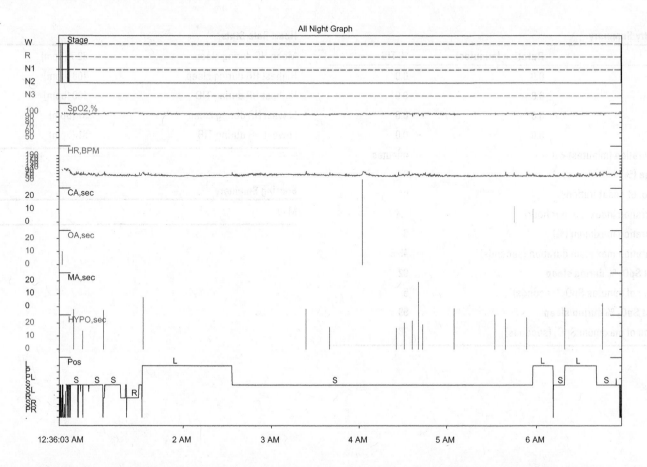

All Night Graph

HST: This home monitoring sleep test did not reveal any definite evidence of a sleep-related breathing disorder. A negative home sleep study does not completely exclude the possibility of a sleep-related breathing disorder such as obstructive sleep apnea. Clinical correlation is advised.

Recommendations: The patient will follow up with her cardiologist.

_____, M.D.

Sleep Specialist

Diplomate, The American Board of Sleep Medicine

Sleep specialist reviewed the raw data in its entirety, including pulse, snore, respiration, oxygen saturation, and body position. The interpretation is based on this information in addition to the available clinical history and physical examination.

TABLE 12-2 HSAT Indeterminate Report

Study Description: Sleep Study, Unattended (95806)		Study Date: 8/29/2016	
Patient name:		**Recording device:**	#1016
Sex:	Male	**Height:**	74 inch
DOB:	1/12/1954	**Weight:**	255 pounds
Age:	62 years	**BMI:**	32.7

Referring Physician:

Indications: Hypersomnolence (G47.10).

Times and Durations

Lights off clock time:	9:02:34 PM	**Total recording time (TRT):**	341.4 minutes
Lights on clock time:	2:41:58 AM	**Time in bed (TIB):**	339.4 minutes
		Monitoring time (MT):	79.5 minutes

Device and Sensor Details

The study was recorded on an approved type III device using 1 RIP effort belt and a pressure-based flow sensor. The heart rate is derived from the oximeter sensor, and the snore signal is derived from the pressure sensor. The device also records body position and uses it to determine the monitoring time (sleep/wake periods).

Summary: REI is the number of respiratory events per hour. OAI is the number of obstructive apneas per hour. CAI is the number of central apneas per hour. Lowest desaturation is the lowest blood oxygen level that lasted at least 2 seconds.

REI	18.9	OAI	4.5	CAI	0.8	Lowest desaturation	85

Please note that the "REI" in the report is consistent with the recommended hypopnea definition according to Medicare.
Criteria where there is a greater than or equal to 4% oxygen desaturation from pre-event baseline.

RESPIRATORY EVENTS

	Index (no. per hour)	Total No. of Events	Mean Duration (seconds)	Maximum Duration (seconds)	No. of Events by Position				
					Supine	Prone	Left	Right	Up
Central apneas	0.8	1	15.5	15.5	1				0
Obstructive apneas	4.5	6	23.8	34.5	5				1
Mixed apneas	0.0	0	0.0	0.0	0				0
Hypopneas	13.6	18	34.1	79.0	18				0
Apneas + hypopneas	18.9	25	30.8	79.0	24				1
RERAs	0.0	0	0.0	0.0	0				0
Total	**18.9**	**25**	30.8	79.0	24				1
Time in position					79.2				0.3
REI in position					**18.2**				**200.0**

Oximetry Summary

	Duration (minutes)	% TIB
<90%	100.2	29.5
<85%	0.0	0.0
<80%	0.0	0.0
<70%	0.0	0.0
Total duration (minutes) < 0		minutes
Average (%)		**91**
Total no. of desaturations		25
Desaturation index (per hour)		19.0
Desaturation maximum (%)		8
Desaturation maximum duration (seconds)		64.0
Lowest SpO₂ % during sleep		**85**
Duration of minimum SpO₂ (seconds)		3
Highest SpO₂ % during sleep		**95**
Duration of maximum SpO₂ (seconds)		14

Heart Rate Stats

Mean HR during sleep	73.9 (bpm)
Highest HR during sleep	102 (bpm)
Highest HR during TIB	102 (bpm)
Lowest HR during sleep	60 (bpm)
Lowest HR during TIB	51 (bpm)

Snoring Summary

Moderate

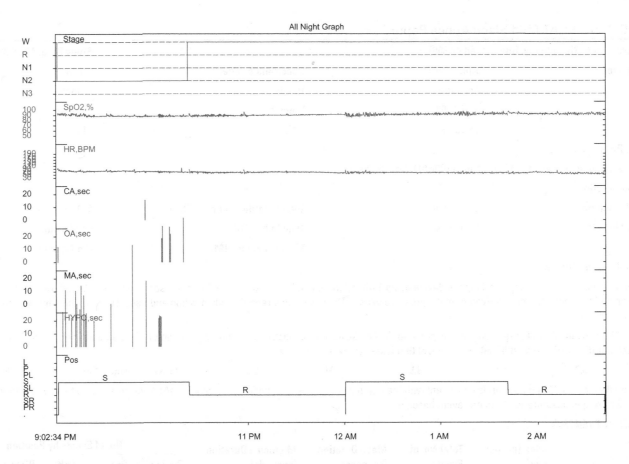

Impression: Hypersomnolence (G47.10). Technically inadequate study.

HST: There were physiologic oxygen desaturations resulting in an REI of 18.9 with a minimum oxygen saturation of 85% during very limited monitoring time. This study was inadequate for formal diagnosis secondary to loss of the nasal pressure monitor. Clinical correlation is advised.

Recommendations: The patient will be scheduled for a repeat home sleep test.

_____, M.D.

Sleep Specialist

Diplomate, The American Board of Sleep Medicine

Sleep specialist reviewed the raw data in its entirety, including pulse, snore, respiration, oxygen saturation, and body position. The interpretation is based on this information in addition to the available clinical history and physical examination.

TABLE 12-3 HSAT Mild Sleep Apnea Report

Study Description: Sleep Study, Unattended (95806)		**Study Date:** 4/16/2016	
Patient name:	Apnea, Mild	Recording device:	#1023
Sex:	Female	Height:	66 inch
D.O.B.:	1/21/1958	Weight:	194 pounds
Age:	58 years	BMI:	31.37

Referring Physician:

Indications: Hypersomnolence (G47.10). Apnea (R06.81). Snoring (R06.83)

Times and Durations

Lights off clock time:	10:14:51 PM	Total recording time (TRT):	430.7 minutes
Lights on clock time:	5:25:33 AM	Time in bed (TIB):	430.7 minutes
		Monitoring time (MT):	426.7 minutes

Device and Sensor Details

The study was recorded on an approved type III device using 1 RIP effort belt and a pressure-based flow sensor. The heart rate is derived from the oximeter sensor, and the snore signal is derived from the pressure sensor. The device also records body position and uses it to determine the monitoring time (sleep/wake periods).

Summary: REI is the number of respiratory events per hour. OAI is the number of obstructive apneas per hour. CAI is the number of central apneas per hour. Lowest desaturation is the lowest blood oxygen level that lasted at least 2 seconds.

REI	9.7	OAI	3.5	CAI	0.8	Lowest desaturation	86

Please note that the "REI" in the report is consistent with the alternative hypopnea definition according to AASM criteria where there is a greater than or equal to a 3% oxygen desaturation from pre-event baseline.

RESPIRATORY EVENTS

	Index (no. per hour)	Total No. of Events	Mean Duration (seconds)	Maximum Duration (seconds)	No. of Events by Position				
					Supine	Prone	Left	Right	Up
Central apneas	0.8	6	13.4	17.0	2	0	4	0	0
Obstructive apneas	3.5	25	14.3	30.5	20	0	5	0	0
Mixed apneas	0.0	0	0.0	0.0	0	0	0	0	0
Hypopneas	5.3	38	33.5	67.0	22	2	9	5	0
Apneas + hypopneas	9.7	69	24.8	67.0	44	2	18	5	0
RERAs	0.0	0	0.0	0.0	0	0	0	0	0
Total	9.7	69	24.8	67.0	44	2	18	5	0
Time in position					111.9	10.3	204.1	99.1	1.0
REI in position					23.6	11.7	5.3	3.0	0.0

Oximetry Summary

	Duration (minutes)	% TIB
<90%	2.0	0.5
<85%	0.0	0.0
<80%	0.0	0.0
<70%	0.0	0.0
Total duration (minutes) < 0		minutes
Average (%)		**94**
Total no. of desaturations		56
Desaturation index (no. per hour)		7.9
Desaturation maximum (%)		7
Desaturation maximum duration (seconds)		74.5
Lowest SpO$_2$ % during sleep		**86**
Duration of minimum SpO$_2$ (seconds)		12
Highest SpO$_2$ % during sleep		**100**
Duration of maximum SpO$_2$ (seconds)		16

Heart Rate Stats

Mean HR during sleep	68.6 (bpm)
Highest HR during sleep	94 (bpm)
Highest HR during TIB	94 (bpm)
Lowest HR during sleep	57 (bpm)
Lowest HR during TIB	57 (bpm)

Snoring Summary: Mild and positional

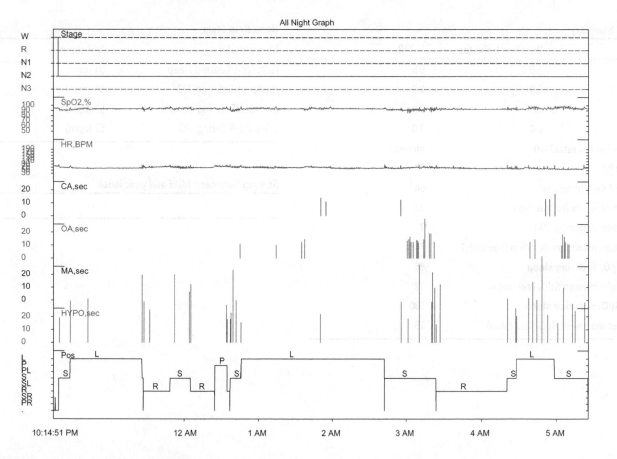

All Night Graph

Impression: Obstructive sleep apnea (G47.33).

HST: There were physiologic oxygen desaturations resulting in an REI of 9.7 with a minimum oxygen saturation of 86%. This is consistent with a sleep-related breathing disorder. Clinical correlation is advised.

Recommendations: The patient will be scheduled for a PAP titration.

_____, M.D.

Sleep Specialist

Diplomate, The American Board of Sleep Medicine

Sleep specialist reviewed the raw data in its entirety, including pulse, snore, respiration, oxygen saturation, and body position. The interpretation is based on this information in addition to the available clinical history and physical examination.

TABLE 12-4 HSAT Severe Sleep Apnea Report

Study Description: Sleep Study, Unattended (95806)		Study Date: 1/10/2017	
Patient name:		Recording device:	#1003
Sex:	M	Height:	74 inch
D.O.B.:	5/12/1967	Weight:	255 pounds
Age:	49 years	BMI:	32.7

Referring Physician:

Indications: Sleep apnea, unspecified (G47.30). Hypersomnolence (G47.10). Snoring (R06.83). Apnea (R06.81). Fatigue. Hypertension (I10). Anxiety.

Times and Durations

Lights off clock time:	11:17:04 PM	Total recording time (TRT):	392.0 minutes
Lights on clock time:	5:49:04 AM	Time in bed (TIB):	392.0 minutes
		Monitoring time (MT):	361.5 minutes

Device and Sensor Details

The study was recorded on an approved type III device using 1 RIP effort belt and a pressure-based flow sensor. The heart rate is derived from the oximeter sensor, and the snore signal is derived from the pressure sensor. The device also records body position and uses it to determine the monitoring time (sleep/wake periods).

Summary: REI is the number of respiratory events per hour. OAI is the number of obstructive apneas per hour. CAI is the number of central apneas per hour. Lowest desaturation is the lowest blood oxygen level that lasted at least 2 seconds.

REI	58.6	OAI	21.7	CAI	2.3	Lowest desaturation	68

Please note that the "REI" in the report is consistent with the recommended hypopnea definition according to Medicare criteria where there is a greater than or equal to a 4% oxygen desaturation from pre-event baseline.

RESPIRATORY EVENTS

	Index (no. per hour)	Total No. of Events	Mean Duration (seconds)	Maximum Duration (seconds)	No. of Events by Position				
					Supine	Prone	Left	Right	Up
Central apneas	2.3	14	16.6	43.5	4		4	6	0
Obstructive apneas	21.7	131	30.6	89.0	128		1	2	0
Mixed apneas	0.3	2	20.3	21.5	0		1	1	0
Hypopneas	34.2	206	38.2	101.5	114		73	17	1
Apneas + hypopneas	58.6	353	34.4	101.5	246		79	26	1
RERAs	0.0	0	0.0	0.0	0		0	0	0
Total	58.6	353	34.4	101.5	246		79	26	1
Time in position					251.2		66.9	65.2	8.1
REI in position					61.2		70.9	34.5	7.8

Oximetry Summary

	Duration (minutes)	% TIB
<90%	90.4	23.1
<85%	13.1	3.3
<80%	5.7	1.5
<70%	0.1	0.0
Total duration (minutes) < 0		minutes
Average (%)		**91**
Total no. of desaturations		341
Desaturation index (no. per hour)		56.7
Desaturation maximum (%)		26
Desaturation maximum duration (seconds)		106.0
Lowest SpO₂ % during sleep		**68**
Duration of minimum SpO₂ (seconds)		2
Highest SpO₂ % during sleep		**98**
Duration of maximum SpO₂ (seconds)		71

Heart Rate Stats

Mean HR during sleep	86.9 (bpm)
Highest HR during sleep	122 (bpm)
Highest HR during TIB	122 (bpm)
Lowest HR during sleep	52 (bpm)
Lowest HR during TIB	52 (bpm)

Snoring Summary

Loud

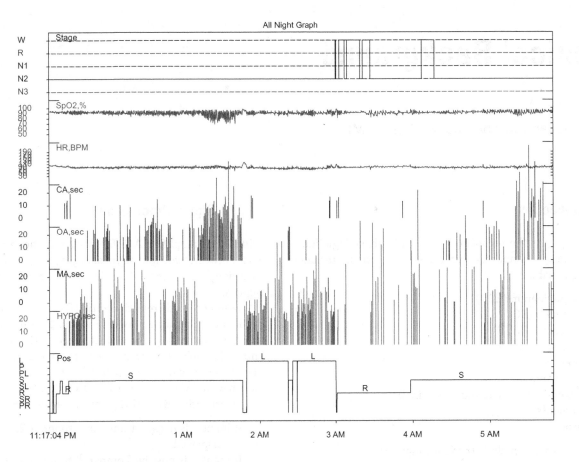

Impression: Obstructive sleep apnea (G47.33).

HST: There were physiologic oxygen desaturations resulting in an REI of 58.6 with a minimum oxygen saturation of 68%. This is consistent with a severe sleep-related breathing disorder. Clinical correlation is advised.

Recommendations: An AutoPAP titration will be ordered with a starting range of 5 to 15 cm.

_____, M.D.

Sleep Specialist

Diplomate, The American Board of Sleep Medicine

Sleep specialist reviewed the raw data in its entirety, including pulse, snore, respiration, oxygen saturation, and body position. The interpretation is based on this information in addition to the available clinical history and physical examination.

Technical Background

James D. Geyer, MD and Paul R. Carney, MD

 ## Introduction

Polysomnography is the recording of multiple physiologic functions during sleep. Standard polysomnography usually includes the following variables:

- Electroencephalogram (EEG)
- Electrooculogram (EOG)
- Electrocardiogram (EKG)
- Electromyography (EMG)
- Pulse oximetry
- Airflow (nasal and oral)
- Respiratory effort (thoracic and abdominal)
- Limb movements
- Snore sensors

Special studies may include the following:

- Expanded EEG
- Esophageal manometry
- CO_2 monitoring
- CPAP/BiPAP
- Esophageal pH

The EEG, EMG, and EOG data are used to identify the sleep stage. Accurate sleep staging is necessary for the diagnosis and management of sleep disorders. In addition to these channels, the other variables listed above are used to identify specific sleep-related disorders.

 ## Signal Processing

Differential amplifier: A differential amplifier amplifies the difference between two input signals. Any potentials shared between the two signals are removed leaving only the difference between the signals.

Common mode rejection ratio (CMRR): This ratio refers to the ability of an amplifier to reject inphase potentials and amplify out-of-phase potentials. The CMRR is measured by connecting both input channels of an amplifier to the same signal source. Ideally, the output would be zero (CMRR would be infinity). Good amplifiers have a CMRR between 1,000 and 10,000.

Polarity: Standard EEG polarity convention is as follows:

If input 1 is negative compared to input 2, an upward signal is displayed.
If input 1 is positive compared to input 2, a downward signal is displayed.
If input 2 is negative compared to input 1, a downward signal is displayed.
If input 2 is positive compared to input 1, an upward signal is displayed.

Filters

Filters allow the technologist and polysomnographer an opportunity to attenuate artifacts.

Low-frequency filter: Ideally, the low-frequency filter attenuates all frequencies below the cutoff frequency of the filter and allows all frequencies above the cutoff frequency to pass unchanged. In reality, the cutoff does not occur at a distinct single frequency but over a range of frequencies with a variable attenuation. For EEG, the cutoff frequency is defined as the frequency at which the output is reduced by 30%. In digital recording, little filtering is performed prior to digitization. Subsequent digital filtering can be performed as needed.

High-frequency filter: Ideally, the high-frequency filter attenuates all frequencies above the cutoff frequency of the filter and allows all frequencies below the cutoff frequency to pass unchanged. In reality, the cutoff does not occur at a distinct single frequency but over a range of frequencies with a variable attenuation. For EEG, the cutoff frequency is defined as the frequency at which the output is reduced by 30%. In digital recording, little filtering is performed prior to digitization. Subsequent digital filtering can be performed as needed.

60 Hz notch filter: Ideally, the 60-Hz notch frequency filter removes 60-Hz noise from electrical sources without affecting other frequencies. In reality, the 60-Hz filter attenuates a range of frequencies around 60 Hz. When 60-Hz noise is attenuated, all EEG activity in that range is also attenuated. Given these and other problems associated with the use of the 60-Hz notch filter, it should be used only when absolutely necessary.

Phase Shift: Shift of a waveform either earlier or later in time caused by filtering.

The low-frequency filter may cause a significant phase shift. Increasing the low-frequency filter attenuates the signal and shifts it to the left or earlier in time. This may have a significant effect on the interpretation of epileptiform discharges in expanded EEG studies.

The phase shift secondary to the high-frequency filter and the 60-Hz notch filter has a minimal effect on the signals recorded during polysomnography. The phase shift caused by decreasing the high-frequency filter is to the right or later in time.

 ## Sleep Montages

Abbreviations used:

EKG	=	electrocardiogram
hff	=	high-frequency filter in Hz
LAT and RAT	=	left and right anterior tibialis surface EMG
LEOG and REOG	=	left and right electrooculogram
lff	=	low-frequency filter in Hz
N/O airflow	=	nasal/oral airflow
Pes	=	intrathoracic (esophageal) pressure monitor
SaO$_2$	=	pulse oximetry
sens	=	sensitivity in microvolts/millimeter

Montage for Standard Polysomnogram

Channel

1. LEOG
2. REOG
3. Chin-EMG
4. F3-M1
5. F4-M1
6. C3-M1
7. C4-M1
8. O1-M1
9. O2-M1
10. LAT-EMG
11. RAT-EMG
12. EKG
13. LAT-A1
14. Snore1-Snore2
15. Nasal pressure
16. N/O airflow
17. Thoracic motion
18. Abdominal motion
19. Backup motion
20. Intercostal EMG
21. SaO$_2$

Montage for Multiple Sleep Latency Test

Channel

1. LEOG
2. REOG
3. Chin-EMG
4. F3-M1
5. F4-M1
6. C3-M1
7. C4-M1
8. O1-M1
9. O2-M1
10. LAT-EMG
11. RAT-EMG
12. EKG

Montage for CPAP Trial

Channel

1. LEOG
2. REOG
3. Chin-EMG
4. F3-M1
5. F4-M1
6. C3-M1
7. C4-M1
8. O1-M1
9. O2-M1
10. LAT-EMG
11. RAT-EMG
12. EKG
13. LAT-A1
14. Snore1-Snore2
15. Mask flow
16. Tidal volume
17. Oral airflow
18. Thoracic motion
19. Abdominal motion
20. Backup motion
21. SaO$_2$

Montage for Suspected Parasomnias or Seizures

Channel

1. Fp1-F7
2. F7-T3
3. T3-T5
4. T5-O1
5. Fp1-F3
6. F3-C3
7. C3-P3
8. P3-O1
9. Fp2-F4
10. F4-C4
11. C4-P4
12. P4-O2
13. Fp2-F8
14. F8-T4
15. T4-T6
16. T6-O2
17. LEOG
18. REOG
19. Chin-EMG
20. F3-M1
21. F4-M1
22. C3-M1
23. C4-M1
24. O1-M1
25. O2-M1
26. LAT-EMG
27. RAT-EMG
28. EKG
29. LAT-A1
30. Snore1-Snore2
31. Nasal pressure
32. N/O airflow
33. Thoracic motion
34. Abdominal motion
35. Backup motion
36. Intercostal EMG
37. SaO$_2$

Montage for Suspected REM Sleep Behavior Disorder

Channel

1. Fp1-F7
2. F7-T3
3. T3-T5
4. T5-O1
5. Fp1-F3
6. F3-C3
7. C3-P3
8. P3-O1
9. Fp2-F4
10. F4-C4
11. C4-P4
12. P4-O2
13. Fp2-F8
14. F8-T4
15. T4-T6
16. T6-O2
17. LAT1-EMG
18. RAT1-EMG
19. LED-EMG
20. RED-EMG
21. LEOG
22. REOG
23. Chin-EMG
24. F3-M1
25. F4-M1
26. C3-M1
27. C4-M1
28. O1-M1
29. O2-M1
30. LAT-EMG
31. RAT-EMG
32. EKG
33. LAT-A1
34. Snore1-Snore2
35. Nasal pressure
36. N/O airflow
37. Thoracic motion
38. Abdominal motion
39. Backup motion
40. Intercostal EMG
41. SaO$_2$

Recording Artifacts and Solving Technical Problems with Polysomnography Technology

James D. Geyer, MD and Paul R. Carney, MD

Artifacts in Polysomnography Recordings
Loose Electrode
Muscle (EMG) Artifact
EKG in the EEG Channel Artifact
Vibration Artifact
Electrode Pop Artifact
Cardio Ballistic Artifact
Blink Artifact
Sweat Artifact
Loose Belt Artifact
Swallow Artifact
Misplaced Thermocouple Artifact
Humidifier Condensation or Drainage in the Continuous Positive Air Pressure Tubing
Rectus Spike Artifact
Sixty-Hertz Artifact
Continuous Positive Air Pressure Complications and Potential Responses

Artifacts in Polysomnography Recordings

Loose Electrode

Description: High-frequency noise superimposed on high-amplitude slow activity with possible superimposed electrode pops.

Method for reducing or eliminating the artifact: Reprep and repaste the electrode to decrease the impedance.

Muscle (EMG) Artifact

Description: Obscuration of the background EEG and occasionally EOG by myogenic (muscle) artifact.

Method for reducing or eliminating the artifact: Ask the patient to relax; opening the jaw slightly can dramatically reduce EMG artifact. Rereferencing electrodes can also decrease artifact.

EKG in the EEG Channel Artifact

Description: A representation of the EKG in the EEG channels secondary to volume conduction of the EKG waveform. The artifact in the EEG channels should be time locked to the EKG.

Method for reducing or eliminating the artifact: Re-reference the EEG channels to A1 + A2.

Vibration Artifact

Description: The vibration caused by leg movements or snoring can result in high-frequency artifacts in other channels. One can see a manifestation of the snore registering in the chin EMG channel.

Method for reducing or eliminating the artifact: This artifact is very difficult to reduce but should be recognized as a normal physiologic occurrence.

Electrode Pop Artifact

Description: Very sharp, spikelike deflection originating from a mechanically or electrically unstable electrode. The deflections should have no electrical field and should be isolated to a single electrode. The deflection may however be seen in multiple channels if that electrode is used as a component of a channel.

Method for reducing or eliminating the artifact: Reprep and repaste the electrode to decrease the impedance.

Cardio Ballistic Artifact

Description: A pulse wave may be seen in the chest belt or abdominal belt that has only a slight delay behind the EKG channel. A representation of the pulse wave may be seen in airflow channels, nasal pressure monitors, and in esophageal pressure-monitoring channels.

Method for reducing or eliminating the artifact: This artifact is very difficult to reduce but should be recognized as a normal physiologic occurrence.

Blink Artifact

Description: An electric dipole is created by the eye, with the cornea being electropositive and the retina being electronegative. Eyelid movement also creates an electrical potential. Eye and eyelid movement creates a frontally (with variable amplitude and field depending upon the direction of gaze) predominate slow wave.

Method for reducing or eliminating the artifact: This artifact is very difficult to reduce but should be recognized as a normal physiologic occurrence.

Sweat Artifact

Description: Slow delta frequency rolling or swaying deflections are superimposed on the background EEG. One can see the sweat artifact most prominently in the O1-A2 channel.

Method for reducing or eliminating the artifact: Decrease the room temperature by lowering the airconditioner temperature or by turning on a fan. Use of filtering to decrease in the artifact can result in alteration of physiologic waveforms.

Loose Belt Artifact

Description: Effort channels begin to flatten without any evident movement despite continued respiratory effort because the belt is no longer tight enough or in the appropriate location to accurately reflect movement.

Method for reducing or eliminating the artifact: Tighten the loose belt.

Swallow Artifact

Description: The glossokinetic potential occurs because the tip of the tongue is more electrically negative than the base of the tongue. Movement of the tongue may result in a slow wave, predominantly in the temporal regions. One can see the swallow occurring during the arousals.

Method for reducing or eliminating the artifact: This artifact is very difficult to reduce but should be recognized as a normal physiologic occurrence.

Misplaced Thermocouple Artifact

Description: The airflow-sensing thermocouple can move from its proper position. When the thermocouple moves, it may no longer be able to monitor changes in temperature between inhalation and exhalation.

Method for reducing or eliminating the artifact: Place thermocouple in proper position.

Humidifier Condensation or Drainage in the Continuous Positive Air Pressure Tubing

Description: In the airflow channels, there may be an M-shaped waveform with each breath as the water moves backward and forward in the tubing.

Method for reducing or eliminating the artifact: Drain water from the tubing.

Rectus Spike Artifact

Description: The electric potential created by the rectus eye muscles can create a small spikelike discharge in the frontal and frontotemporal EEG derivations.

Method for reducing or eliminating the artifact: This artifact is very difficult to reduce but should be recognized as a normal physiologic occurrence.

Sixty-Hertz Artifact

Description: Lighting, electrical wiring, and machinery can produce electrical artifact, which occurs at approximately 60 Hz. This may be superimposed on baseline EEG, EKG, EOG, and EMG waveforms.

Method for reducing or eliminating the artifact: Reprep or reattach electrodes. Check ground lines. Turn off lighting and any unnecessary electrical equipment.

 ## Continuous Positive Air Pressure Complications and Potential Responses

- Nasal drainage—treat with nasal saline spray, nasal steroid spray, or over-the-counter nasal decongestant sprays.
- Nasal congestion—increase heated humidity, nasal spine saline spray, nasal steroid spray, and, when occurring on an infrequent basis, over-the-counter nasal decongestant sprays.
- Poor seal/mask leak—tighten headgear, refit mask, and try a new style of mask.

- Sore nose—loosen headgear; if no improvement, try a new mask style; topical antibiotic ointment.
- Nasal dryness—increase heated humidification and nasal saline spray.
- Nosebleeds—increase heated humidification and nasal saline spray.
- Allergy to mask material—change to a hypoallergenic mask.
- Patient reports pressure feels too high, but study shows that setting is correct—change to C-flex produced by Respironics.
- Difficulty exhaling—use lowest possible CPAP setting, change to a bilevel pressure system, and change to C-flex by Respironics.
- Claustrophobia—educate patients on the possibility of claustrophobia and that it will likely improve over time, select mask for patient comfort, meditation, CPAP adjustment periods during wakefulness, sedative medications, or anxiolytic medications at bedtime if necessary.
- Air swallowing (aerophagia) and gas—chin strap and bilevel pressure; educate patients on the possibility that this may occur.

Electrode Placement

1.1. All material should be assembled on a tray and positioned for easy access during hook-up.

1.2. The patient's head is measured, and electrode placement sites are plotted according to the International 10/20 system of electrode placement. The nasion is the indentation above the bridge of the nose, below the forehead. The inion is the small bony protrusion at the back of the head. The preauricular points are the small indentations in the front of the ears.

1.2.1. The first measurement is made by applying the tape across the top of the head measuring the distance from the nasion to the inion. A mark is made at the top of the head.

1.2.2. Calculate 10% of the distance between the nasion and the inion and make a mark 10% above the nasion.

1.2.3. Look down the bridge of the patient's nose and center the 10% mark in line with the nose. This location is called FPz.

1.2.4. Make a mark 10% above the inion.

1.2.5. Measure the patient's head across from left to right preauricular points, holding the measuring tape directly through the center mark at the top of the head. The midpoint between the two preauricular points is identified as Cz.

1.2.6. Calculate 10% of the distance between the two preauricular points and make a mark 10% above the left preauricular point. Then, locate the 30% mark by measuring half the distance between the 10% mark above the preauricular points and the center mark at the top of the head (Cz). Repeat the same procedure on the opposite side of the head.

1.2.7. At this time, you should have a 10% mark above the nasion, a 10% mark above the inion, and 10% marks above each preauricular points. Holding the tape through these four landmarks, measure the circumference of the patient's head.

1.2.8. Calculate 5% of the head circumference and make a mark 5% to the left and 5% to the right of the FPz on the patient's forehead. These locations are designated Fp1 and Fp2. This spacing should be 10% of the total head circumference.

1.2.9. Center the 10% mark above the inion by calculating one-half the head circumference and vertically intersecting that 10% mark. This location is called Oz. Then, measure 5% over to the left and 5% over to the right. These locations are designated O1 and O2.

1.2.10. Locate C3, measure the distance between Fp1 and O1 holding the tape through the 30% mark above the left preauricular point. Calculating half of that distance, intersect the 30% mark. This intersect site is the placement for electrode C3.

1.2.11. To locate electrode site C4, repeat the same procedure on the right side of the head, measuring from Fp2 to O2, holding the tape through the 30% mark above the right preauricular point.

1.3. Gloves should be worn.

1.4. Examine the condition of the electrodes.

1.4.1. Check for frayed or loose connections.

1.5. Electrode application

    1.5.1. The electrode cups are filled with conductive gel, which serves as an interface between the patient and the electrode providing a pathway for the electrical signals.

    1.5.2. Surface electrodes are applied by using electrode paste. Electrode paste is a thick substance, which holds electrodes in place and is easily removed after the study. The paste should be squeezed from the tube onto the gauze pad for each electrode. Press the electrode into the paste to obtain a cap full leaving the remainder on the gauze to cover the entire electrode. Press this on the patient's scalp with the gauze over the electrode. Too much paste can cause the electrode to shift during the study.

1.6. Facial electrodes are applied using infant pellet electrodes.

1.7. Respiratory sensors include nasal/oral thermocouple and piezo-crystal respiratory effort bands. The leads from these devices are plugged directly into the electrode jack box. The thermocouple should be placed directly in the path of the patient's oral and nasal outflow tracts. They should be secured in place with tape.

1.8. The pressure transducer should be applied in a fashion similar to nasal cannula oxygen in order to monitor nasal pressure. Exact sensor location should be obtained from the transducer package instructions.

1.9. Leg EMG electrodes are placed in close proximity of the ridge of the anterior tibialis muscle. The leads are taped to the patient's leg and routed through the patient's bedclothes. They are then plugged into the jack box.

1.10. Oximetry is used for measuring and recording blood oxygen saturation levels. A probe is attached to the patient's finger. It is then plugged into the appropriate socket.

1.11. Intercostal EMG electrodes (if used) are placed in the area over the respiratory muscles. They should be placed in close proximity to each other.

1.12. The snoring sensor should be placed to the side of the larynx.

1.13. Electrode leads should be plugged into the electrode jack box in the appropriate pen sockets. The jack box should be placed in the jack box holder.

1.14. Impedances should be checked. If unable to achieve readings below 30 kΩ without over scrubbing the electrode sites, try to balance the impedances between the two locations. This will help minimize artifact caused by voltage imbalances between two similar electrode locations.

Patient Calibrations for Night Time Polysomnography

1. Patient calibrations are performed before the start of each test to verify that all the channels being recorded are working properly. The patient should be instructed to do these simple exercises. As these are done, the commands should be clearly documented on the recording. If a piece of equipment is malfunctioning, it should be repaired prior to the start of the test. Occasionally, a patient may be so sleepy that they are unable to stay awake during the pretrials, when these situations occur the technician should document that the patient is unable to complete the pretrials and use their better judgment as to what pieces of equipment need to be repaired.

   1.1. Ask the patient to relax with the eyes open and stare straight ahead for 30 seconds.

   1.2. With eyes open, move your eyes to the L, R, L, R, U, D, U, D.

   1.3. Ask the patient to close the eyes for 30 seconds.

   1.4. With eyes closed, move your eyes to the L, R, L, R, U, D, U, D.

   1.5. Ask the patient to open the eyes and then to blink three times.

   1.6. Ask the patient to smile, or grit his or her teeth, or make a chewing motion.

   1.7. Ask the patient to point the toes on his or her left foot only, toward the end of the bed.

   1.8. Ask the patient to point the toes on his or her right foot only, toward the end of the bed.

   1.9. Ask the patient to breathe through the nose only for 30 seconds.

   1.10. Ask the patient to breathe through the mouth only for 30 seconds.

   1.11. Ask the patient to hold the breath for 10 seconds.

   1.12. If a snore sensor is being used, ask the patient to make three snoring noises.

   1.13. Abbreviations

      1.13.1. L = left

      1.13.2. R = right

      1.13.3. U = up

      1.13.4. D = down

Multiple Sleep Latency Test (MSLT) Protocol

1. Stimulant medications, including modafinil and traditional amphetamine-based medications, should be withdrawn 2 weeks prior to the study if possible.
2. Sleep logs should be obtained for 1 week prior to the MSLT to assess the sleep–wake schedule.
3. The MSLT should be conducted in the sleep laboratory following the polysomnogram or CPAP retitration.
4. The patient's arising time should be noted on the night summary sheet, which is completed by the night technologist near the end of the overnight polysomnogram or CPAP retitration.
5. After completion of the polysomnogram, airflow, chest respiration belts, oximeter probe, and leg EMG leads are removed.
6. The night postsleep questionnaire should be completed.
7. No caffeine should be ingested on the day of the test.
8. Technologist to perform MSLTs should be experienced in conducting the studies.
9. The daytime technologist conducting the MSLT upon arriving should introduce his/her self, explain the day's itinerary and other necessary information, and answer any appropriate questions the patient may have.
10. Patients may "freshen up" and attend to minimum daily personal routines.
11. A urine drug screen should be obtained.
12. The MSLT procedure is explained to the patient.
13. Breakfast is recommended at least 1 hour prior to the first nap. Lunch is recommended immediately following the termination of the second nap. The patient should be asked if he/she needs to use the bathroom prior to each nap.
14. The first nap begins 1.5 to 3 hours after the ending of the patient's nighttime sleep study and every 2 hours afterward.

15. Perform five nap opportunities at 2-hour intervals.
16. Between naps, the patient should be out of bed and continuously monitored visually by technicians to ensure that no napping occurs.
17. Suspensions.
18. No smoking 30 minutes prior to nap.
19. Physical activity 15 minutes prior to nap.
20. The technologist conducting the MSLT is responsible for replacing necessary electrodes, 10 minutes prior to nap.
21. *MSLT Montage*
    21.1. LEOG-M2
    21.2. REOG-M1
    21.3. SUBMENTAL EMG
    21.4. F3-M2
    21.5. F4-M1
    21.6. O1-M2
    21.7. O2-M1
    21.8. C3-M2
    21.9. C4-M1
    21.10. EKG
22. The patient should be in bed at naptime, equipment plugged in, and using CPAP if appropriate, 6 minutes prior to nap.
23. A quiet and dark room, conducive to sleep and with minimal interruptions, should be used. Any noise interruptions especially those producing arousals or delayed sleep should be documented.
24. Perform machine and patient calibrations, 3 minutes prior to each nap.
25. Bio-cals
    25.1. A 50-mV standard calibration is performed for all recording channels.

25.2. An impedance check will be performed—the impedance will vary between signals—but EEG values greater than 5 kΩ of resistance require corrective measures. (If necessary, electrodes will be replaced and rechecked.)

26. Patient calibrations. When tracing is acceptable, technologist performs the following patient biocalibrations:

26.1. Eyes open for 30 seconds

26.2. Eyes closed for 30 seconds

26.3. Moving eyes only, look right

26.4. Moving eyes only, look left

26.5. Moving eyes only, look up

26.6. Moving eyes only, look down

26.7. Blink 10 times

26.8. Act like you are chewing gum

27. Phrase good night, lights out, and begin test.

28. Guidelines during the nap:

28.1. End nap after the following:

28.1.1. 20 minutes if no scorable epochs of sleep.

28.1.2. 15 minutes after first scorable epoch of sleep (even if not until the second epoch of 19th minute) with no REM.

28.1.3. 5 minutes after the first epoch of REM. The maximum nap time in this scenario could be as long as 40 minutes.

28.2. *Sleep onset* is defined as the first page of the first epoch of sleep.

28.3. The absence of sleep on a nap opportunity is recorded as a sleep latency of 20 minutes.

28.4. In order to assess the occurrence of REM sleep, the test continues for 15 minutes after the first recorded epoch of sleep. The duration of 15 minutes is determined by "clock time" and is not determined by a sleep time of 15 minutes. REM latency is the time from the first epoch of sleep to the beginning of the first epoch of REM sleep, regardless of the intervening stages of sleep or wakefulness.

28.5. At the end of the nap, do posttest calibrations.

28.5.1. Knock and enter the patient's room, disconnect jack box from the head of bed and get the patient out of bed. Inform them that they must stay out of bed and awake until the start of the next nap at approximately (time).

29. End of Study:

29.1. Gently remove all sensors from the patient. Take care to avoid irritation of patient's skin.

29.2. Remove and discard any remaining tape and gauze.

29.3. Assure that all paste residues have been removed by using a wet washcloth on the skin and scalp.

29.4. Allow electrodes to soak in soap and hot water. Rinse well and allow to dry. Clean and disinfect all reusable equipment per manufacturer instructions. Inspect wires at this time to ensure their integrity. Return equipment to their storage area for future use.

29.5. If CPAP and/or oxygen equipment was used, remove and place it in designated "dirty equipment area" for cleaning and disinfecting. Always discard disposable items.

29.6. Clean CPAP equipment filter.

29.7. Stock patient preparation box as needed.

29.8. Return patient preparation box to appropriate area.

29.9. Leave patient suites in clean and orderly condition.

30. Scoring:

30.1. Data will be scored by the senior technologist.

30.2. Sleep stage scoring should be based on the AASM scoring guidelines. The sleep latency is determined from lights out to the first scored epoch of any stage of sleep. REM latency is scored from sleep onset to the first epoch of REM.

30.3. All scoring is based in The AASM Manual for the Scoring of Sleep and Associated Events: Rules, Terminology and Technical Specifications, version 2.2.

31. The study will then be reviewed and interpreted by the medical director.

32. The study results are then sent to the referring provider.

33. The study shall be archived into the sleep archive hard drive and kept on file at the sleep center.

34. MSLT reports should include the start and end times of each nap or nap opportunity, mean sleep latency, and number of sleep-onset REM periods (defined as >15 seconds of REM sleep in a 30-second epoch).

35. References

AASM Manual for the Scoring of Sleep and Associated Events: Rules, Terminology and Technical Specifications, version 2.2.

Standards of Practice Committee of the AASM. Practice parameters for clinical use of the multiple sleep latency test and the maintenance of wakefulness test. *Sleep* 2005;28(1):113–121.

Maintenance of Wakefulness Test (MWT) Protocol

1. Stimulant medications, including modafinil and traditional amphetamine-based medications, should be withdrawn 2 weeks prior to the study of possible, unless the study is being performed to assess the effectiveness of treatment.

2. The use of medications and tobacco should be decided on an individual basis by the sleep specialist.

3. The MWT should be conducted at the sleep laboratory following the polysomnogram or CPAP retitration (based on the clinical considerations as decided by the medical director).

4. The patient's arising time should be noted on the night summary sheet, which is completed by the night technologist near the end of the overnight polysomnogram or CPAP retitration.

5. Respiratory monitoring devices and tibialis electrodes should be removed from the patient.

6. The night postsleep questionnaire should be completed following the patient's arising in the morning.

7. No caffeine should be ingested on the day of the test.

8. The MWT study should be performed by a sleep technologist who is experienced in conducting the study.

9. The daytime technologist conducting the MWT upon arriving should introduce his/her self, explain the day's itinerary and other necessary information, and answer any appropriate questions the patient may have.

10. Patients may "freshen up" and attend to minimum daily personal routines.

11. A urine drug screen should be obtained prior to the MWT. Breakfast is recommended at least 1 hour prior to the first nap. Lunch is recommended immediately following the termination of the second nap.

12. The first trial should begin 1.5 to 3 hours after the patient's usual wake-up time.

13. The patient will be served breakfast prior to the first nap trial and lunch following the noon trial per individual dietary requirements. Subdue physical activity 15 minutes before nap.

14. Trials should be run every 2 hours for a total of four nap trials. Four 40-minute trials should be run.

15. The technologist conducting the MWT is responsible for replacing necessary electrodes.

16. MWT Montage
    16.1. LEOG-M2
    16.2. REOG-Ml
    16.3. SUBMENTAL EMG
    16.4. F3-M2
    16.5. F4-Ml
    16.6. O1-M2
    16.7. O2-Ml
    16.8. C3-M2
    16.9. C4-M1
    16.10. EKG

17. A quiet and dark room, conducive to sleep, with a light source (a 7.5-W night light) positioned slightly behind the patient's head, placed one foot off the floor, 3 feet laterally removed from the patient's head, just out of vision, should be utilized. The patient should be seated upright in bed, with the back and head supported by a bed rest (bolster pillow) such that the neck is not uncomfortably flexed or extended. Patients are not permitted to use extraordinary measures to stay awake such as slapping the face or singing.

18. The room should have minimal interruptions. Any noise interruptions, especially those producing arousals or delayed sleep, should be documented.
19. Prior to each trial, the patient should be asked if he or she needs to go to the bathroom or needs other adjustments for comfort.
20. Perform machine and patient calibration's prior to each nap, about 2 minutes prior to the start of the nap. *Patient calibration* is conducted the same as the night time polysomnogram with the exception of leg movement and respiratory documentation. An impedance check will be performed. The impedance will vary between signals, but EEG values greater than 5 kΩ of resistance require corrective measures (if necessary, electrodes will be replaced and rechecked).
21. Guidelines during testing:
    21.1. End test after 40 minutes with no scorable epochs of sleep.
    21.2. *Sleep onset* is defined as the first page of the first epoch of sleep. Sleep is defined as greater than 15 seconds of cumulative sleep in a 30-second epoch.
    21.3. Trials are ended after unequivocal sleep, defined as three consecutive epochs of stage I sleep or one epoch of any other stage of sleep.

21.4. All scoring is based in The AASM Manual for the Scoring of Sleep and Associated Events: Rules, Terminology and Technical Specifications, version 2.2.
22. *MWT Report*: The following data should be noted:
    22.1. Start and stop times for each trial
    22.2. Sleep latency
    22.3. Total sleep time
    22.4. Stages of sleep achieved for each trial
    22.5. Mean sleep latency (the arithmetic mean of the four trials)
23. The study will be reviewed and interpreted by medical director.
24. The interpreted study results are then sent to the referring provider.
25. The study shall be archived onto the sleep archive database and kept on file at the sleep center. Reports and all other patient records will be archived in their file.
26. References

AASM Manual for the Scoring of Sleep and Associated Events: Rules, Terminology and Technical Specifications, version 2.2.
Standards of Practice Committee of the AASM. Practice parameters for clinical use of the multiple sleep latency test and the maintenance of wakefulness test. *Sleep* 2005;28(1):113–121.

Adult and Pediatric Preparation for Recording

1. Guidelines for patient preparation for recording.
   1.1. The following materials will be needed for the hookup.
       1.1.1. Clean electrodes
       1.1.2. Scissors
       1.1.3. Electrode cream
       1.1.4. China marker
       1.1.5. 2 RIP belts
       1.1.6. Ample tape (silk, Transpore, paper)
       1.1.7. 1 channel N/O thermocouple
       1.1.8. Skin prep
       1.1.9. Cotton-tipped swabs
       1.1.10. 2-inch gauze squares
       1.1.11. Oximeter probe
       1.1.12. Pressure transducer
       1.1.13. 6 EKG pads
       1.1.14. Snore sensor
   1.2. All EEG, EOG, EMG, EKG electrodes should be of the same metal.
   1.3. Patients are previously instructed to wash their hair prior to arrival. If they fail to do so, extra care should be given in preparing the scalp for electrode application.
   1.4. The technologist should first review the patients chart for the diagnosis and other relevant information, this will determine the montage that will be used for polysomnogram.
   1.5. The sampling rates and filtering parameters are listed in the Policy: Parameters to be Reported for Polysomnography. This is based on The AASM Manual for the Scoring of Sleep and Associated Events: Rules, Terminology and Technical Specifications, version 2.2.
   1.6. The location of the EEG electrodes is determined by the International 10-20 system of electrode placement. Reference electrodes are placed on the bony surface of the mastoid process. (Reference electrodes may also be placed on the earlobes.) F3, F4, C3, C4, O1, O2, A1, A2, and Ground electrode are used. Central leads are used because markers for sleep stages are prominent over these regions (sleep spindles, K-complexes). Amplifier settings commonly used are as per the Policy: Parameters to be Reported for Polysomnography.
   1.7. After measurements have been made and marked, each electrode site should be cleaned with skin prep. To do this, use a cotton-tipped swab dipped in the skin prep and gently abrade the scalp taking care not to break the skin. Failure to do so will impede the electrode adherence.
   1.8. After the electrode sites have been prepped, take the electrode that is to be applied and fill the cup with electrode paste. Now cut a cotton gauze in half inch by half inch squares and apply a small amount of electrode paste to the cotton gauze and place the back of the electrode cup (convex) into the paste and cotton gauze. Part the hair at the site and gently but firmly press the electrode and cotton gauze onto the scalp. Tape the electrode in place to keep the electrode from being displaced.
   1.9. The EOG and EMG electrodes are applied in the same manner (all electrodes must be filled with electrode paste).
   1.10. The EOG is a recording of the movement of the cornea–retinal potential difference that exists in the eye. It is important to recognize that it is the movement of this dipole that is recorded, not muscle activity.

1.11. The EOG electrode is typically applied at the outer canthus of the right eye (ROC) and is offset 1 cm above the horizontal plane. The other electrode is applied to the outer canthus of the left eye and 1 cm below the horizontal plane (LOC). The EOG tracings are used to aid in the scoring of sleep onset (rolling eye movements) and stage REM (rapid eye movements).

Amplifier settings commonly used are as per the Policy: Parameters to be Reported for Polysomnography.

1.12. The chin EMG (electromyography) electrodes are applied to record the mentalis and submentalis muscle activity. Three electrodes should be applied (one as a backup as the chin electrodes are most likely to fall off during recording). One electrode is placed directly under the chin and the other two are placed under the jaw bone. Interelectrode distance should not exceed an inch, and care should be taken not to place the electrodes too far down on the neck as this could result in excessive EKG artifact in the tracing. The chin EMG tracing is used to determine arousals, the onset of stage REM, bruxism, and in infant studies sucking motions. Amplifier settings commonly used are as per the Policy: Parameters to be Reported for Polysomnography. Adult electrode derivations for EEG, EOG, and chin EMG are acceptable for recording sleep except that the distance between the chin EMG electrodes often needs to be reduced from 2 to 1 cm and the distance from the eyes in EOG electrodes often need to be reduced from 1 to 0.5 cm in children with small head size.

1.13. Two EKG electrodes are applied. One is placed on the left side of the body just below the left clavicle bone, the other just under the right clavicle bone. In order to rule out artifacts, another EKG channel is used on the recording by referencing an LEG-EMG electrode to the A1. EKG channels are used to determine heart rates during both REM and NREM sleep, determine if there is a slowing of the heart rate in association with respiratory events, and EKG abnormalities that may occur in association with or without respiratory events. Amplifier settings commonly used are as per the Policy: Parameters to be Reported for Polysomnography.

1.14. Leg EMG electrodes are placed over both the left and right anterior tibialis muscle sites, two electrodes on each leg are referenced to one another (left to left, right to right).

Interelectrode distance should not exceed 2 inches. The leg EMG electrodes are used to determine the presence of and scoring of periodic leg movements (PLMs) during sleep. They are also used in determining arousals, and abnormal limb movements that occur in patients who have REM behavior disorder (RBI). Amplifier settings commonly used are as per the Policy: Parameters to be Reported for Polysomnography.

1.15. Respiratory Effort

    1.15.1. Two channels of respiratory effort are recorded and are used to determine the presence of and classification of respiratory events.

        1.15.1.1. Two respiratory belts are applied, one around the thoracic area and the other around the abdominal area. The belts should be applied, so they are snug but not too tight as to cause the patient discomfort. The RIP belts are placed on both the thorax and the abdomen to monitor respiratory effort. One is placed on the upper chest at the area of maximum chest excursion during normal respiration with the patient lying supine. Similarly, the other belt is placed on the patient's abdomen at the area of maximal excursion during normal respiration. Impedance Pneumography Electrodes are also used to measure respiratory effort. These electrodes are placed one on the left side of the chest cavity and one on the right side (another highly reliable method of application is to place one electrode above the diaphragm and one below). The pneumograph electrodes are plugged into an amplifier box that is interfaced with the headboard. The measurement that is appearing on the tracing is actually measurement of the changing impedances between the electrodes. As the patient breaths, there is change in the distance between the electrodes and the change in distance corresponds to a change in impedance, that is, as the patient inhales, the distance increases, and the impedance increases. The change is measured, and a voltage equivalence of the change is sent to the polygraph. Amplifier settings commonly used are as per the Policy: Parameters to be Reported for Polysomnography.

1.15.1.2. Three intercostal EMG electrodes (I-C EMG) may be applied over either the left or the right side of the rib cage (usually the side that will be closest to the headboard). The I-C EMG tracing at times can be difficult to record, but when a clean signal can be obtained, they are extremely valuable in determining the presence of respiratory effort and distinguishing between central and obstructive respiratory events. A fairly reliable method of application is to ask the patient to raise his or her arm and to feel with your fingers the rib cage muscles working as the patient is breathing in and out, then apply to the electrodes to the site you feel the muscles working. Amplifier settings commonly used are as per the Policy: Parameters to be Reported for Polysomnography.

1.16. Respiratory Airflow

1.16.1. The nasal/oral thermocouple is applied just under the nose and held in place with a piece of tape. The wires are looped back around the ears in a "cannula" fashion. The nasal beads should be sitting just at the opening of the nostrils. Care should be taken to ensure the beads are not touching the skin or poking into the nostrils. The oral bead should positioned, so that it is directly in line with the oral airflow. A thermocouple is a junction of two different metals that when joined generate a small current. As the junction of metal is heated (warm air from exhalation), there is an increase in current, and as the junction is cooled (cool air from inhalation), there is a decrease in current. The polarity of the tracing is set, so there is an upward deflection during inhalation. The respiratory airflow tracing is used to distinguish between apnea events (cessation of airflow for ≥10 seconds) and hypopnea events (decrease in airflow

for ≥10 seconds). Amplifier settings commonly used are as per the Policy: Parameters to be Reported for Polysomnography.

1.16.2. A nasal/oral pressure transducer will also be used with the thermocouple.

1.16.2.1. Hook the pressure transducer cannula into the positive input located at the top of the PTAF.

1.16.2.2. The AC cable should be inserted into the filter port.

1.16.2.3. Press the gain set for the machine to set itself to recognize the wave form.

1.17. An oximeter probe is placed on the finger or another appropriate location and held in place with tape. Finger probe oximetry is a noninvasive method of measuring saturated oxygen. They use an infrared and near infrared light source and detector to measure the amount of arterial oxygen that is saturated by passing this light through a vascular bed and measuring how much of the light is absorbed. Two different types of light are used to measure the total hemoglobin and the oxygenated hemoglobin, thus a percentage value of saturation can be calculated.

1.17.1. An oximeter probe is placed on a finger and held in place with a "Band-Aid" made for the probe. The oximeter signal is a slow signal with a voltage range between 0 and 1 V and has to be calibrated and recorded with a DC amplifier.

1.18. Intercostal electrodes. Two intercostal electrodes should be placed on the right side of the chest as described in the section under respiratory monitoring.

1.19. After all the devices are applied to the patient, ask the patient if he or she needs to use the bathroom or take care of any last items before you plug the electrodes into the jack box. After the electrodes are plugged in, test the resistances (≤10 kΩ); if any of the electrodes are above this limit, they should be reapplied to meet these criteria.

1.20. Group wires together and secure.

1.21. Exit the patient room, turn off the room lights, and turn on the camera and the infrared lights.

1.22. Turn on the polysomnography, make adjustments, and begin patient pretrials (see routine responsibilities and patient pretrials).

1.23. Impedance: An impedance test can be run at this time to determine good electrode hook up. The impedance will vary between signals, but EEG values greater than 5 kΩ of resistance require corrective measures.

1.24. General Cleanup Checklist

1.24.1. Discard all used tape, collars, gauze, etc.

1.24.2. Clean and disinfect thermocouples/thermistors, if not disposable.

1.24.3. Return patient preparation kit to appropriate area.

1.24.4. Stock patient preparation kit as needed.

1.24.5. If CPAP and/or oxygen equipment was used, remove and empty humidifier, connecting tubing, nasal cannula, patient bore tubing, and any other equipment and place in designated "dirty equipment area" for cleaning and disinfecting.

1.24.6. Discard disposable equipment such as the nasal cannula or disposable oximeter probe.

1.24.7. Remove any lint from CPAP equipment filter.

Oral Appliance (OA) Titration

1. Follow Polysomnogram Protocol.
2. Oral appliance–specific instructions/protocol for titration is recommended.
   2.1. Instructions protocol should be obtained from the dentist who has fit patient with the device or the ordering provider.
3. Sleep center standard protocol for titration of oral appliance.
   3.1. Oral appliance will be advanced until the AHI is less than or equal to 5.
   3.2. The patient should be asleep and observed at each advancement for a minimum of 30 minutes.
   3.3. The oral appliance will eventually limit out on advancements possible.
   3.4. If the patient experiences any jaw and/or muscle pain, do not advance the oral appliance further.
4. The patient must be instructed by his or her dentist on adjustment of the oral appliance prior to sleep study.
5. The patient must bring the tool needed to adjust oral appliance with to sleep study.
6. Follow the instructions/protocol to titrate the oral appliance.
   6.1. The patient must adjust the oral appliance.
      6.1.1. The technician can assist them by reading instructions/protocol to them, holding flashlight, or using a magnifying glass.
7. Documentation
   7.1. File section should be marked as "Treatment."
   7.2. Document adjustments using the CPAP numeric tags in the sleep study recording/raw data.
      7.2.1. CPAP "0" = start of study, prior to any adjustments.
      7.2.2. CPAP "1, 2, 3, etc." = adjustment made. CPAP "1" would be for the 1st adjustment, CPAP "2" for the 2nd adjustment, and CRAP "3" for the 3rd adjustment, etc.
   7.3. Document all adjustments made on the observation log.
   7.4. Document number of turns made in total in the final collection notes.

Protocol for Unattended Sleep Studies/ Portable Monitoring

1. Technology for unattended sleep studies/portable monitoring (PM)
   1.1. Minimum requirements
      1.1.1. Airflow—The sensor to detect apnea is an oral/nasal thermal sensor and to detect hypopnea is a nasal pressure transducer. Ideally, unattended sleep studies/PM should use both sensor types.
      1.1.2. Respiratory effort—The sensor for identification of respiratory effort is either calibrated or uncalibrated respiratory inductance plethysmography (RIP belts).
      1.1.3. Blood oxygenation—The sensor for the detection of blood oxygen is pulse oximetry.
         1.1.3.1. With the appropriate signal averaging time
         1.1.3.2. With accommodation for motion artifact
   1.2. The biosensors used to monitor these parameters for an in-laboratory PSG are recommended for use in unattended sleep studies/PM/HSAT/OCST.
2. After a comprehensive sleep evaluation, an unattended sleep study/PM/HSAT/OCST can be ordered or approved by the medical director. The patient will be scheduled through the sleep center for an unattended sleep study/PM/HSAT/OCST. Unattended sleep studies/PM/HSAT/OCST are offered Monday to Friday and are ordered on an outpatient status. The use of unattended sleep studies/PM follows AASM practice parameters, Clinical Guidelines for the use of unattended Portable Monitors in the Diagnosis of OSA in Adult Patients.
3. Patients will arrive at the sleep center at a scheduled time and will be greeted in a professional and courteous manner by the sleep center staff.
4. The patient will complete any necessary paperwork.
   4.1. Admission paperwork (consent for treatment and off-site liability form).
   4.2. Product Responsibility Agreement, which includes the HST units ID device number. This will be part of the patient's medical record. The ID device number will be used to assist in failure investigation and quality reporting.
5. The senior technician, who is trained and familiar with the equipment, a certified RPSGT/RST, will educate patient on set up of equipment.
   5.1. Educate patient on the study and the procedure. Answer any questions they may have about the study.
   5.2. The patient will watch an educational video about home sleep testing.
   5.3. Instruct patient on application of sensors. Have patient demonstrate proper set up.
   5.4. Discuss some troubleshooting techniques.
   5.5. If patient is having issues, he or she can call the senior technologist at 205-367-2400.
   5.6. All calls received during testing hours (nighttime) will be logged and reviewed to identify and monitor for trends of sensor, service, or device issues. The log sheet shall be kept in the control room. Log will include:
      5.6.1. Date and time of call.
      5.6.2. Name of the patient and person calling.
      5.6.3. Issue identified or nature of problem.
      5.6.4. Device ID #.
      5.6.5. Resolution or recommendation for change.

5.6.6. The log sheet should be used to identify trends of device, or sensor or service issues, and to facilitate the quarterly QA audit of equipment performance.

5.7. Instruct patient to call emergency services 911 in the event of an emergency.

5.8. Instruct patient that he or she needs to return the equipment the following morning, unless otherwise notified.

6. All patient data will be deleted from machine immediately upon device return and after data are downloaded to the appropriate server. The HST device is set up to automatically delete all PHI and study data after download of data to server.

7. Sleep montage

   7.1. *Respiratory effort*: LFF 0.1 Hz and HFF 15 Hz

      7.1.1. The RIP belt is placed on the thorax to monitor respiratory effort.

   7.2. *Airflow*: LFF 0.1 Hz and HFF 15 Hz

      7.2.1. Oral/nasal thermal sensor or thermocouple—Place on patient, so that it is anchored firmly and centered in the direct path of oral/nasal airflow to record air temperature changes.

      7.2.2. Nasal pressure transducer—Place the pressure transducer cannula into the nares with the cannula anchored on top of the thermistor to record pressure changes.

   7.3. *Blood oxygenation/oximetry*

   7.4. Place pulse oximeter on the finger.

8. Raw data will be scored by a senior technician. Scoring personnel include RST, RPSGT, CPSGT, CRT-SDS, RRT-SDS, sleep specialists, or other AASM-recognized certifications.

   8.1. All scoring is based on The AASM Manual for the Scoring of Sleep and Associated Events: Rules, Terminology and Technical Specifications, version 2.2.

   8.2. We use Hypopnea Rule 4A.

9. Unattended sleep study/PM reports include:

   9.1. AHI or RDI

   9.2. Evaluation of oxygen saturations during recording

   9.3. Recording duration of test

   9.4. Technical adequacy of test

      9.4.1. Technical failures due to equipment malfunction must be documented, and the study could be repeated.

10. The study will then be reviewed and interpreted by a designated board certified sleep physician.

11. The interpreted study results are then sent to the ordering provider.

12. Patient interpretations, reports, paperwork, and all other patient records will be in the EMR. All scanned paper patient records will be kept in the Medical Records Department. A database will be maintained using the most current ICD-10 codes.

13. All patient data will be deleted from machine immediately upon device return and after data are downloaded to the appropriate server.

14. A follow-up in-person visit with a sleep staff provider must be offered to all patients undergoing an unattended sleep study/PM to discuss the results of the test and treatment options. Documented evidence of attempts at follow-up must be in patient's medical record.

   14.1. PAP titration or split night study

   14.2. APAP home trial

   14.3. Determination of an alternate to PAP therapy

15. An in-laboratory PSG should be performed in cases where an unattended sleep study/PM/HSAT/OCST is inadequate or fails to establish the diagnosis of OSA in patients with a high pretest probability.

16. Equipment maintenance

   16.1. All equipment will be cleaned and inspected after each use. All patient data will be deleted from machine immediately upon device return and after data are downloaded to the appropriate server.

   16.2. Adhere to manufacturers recommendations for monitoring and maintenance.

   16.3. Follow Infection Control Policy for cleaning.

17. Policy Equipment Management Plan

   17.1. Yearly inspection of patient-related equipment for electrical and mechanical safety.

   17.2. All units or sensors associated with a failed test must be removed from service and tested for proper function prior to its next use.

18. References

National Guidelines/National Standards/Regulatory AASM Manual for the Scoring of Sleep and Associated Events: Rules, Terminology and Technical Specifications, Version 2.2.

Standards of Practice Parameters. Clinical guidelines for the use of unattended portable monitors in the diagnosis of obstructive sleep apnea in adult patients. *J Clin Sleep Med* 2007;3(7):737–747.

Collop NA, Tracy SL, Kapur V, et al. Obstructive sleep apnea devices for out-of-center (OOC) testing: Technology evaluation. *J Clin Sleep Med* 2011;7(5):531–548.

Berry RB, Brooks R, Gamaldo CE, et al.; for the American Academy of Sleep Medicine. *The AASM Manual for the Scoring of Sleep and Associated Events: Rules, Terminology and Technical Specifications, Version 2.2.* www.aasmnet.org. Darien, IL: American Academy of Sleep Medicine, 2015.

Technical Specifications for Routine Polysomnography Recordings

In the absence of clear preferences, use similar settings among leads to simplify technical implementation.

1. Maximum Electrode Impedances: 5 kΩ

This applies to measured EEG and EOG electrode impedance. Electrode impedances should be rechecked during a recording when any pattern that might be artifactual appears.

2. Minimum Digital Resolution: 12 bits per sample

3. Sampling Rates

	Desirable	Minimal
EEG	500 Hz	200 Hz

For EEG, 500 Hz sampling rate could improve resolution of spikes in the EEG and better maintain details of the waveform.

For more detailed EEG analysis, sampling rate and high-frequency filter settings may be increased. In these circumstances, the sampling rate should be at least three times the high-frequency filter settings.

	Desirable	Minimal
EOG	500 Hz	200 Hz

For EOG, using the 500 Hz desirable EEG sampling rate also allows the reflection of the EEG in this lead as an EEG backup and may better define some artifacts in these leads.

	Desirable	Minimal
EMG	500 Hz	200 Hz

This applies to submental and leg EMG. Higher sampling rates better define waveforms; while the waveform itself is not an issue, a better-defined waveform can help avoid amplitude attenuation as the envelope of the rapidly oscillating signal is interpreted.

	Desirable	Minimal
ECG	500 Hz	200 Hz

For ECG, 500 Hz sampling rate can better define pacemaker spikes and ECG waveforms; however, pacemaker spikes can be seen at 200 Hz, and the evaluation of cardiac ischemia by ECG waveform is not a common PSG issue. Higher frequencies may be required for complex waveform analysis and research applications.

	Desirable	Minimal
Airflow	100 Hz	25 Hz
Oximetry, Transcutaneous PCO_2	25 Hz	10 Hz

For oximetry, 25 Hz sampling is desirable to assist with artifact evaluation.

	Desirable	Minimal
Nasal Pressure, End-Tidal PCO$_2$, PAP Device Flow	100 Hz	25 Hz

For nasal pressure transducer technology (especially with settings that identify snoring occurring on top of the airflow waveform), this higher frequency may be of benefit for better definition of flattening, plateauing, and/or fluttering in the airflow waveform.

	Desirable	Minimal
Esophageal Pressure	100 Hz	25 Hz
Body Position	1 Hz	1 Hz

The body position channel is exempt from the digital resolution standard. However, the recommended sampling rate of 1 Hz remains in effect.

	Desirable	Minimal
Snoring Sounds	500 Hz	200 Hz

For snoring sound, 500 Hz sampling rate can better define amplitude variation by clearer waveforms with more accurate amplitude determination as the envelope of the rapidly oscillating signal is interpreted (as for EMG). If a preprocessing of snoring results in a continuous sound loudness level or in a sound intensity level, then a much lower sampling rate is acceptable. That sampling rate is not specified because it depends on the preprocessing of the sound in order to produce loudness.

	Desirable	Minimal
Rib Cage and Abdominal Movements	100 Hz	25 Hz

For rib cage and abdominal movements using inductance plethysmography, cardiogenic oscillations can be better seen and may result in better artifact assessment at a higher sampling rate.

4. Reference

Berry RB, Brooks R, Gamaldo CE, et al.; For the American Academy of Sleep Medicine. *The AASM Manual for the Scoring of Sleep and Associated Events: Rules, Terminology and Technical Specifications, Version 2.2.* www.aasmnet.org. Darien, IL: American Academy of Sleep Medicine, 2015.

Guidelines for CPAP Titration

1. Initiation
   1.1. Review the patient's clinical note for pertinent history.
   1.2. Review the patient's previous sleep study or studies to assess the severity of sleep-disordered breathing, the type of respiratory events, and the position and stage at which the events were most severe. This will help to attain a better titration.
   1.3. Application of electrodes, montages, filters, sensitivities, and scoring will be performed according to The AASM Manual for the Scoring of Sleep and Associated Events: Rules, Terminology and Technical Specifications, version 2.2.
   1.4. The goal of CPAP therapy is to eliminate all traces of upper airway obstruction. This is to be accomplished by reaching the appropriate level of CPAP, which will act as a splint on the patient's upper airway. The technologist must be vigilant to recognize events and resultant arousals that may sometimes be quite subtle.
   1.5. Mask options should be reviewed. The patient should be assessed for special mask interface needs. In conjunction with patient desires, a mask interface system (mask and headgear) should be selected as the initial mask to be tried.
   1.6. If necessary, during the study, the mask should be changed or the fit adjusted.
   1.7. Before the actual study, the patient should be given a CPAP trial at 5 cm of H_2O while awake. This is to allow the patient to adjust to CPAP. The patient should be encouraged to keep his/her mouth closed and breathe through the nose only if using nasal device. The technician must make sure that there is an open exhalation port in the CPAP delivery system. The technician should observe the patient's tolerance to CPAP and address any fears or concerns the patient may have.
   1.8. Just before lights are out, the technician should double check the mask fit and be sure that there are no leaks. The patient is to be on 5 cm of H_2O at this point. The patient should be observed at this and each successive level for at least 15 minutes. If apneas have been observed at a pressure, CPAP should be increased by 2 cm of H_2O. If a patient still shows respiratory events at 18, bilevel may be tried. By moving the patient up quickly and aggressively in 2-cm increments, the elimination of respiratory arousals will be expedited, thus deepening sleep and increasing tolerance to CPAP.
   1.9. However, it should be noted that this can sometimes cause central events, and these are not to be confused with or treated as obstructive events.
   1.10. In general, the optimal CPAP level is the pressure that eliminates obstructive respiratory events even while supine in REM. The monitoring technician should strive to document all pressures used during the night.
2. Demonstrating CPAP to a patient
   2.1. The routine for initiating patients to nasal CPAP includes a consultation with the ordering physician followed by a demonstration of the unit by the polysomnographic technologist. During this routine, the patient is evaluated and is given an opportunity to try to breathe through the nasal mask to become accustomed to the sensation it produces.

2.2. It is important to emphasize relaxation and regular breathing during this trial so that the patient learns to be comfortable with the system from the start. The technologist explains how the system works, and the patient is encouraged to ask any questions he/she may have regarding the treatment.

3. Titration Procedure

3.1. Begin the patient at 4 or 5 cm of water of pressure.

3.2. Increase in increments of 2 cm of water pressure until events are eliminated or minimized. In general, the pressure should be adjusted for the following reasons.

3.2.1. 2 obstructive apneas

3.2.2. 3 hypopneas

3.2.3. 3 minutes of loud unambiguous snoring

3.3. Do not go above 18 cm of water.

3.4. Aim to eliminate apneas and hypopneas.

3.5. Central apneas are not necessarily a reason to increase CPAP pressure (except under special circumstances, i.e., the patient has specifically been sent for a trial of CPAP for known central apnea). A brief increase in pressure can be attempted to assess the possibility that the apparent central apneas are a component of the obstructive sleep apnea.

3.6. Maintain all CPAP pressures for at least 15 minutes before increasing them. An exception to this might be the case in which the patient is in REM and still desaturating even though the CPAP was increased. The technician may want to increase CPAP more quickly in this situation, so that he or she can evaluate a higher pressure before the REM period ends.

3.7. Ideally, you should obtain REM when evaluating your optimal CPAP pressure. This may mean allowing the patient to sleep a bit longer in the morning. Also, optimally, the patient should be studied in the position that was determined to be worst for them on the routine PSG. Please refer to the previous study. If necessary, ask the patient to assume this position, if it is already late in the evening.

3.8. After determining the CPAP pressure at which events are minimized, decrease the pressure by 1 cm of water to see whether a slightly lower pressure would be as effective.

3.9. If the patient awakens (i.e., restroom break, etc.), do not decrease the CPAP pressure on attempted return to sleep unless:

3.9.1. The patient remains awake for 15 minutes or more.

3.9.2. The patient specifically requests a lower pressure. Remember, the patient will need to be able to fall asleep at home without adjusting CPAP.

3.10. Optimal CPAP therapy is an AHI less than 5 per hour for at least 15 minutes at the selected pressure and with minimal mask leak.

3.11. Patients who are scheduled for split night studies in the laboratory should have CPAP added only after it has been determined that the patient has at least moderate obstructive-related breathing. If the situation arises that one is unsure about adding CPAP, consult the senior technician on call.

3.12. CPAP follow-up retitration protocol:

3.12.1. Patients who are scheduled for CPAP retitration or follow-up are instructed to bring their machines with them. The technician should verify what the pressure setting is with a water column manometer. The mask and headgear should also be inspected for proper fit.

3.12.2. Based on the pressure reading from the water column manometer if the pressure is greater than or equal to 10 cm of water, the polysomnogram should be started with the CPAP set at 5 cm of water below the pressure reading. For example, if the patients machine = 12 cm of water, start the polysomnogram at 7 cm of water.

3.12.3. When the CPAP pressure is less than 10 cm, start the polysomnogram with the CPAP pressure = 5 cm of water.

3.12.4. If patients do not bring their machine with them, review the chart and find what the prescribed pressure was and start 5 cm of water below that pressure. If no previous documentation of prescribed CPAP pressure can be located, start at 5 cm of water.

3.13. In the severely obese patient, or when high CPAP pressures are not advisable (or insufficient), it may help to elevate the head of the bed for better response.

4. Trouble Shooting
   4.1. Intolerance: If the patient cannot tolerate CPAP and different masks and pressures have been tried, it is recommended that the patient be offered the bed for the night anyway, and details of the trial documented and discussed with the physician. Possible desensitization may be needed by having the physician prescribe CPAP at a low pressure to be tried at home for a while. And then have the patient come back to have a CPAP titration night.
   4.2. Central apneas: If the patient begins to have central apneas that were not documented on the previous study and are not accompanied by snores or arousals, watch the patient closely. If he or she begins to have snores and arousals at the end of the apnea, it is more than likely obstructive and needs to have the pressure increased. If he or she is true central apneas, follow the protocol for bilevel and O_2 administration. Keep in mind that *some* centrals can be normal when the patient is adjusting to CPAP. Always document when someone is intolerable of CPAP.
   4.3. Mouth leaks: If the patient, after being seemingly fixed, begins to have events, it is possible that he or she has a mouth leak. This needs to be fixed immediately. A mouth leak can be heard, and at some stations, it is measured. You can also tell a mouth leak from the airflow channel, which tends to look "hypopneic" but for very long periods of time. Your options for a mouth leak are limited, but it needs to be taken care of. Some options are (1) chin strap, a cloth strip that goes under the chin and Velcro's over the head to keep the mandible together; (2) full face mask; (3) total face mask; (4) pressure changes; and (5) increase heated humidification.

5. Follow-up
   5.1. The patient will generally be evaluated by the medical director or the physician in 2 to 4 weeks for a follow-up after PAP is prescribed.

6. References

National Guidelines/National Standards/Regulatory.

AASM Manual for the scoring of Sleep and Associated Events: Rules, Terminology and Technical Specifications, Version 2.2.

AASM Clinical Guidelines for the Manual Titration of PAP in Patients with OSA.

Index

Page numbers in *italics* denote figures; those followed by "t" denote tables.